Financing Medicaid

Medicaid has evolved over the past five decades from a tiny "welfare medicine" program into the single largest health insurance program in the United States. Contrary to the conventional wisdom that programs for the poor are vulnerable to instability and retrenchment because they lack a powerful constituency, Shanna Rose finds that, as a result of its unique institutional structure, Medicaid does, in fact, have an organized, influential interest group: the nation's governors. Although governors routinely criticize Medicaid for its mounting cost to the states, they have found it difficult to resist the powerful expansionary incentives created by the program's open-ended federal matching grants. Throughout the program's history, state leaders have used a variety of methods ranging from lobbying and negotiation to creative financing mechanisms and waivers to maximize federal aid, thereby fueling Medicaid's growth. And, perceiving federal retrenchment efforts as a threat to their states' financial interests, the governors have repeatedly worked together in bipartisan fashion to defend the program against cutbacks. Indeed, Rose argues, Medicaid has been a driving force behind the mobilization of the intergovernmental lobby, and specifically the National Governors Association—one of the most powerful interest groups in Washington. *Financing Medicaid* engagingly intertwines theory, historical narrative, and case studies, drawing on a variety of sources including archival materials from gubernatorial and presidential libraries and the National Governors Association.

Shanna Rose is Assistant Professor at New York University's Robert F. Wagner Graduate School of Public Service.

Financing Medicaid

FEDERALISM AND THE GROWTH OF AMERICA'S HEALTH CARE SAFETY NET

Shanna Rose

The University of Michigan Press
Ann Arbor

Published in the United States of America by
The University of Michigan Press
Manufactured in the United States of America
⊗ Printed on acid-free paper

2016   2015   2014   2013   4   3   2   1

A CIP catalog record for this book is available from the British Library.

Library of Congress Cataloging-in-Publication Data

Rose, Shanna, 1975–
    Financing medicaid : federalism and the growth of America's health care safety net / Shanna Rose.
       pages   cm
    Includes bibliographical references and index.
    ISBN 978-0-472-07197-5 (cloth : alk. paper) — ISBN 978-0-472-05197-7 (pbk. : alk. paper) — ISBN 978-0-472-02941-9 (e-book)
    1. Medicaid—Finance.   2. Health care reform—United States.   3. Health insurance—Government policy—United States.   I. Title.
    RA412.4R67   2013
    368.4'200681—dc23

2013015658

Contents

Acknowledgments

I AM EXTREMELY GRATEFUL for the generous guidance and support I received from numerous individuals throughout the course of this project. I benefited immensely from enlightening conversations with, and thoughtful suggestions from, my colleagues at New York University's Wagner School of Public Service, particularly Charles Brecher, Rogan Kersh, and Tony Kovner, as well as many scholars of health policy, political science, and economics around the country including—but not limited to—James Alt, Andrew Karch, Thad Kousser, Ilyana Kuziemko, James Morone, Laura Katz Olson, Eric Patashnik, Mark Rom, Raymond Scheppach, Michael Sparer, Frank Thompson, Bruce Vladeck, Kent Weaver, Tim Westmoreland, seminar participants at the University of Minnesota and NYU-Wagner, and conference participants at UCLA, the American Political Science Association, the Association for Public Policy Analysis and Management, and the Association for Budgeting and Financial Management. I am also very grateful to three anonymous referees for their insightful and constructive suggestions, which have helped make this a substantially better book.

I owe an enormous debt to the many individuals who helped make this book a reality. For superb research assistance, I thank Hannah Caporello, Dan Han, Maggie Gribben, Megan Meagher, Caroline Ross, Anne Lu, and Susan Au. For exceptional administrative assistance, I thank Ann Lin. My outstanding developmental editor, Leslie Kriesel, was a constant source of insight and encouragement. I am extremely grateful to the University of Michigan editorial team, particularly Melody Herr for believing in this project from the very beginning and ushering it through to completion, as well as Susan Cronin for deftly handling its production. For financial support, I am indebted to NYU's University Research Challenge Fund, NYU's Goddard Junior Faculty Fellowship, and NYU-Wagner's Faculty Research Fund.

Most of all, I am deeply grateful to my family. This book never would have happened without the unwavering love and support of my parents, Joan (who taught me how to write) and Lou (who taught me how to think analytically, despite much resistance on my part). Meeting my husband, Peter, while writing this book may have slowed its progress by several months, but his probing questions and insightful comments contributed to its improvement in innumerable ways. Countless conversations are etched in my memory forever: arguing about the two Wilburs on the streets of Miami, discussing open-ended matching grants at the gym, and poring over the reviewers' comments together on the train to Connecticut. I am immensely grateful for his curiosity, patience, encouragement, and love.

Introduction: Medicaid, Federalism, and Policy Feedback

IN 1965, CONGRESS AMENDED the Social Security Act to create two new health-care programs: Medicare for the elderly, and Medicaid for the poor. Despite their common legislative origins and similar names, the two programs—and the story of how each came to exist—could hardly be more different.

Medicare evolved from the struggle for national health insurance. Throughout the 1940s and 1950s, liberal reformers had tried to enact a compulsory, comprehensive health insurance program for all Americans financed through payroll taxes, but had been stymied by powerful opponents including the American Medical Association (AMA), insurers, employer groups, and congressional conservatives. Repeated setbacks led reformers to scale back their ambitions, targeting the elderly and limiting coverage to hospital care while retaining the payroll-tax financed social-insurance model. They hoped this Medicare program would be a foot in the door—establishing a precedent that would ultimately pave the way for national health insurance.

In order to win congressional approval, Medicare first had to make it through the House Ways and Means Committee. The committee's powerful and fiscally conservative chairman, Wilbur Mills, worried that creating a payroll-tax-financed hospital insurance program for the elderly might lead to subsequent pressure for costly expansions of coverage, straining the Social Security system. For years, he refused to report the bill out of committee, earning him the nickname "the one-man veto on Medicare."[1]

However, a window of opportunity opened for Medicare in the mid-1960s. After President Kennedy was assassinated, the American public's grief translated into strong support for Kennedy's vice president, Lyndon Johnson, who won a landslide victory in the 1964 presidential election. This support carried over to Congress, where voters elected wide Democratic majorities in both the House and the Senate. Suddenly, Medicare's passage seemed all but inevitable.

At the Johnson administration's urging, Wilbur Mills finally reported out the Medicare legislation, along with a rider creating a second health-care program—Medicaid—for particularly vulnerable groups of poor Americans, including the disabled, blind, elderly, and children and mothers on welfare.[2] Mills hoped that by providing comprehensive coverage to key groups of the poor, Medicaid would serve as a firewall around Medicare, alleviating subsequent pressure for costly coverage expansions (Marmor 1973; Cohen 1983). Moreover, by modeling Medicaid on preexisting voluntary state-administered welfare programs and requiring participating states—with their limited fiscal capacity and political commitment—to share responsibility for designing eligibility and benefit policies and paying the program's costs, the fiscally conservative chairman hoped the program would remain small and unobtrusive.

Whereas the battle for Medicare had been fought in the front-line trenches over the course of two decades, the Medicaid provision was tacked on at the last minute and rushed through Congress with little floor debate.[3] Upon signing the legislation, President Johnson spoke at length about Medicare's historic significance, but did not mention Medicaid even once. The program was uniformly overlooked by national policy makers, interest groups, and the media—all of whom seemed to share Mills's presumption that, like existing state-administered welfare programs, Medicaid had limited potential for growth.

However, Medicaid's enormous potential became apparent almost immediately. Within the program's first year, the news media were already exclaiming over the explosive growth of the law's "least known but potentially most revolutionary provision"[4] and predicting that "Medicaid would eventually be a far greater and more significant program than Medicare."[5]

MEDICAID TODAY

Today's Medicaid program stands in stark contrast to its humble origins. In recent years, Medicaid has been called a colossus, a behemoth, a monster, an 800-pound gorilla, a sleeping giant, and the workhorse of the U.S. health system.[6] Since its inception, Medicaid has grown so dramatically that it has surpassed Medicare as the nation's largest health-care program, enrolling an average of 56 million individuals in 2011, compared to Medicare's 48 million (these figures include 9 million "dual eligible" beneficiaries who are enrolled in both programs).[7]

Medicaid covers an increasingly broad range of people and services. The program covers nearly half of all poor Americans, more than one-quarter of near-poor Americans, one-quarter of all children, 40 percent of all births, and nearly two-thirds of all nursing-home residents in the United States.[8] It also covers a wide variety of services that are excluded by Medicare, includ-

TABLE 1. Medicaid and Medicare

	Medicaid	Medicare
Structure	Federal-State program	Federal Program
Eligibility[a]	Low-income individuals who fall into a "categorically eligible" group: children; parents with dependent children; pregnant women; people with severe disabilities; senior citizens	All individuals aged 65 and older, regardless of income; certain permanently disabled individuals under 65; individuals with end-stage renal disease or amyotrophic lateral sclerosis
Number of enrollees	56 million	48 million
Covered services	Inpatient and outpatient hospital services; physician, midwife, and nurse practitioner services; laboratory and x-ray services; nursing facility and home health care; early and periodic screening, diagnosis, and treatment (EPSDT); family-planning services and supplies; rural health clinic/federally qualified health center services; plus many "optional" benefits including dental services, eyeglasses, hearing aids, etc. (see table 2)	Inpatient hospital stays; outpatient services; physician visits; preventive services; skilled nursing facility stays; home health visits; hospice care; and a voluntary, subsidized outpatient prescription drug benefit
Total benefit payments	$432 billion	$565 billion
Financing	Federal and state general revenues	Federal payroll tax, federal general revenues, beneficiary premiums

Source: Data from U.S. Department of Health and Human Services and Kaiser Family Foundation.
[a]Eligibility was extended under the Patient Protection and Affordable Care Act, as discussed in chapter 8.

ing long-term care, dental services, eyeglasses, and routine checkups, among others—although coverage varies considerably from state to state (see table 1 for a comparison of Medicare and Medicaid).

Medicaid has contributed to substantial improvements in the health and well-being of low-income Americans over the past five decades. The program has greatly increased access to health care, and has significantly improved the health outcomes of low-income Americans by virtually every conceivable measure—including infant mortality, maternal mortality, disease incidence, and life expectancy (Engel 2006). A recent study found that the expansion of Medicaid eligibility is associated with significant reductions in mortality and increased rates of self-reported health status of "excellent" or "very good" (Sommers, Baicker, and Epstein 2012; see also Meyer and Wherry 2012). In a recent randomized experiment, Medicaid beneficiaries reported substantial increases in overall health and happiness, and reduced financial strain after enrolling in the program (Finkelstein et al. 2011).

Medicaid's cost, which is shared by the federal and state governments, has grown dramatically over time due to increased enrollment and increased spending per enrollee. The typical state now spends more on Medicaid than it does on any other program—including K–12 education, higher education, corrections, and transportation (fig. 1). In fact, Medicaid has grown so rapidly as a share of total state spending that it has earned another nickname: the Pac-Man of state budgets (Weissert 1992). Medicaid is also a major outlay for the federal government, comprising nearly half of all federal grants to state and local governments (fig. 2).

Medicaid's total cost to federal and state governments was $432 billion in 2011. Despite covering more people, Medicaid's cost is lower than Medicare's ($565 billion) due in large part to the relatively low cost of covering children, who comprise just over half of the program's enrollees, but only 20 percent of its expenditures. By contrast, low-income elderly, disabled, and blind individuals—who collectively make up only 27 percent of Medicaid enrollees—account for two-thirds of the program's expenditures, due in part to the high cost of institutional and home-based care (fig. 3). Since Medicare and private health insurance furnish only limited coverage of long-term care, Medicaid has become the nation's main provider of such coverage. Whereas Medicaid accounts for roughly 16 percent of total U.S. health expenditures, it accounts for 36 percent of total home health-care expenditures, and 32 percent of total nursing home expenditures in the United States.[9]

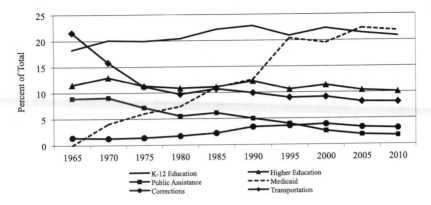

Fig. 1. State spending by function as a percentage of total state spending, 1965–2010. (Data from U.S. Census Bureau and National Association of State Budget Officers.)

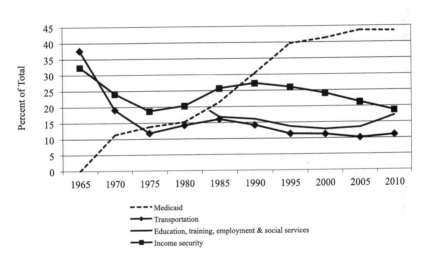

Fig. 2. Federal grants by function as a percentage of total federal grants to state and local governments, 1965–2010. (Data from U.S. Census Bureau.)

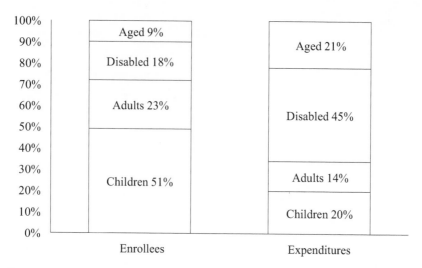

Fig. 3. Medicaid enrollees and expenditures by enrollment group, as a share of total. (Data from U.S. Department of Health and Human Services.)

Medicaid's dramatic expansion is particularly striking when compared with Medicare's relative stability. Whereas Medicaid's eligibility criteria have been repeatedly relaxed to include tens of millions of additional individuals, and its benefits expanded to include dozens of additional services, the nation's health-care program for the elderly has seen only one major eligibility expansion—the addition in 1972 of certain permanently disabled individuals and sufferers of end-stage renal disease—and only two major benefit expansions in its history (Oberlander 2003). The first benefit expansion (catastrophic coverage), which occurred in 1988, was repealed by Congress almost immediately, and the second (prescription drugs) did not occur until 2006, despite enjoying strong public support in the previous four decades. That Medicaid would be more prone to expansion than Medicare is surprising both because universal programs typically have broader political support than means-tested programs (Moene and Wallerstein 2001), and because Medicaid's low-income clientele has lower rates of political participation, fewer resources, and less political influence than the elderly (see for example Oberlander 2003).

Although liberal reformers initially pinned their hopes on Medicare as a foot in the door to national health insurance, it has been Medicaid—the would-be firewall designed to forestall the expansion of coverage—that has served as a springboard for comprehensive reform at both the state and federal levels. In 2006, Massachusetts enacted a groundbreaking universal health-care plan which expanded Medicaid eligibility well beyond the minimum level established by the federal government, and relied on federal Medicaid funds for more than half of its financing. In 2010, President Barack Obama signed into law the Patient Protection and Affordable Care Act, which (among other measures) expanded Medicaid eligibility to include almost all individuals under the age of 65 in families with income below 133 percent of the federal poverty line, bringing millions of new individuals into the program.[10]

How has Medicaid defied expectations—and its creator's intentions—by not only failing to relieve pressure for the expansion of coverage, but also becoming the primary vehicle for that expansion? As I argue in this book, the very institutional design Wilbur Mills hoped would limit Medicaid's scope—joint federal-state responsibility—has, in fact, fueled the program's growth since its inception.

FISCAL FEDERALISM

At first glance, it might seem surprising that Medicaid's federal-state structure could be an engine of growth. There are many reasons to believe that redistributive programs whose eligibility and benefits are largely determined at the state level should be smaller and more unstable than national programs. First, interstate competition for businesses and taxpayers is often said to set off a race to the bottom, whereby state officials adopt "lowest common denominator" programs (Oates 1972). Second, federalism increases the number of veto players, or political actors whose approval is required to change the status quo, potentially impeding policy expansions (Tsebelis 1995). In fact, the Founding Fathers viewed institutional fragmentation as check on government action. Third, the dispersion of policy-making authority may weaken pro-welfare-state coalitions, making it difficult for interest groups and parties to establish coherent national policy strategies since they are geographically diffuse, and focused on narrow jurisdictional issues (Swank 2002). Fourth, federalism is often said to dilute accountability, increasing the scope for blame avoidance, and thus the political feasibility of retrenchment (Weaver 1986). In summary, the consensus that federalism inhibits the welfare state is so strong that, in the words of one scholar: "one might point

to the federalism/social policy linkage as one of the very few areas of una-
nimity in the literature, with writers from all the main competing explanatory paradigms arguing that federal institutions are inimical to high levels of
social spending" (Castles 1999, 82).

Yet this well-established empirical pattern does not appear to apply to
Medicaid. Instead of engaging in a race to the bottom, most states voluntarily adopt more generous policies than federal standards require. For example, federal law does not require states to provide optional services such as
dental care and eyeglasses, but nearly all states do so anyway (table 2). Similarly, federal law only mandates that states cover pregnant women and infants with family incomes up to 133 percent of the federal poverty level, but
nearly all states choose to extend coverage to those with higher incomes—in
some cases as high as 300 percent of the poverty level (table 3). In fact, only
40 percent of Medicaid spending is mandatory; the other 60 percent is undertaken at state discretion.[11] And although the states often cut optional
coverage in times of fiscal austerity, such cuts are typically temporary and
relatively small when compared to Medicaid's rapidly rising baseline (Brown
and Sparer 2003).

The key to understanding how federalism has promoted Medicaid's
growth is its financing mechanism. The remainder of this section explains
how Medicaid is financed and what the existing literature can tell us about
how this arrangement has shaped individual states' Medicaid policies.
The rest of this chapter then outlines this book's central argument: that

TABLE 2. Medicaid Coverage of Selected Optional Services

Optional Services	Number of States Providing Coverage
Prescription drugs	51
Dental services	48
Prosthetic and orthotic devices	50
Eyeglasses	45
Hearing aids	32
Rehabilitation services	51
Physical therapy	36
Nonemergency medical transportation services	51
Hospice care	51
Intermediate care facilities for the mentally retarded	48
Inpatient psychiatric services for children under 21	51

Source: Data from Kaiser Family Foundation.
Note: Numbers include the 50 states and the District of Columbia (total = 51) as of October 2010.

Medicaid's institutional design has also had feedback effects on state leaders' political mobilization, with enormous implications for federal Medicaid policy.

The federal government provides the states with matching grants—meaning the amount of federal assistance depends on how much the state spends on Medicaid. These grants are open-ended—meaning there is no maximum state spending level at which the federal government stops contributing. The rate at which the federal government matches state spending, known as the Federal Medical Assistance Percentage (FMAP), varies inversely with the state's per capita income—a proxy for differences in state resources and needs.[12] The statutory minimum FMAP is 50 percent—meaning the federal government pays half of the Medicaid costs of high-income states like Connecticut, while the maximum is 83 percent—meaning the federal government pays up to 83 percent of the Medicaid costs of low-income states like Mississippi. In practice, however, the distribution of incomes relative to the national average is such that the top rate is typically less than the statutory maximum—around 77 percent. At the time Medicaid was enacted, this matching formula was considerably more generous than that of any existing federal grant program, as is discussed in greater detail below.

The economic effects of open-ended matching grants are by now fairly well understood. Open-ended matching grants give the recipient government an incentive to shift spending toward the targeted program at the expense of other programs. A state can spend a dollar on education or public safety and get a dollar's worth of benefits—or spend a dollar on Medicaid and get a total of two to four dollars' worth of benefits, depending on the federal matching rate. Conversely, during economic downturns, matching grants discourage states from scaling back Medicaid benefits and eligibility

TABLE 3. Medicaid Coverage of Selected Optional Eligibility Groups

Optional Eligibility Groups	Number of States Providing Coverage
Pregnant women above 133% of FPL	42
Infants above 133% of FPL	41
Children aged 1–5 above 133% of FPL	26
Children aged 6–19 above 100% of FPL	32

Source: Data from Kaiser Family Foundation.

Note: FPL = federal poverty level. Numbers include the 50 states and the District of Columbia (total = 51) as of January 2012 and include Medicaid expansions funded by the Children's Health Insurance Program.

because cutting one dollar of state spending means forgoing one to three dollars of federal aid at a time when external sources of funding are most urgently needed.

In the language of economics, matching grants have not only an income effect—whereby the grant increases the recipient government's total resources, leading to increased spending on all programs—but also a substitution effect, whereby the grant lowers the targeted program's relative price, leading the recipient government to redistribute spending away from other programs and toward the targeted program. By contrast, if Medicaid were instead funded with a block grant—a lump sum that does not depend on the amount of state spending—there would only be an income effect, resulting in relatively less state Medicaid spending.[13]

These income and substitution effects arise in the traditional neoclassical economic framework, which assumes that policy makers are benevolent public servants who seek to maximize social welfare. In recent years, economists have increasingly relaxed this assumption, assuming instead that politicians are self-interested maximizers of votes, budgets, or power. These alternative frameworks—part of the so-called public choice literature—yield potentially stronger predicted incentive effects of federal matching grants on state spending.

For instance, since the benefits of grant-funded programs are concentrated, but the costs are diffuse, self-interested state officials may have a tendency to overgraze the "fiscal commons" (Buchanan 1975; Weingast, Shepsle, and Johnsen 1981). Open-ended matching grants in particular present opportunities for one state to export the tax burden to residents of other states because the amount of the grant depends on the state's own actions (McLure 1967; Oates 2005). For instance, state officials can consolidate preexisting state health programs into Medicaid in order to qualify for additional matching dollars, or develop creative financing mechanisms to secure additional federal funding without actually spending state funds (as is discussed in chapter 5).

Similarly, the possibility of a federal bailout may motivate states to expand matching-grant-funded programs beyond a sustainable level. Kornai (1979) coined the term "soft budget constraint" to describe situations in which an economic entity (a state, in this case) anticipates financial rescue by a supporting organization (the federal government) in the event of fiscal distress. The federal government could warn states *ex ante* that bailouts are not available, but to the extent that states are considered too big to fail, this claim is not credible—particularly when there is a precedent of bailouts. In the case of Medicaid, Congress's recent pattern of temporarily increasing federal matching rates during recessions—discussed in chapter 7—may reduce states' incentives to spend prudently during good times.

Empirically estimating the sensitivity of state Medicaid spending to federal matching grants is difficult because the matching rate is a function of state income, and high-income states have more resources—and often stronger preferences—for generous eligibility and benefit policies, relative to low-income states. As a result, the literature finds a fairly wide range of estimates depending on the methodology used, but most studies conclude that state Medicaid spending is quite sensitive to the federal matching rate (see for example Granneman and Pauly 1983; Sloan 1984; Stotsky 1991; Grogan 1994; Chernick 1999; Chernick 2000; Adams and Wade 2001; Kronebusch 2004). For instance, Kousser (2002) finds that a state that receives a 79 percent match spends about 22 percent more on optional services per capita than a state that receives a 50 percent match, all else equal. McGuire and Merriman (2006) find that Medicaid spending is quite resilient during recessions—consistent with the hypothesis that generous federal matching grants diminish the incentive to cut eligibility and benefits during hard times.[14]

In summary, Medicaid's federal-state cost-sharing structure promotes the program's growth by giving state officials powerful financial incentives to adopt expansive programs, as numerous scholars have observed (see for example Gilman 1998; Brown and Sparer 2003; Weil 2003; Nathan 2005; Smith and Moore 2008; Grogan and Smith 2008; Sparer, France, and Clinton 2011; Thompson 2012).

POLICY FEEDBACK

Although Medicaid's economic effects are fairly well understood, less is known about the program's political implications; that is, we know how the program's financing mechanism affects state-level policy choices, but not how it has shaped strategic interactions among the states, or between the states and the federal government. This is surprising since, as the single largest and most complex federal-state program, Medicaid is at the heart of American intergovernmental relations. It is also surprising because political scientists have long understood that public policies are not only a product of the political process, but also a potentially important determinant of political dynamics—a concept known as policy feedback.

The literature on policy feedback can be traced back to 1935, when political scientist E. E. Schattschneider famously observed that "new policies create a new politics." Building on this idea, Theodore Lowi (1964) and James Q. Wilson (1973) argued that public policies allocate benefits and costs among various stakeholders, thereby setting off distinct patterns of interest group mobilization. In recent decades, this idea has become increasingly central to the study of policy making. Paul Pierson attributes the burgeoning policy feedback literature to the explosive growth of government in the twentieth century, which "made it harder to deny that public policies were not only outputs of but important inputs into the political process" (Pierson 1993, 595).

Policy feedback can occur through several distinct mechanisms (Skocpol 1992; Pierson 1993; Ikenberry 1994). First, policies may shape political actors' incentives by altering the payoffs associated with alternative strategies. For example, a policy may confer benefits or costs on a latent group, thereby motivating its members to overcome collective action problems and mobilize into an organized interest group. Second, public policies may confer resources on certain individuals or groups, thereby creating privileged positions from which beneficiaries can work to perpetuate those policies. These resources may be material, as when the government provides financial support to a social group, or nonmaterial, such as information or access to policymakers. Third, policies may have interpretive effects. For example, government action may redefine a policy issue in a new way, changing individuals' perceptions of what their interests are and who their allies might be.

By strengthening supportive constituencies, the introduction of a new policy has the potential to reconfigure political dynamics in ways that both promote that policy's continuation and hinder the adoption of previously plausible policy alternatives (Skocpol 1992; Weir 1992). Policy feedback is thus a specific variety of path dependence, whereby decisions made at a critical juncture can lead a polity down a certain path and, through a self-reinforcing process, make it difficult or costly to reverse course (Pierson 1993). One of the most notable characteristics of path dependence is non-ergodicity, whereby accidental or seemingly small events early in a sequence have potentially important long-term implications because they constrain future choices (Arthur 1994). Once a positive feedback loop is set in motion, "the path not taken" becomes increasingly distant and difficult to reach, even after the triggering events have ceased to exist (Pierson 2000). The claim is not that path dependence permanently or irrevocably locks in existing arrangements, but rather that it imposes constraints on policy makers' subsequent choices, and thus helps to explain why some institutions are extremely persistent (North 1990; Pierson 2004).

One common criticism of path dependence (and, by extension, policy feedback) is that it is potentially such a broad and all-encompassing concept that it offers little analytical leverage. Critics contend that according to the minimalist definition adopted by some scholars, path dependence simply means that "the past affects the future," resulting in "a vague conceptualization in which any causal chain could be seen as exhibiting path dependence; every outcome in the social world is, after all, preceded by a series of historical events" (Mahoney and Schensul 2006, 458; see also Brown 2010). A number of scholars have recently called for a "finer unpacking of historical causality," including theoretical refinements that "identify conditions that are necessary and/or sufficient for past choices and outcomes to influence the present" (Page 2006, 87).

Recent scholarship has thus sought to develop more precise conceptualizations of path dependence and policy feedback. For instance, Eric Patashnik and Julian Zelizer observe that theories that fail to account for the absence of positive feedback have little explanatory force: "if policy feedback is everywhere, it is nowhere" (Patashnik and Zelizer 2010, 2). They develop a framework in which the likelihood of feedback depends on three factors: policy design, timing, and institutional support. First, the authors point out that "policy designs may simply not provide enough material resources to facilitate the emergence of a supportive constituency to defend the policy" (10). Second, because the historical context is so crucial to feedback processes, a policy introduced at the wrong time might not have the potential to reproduce itself; for instance, a new policy might be inconsistent with the social norms prevailing at the time of enactment. Third, feedback effects may not occur when there are "inadequate or conflicting institutional supports," as when state capacities are limited, or in complex institutional environments in which the supportive constituency has multiple identities that are in tension with one another (18). This theoretical framework helps to explain why Medicaid has generated feedback effects while other federal-state programs have not, as I argue in this book.

Another limitation of the literature on policy feedback is its emphasis on the impact of public policies on social groups and mass publics, to the exclusion of government elites. Much of the literature focuses on how policies affect their proximate targets, such as Campbell's 2003 study of the effect of

Social Security and Medicare on the political participation of senior citizens and Mettler's 2005 study of the effect of the GI Bill on veterans. Other research has focused on private-sector interests, such as Hacker's 2002 study of businesses, insurers, and medical providers and the welfare state, or on mass opinion, such as Soss and Schram's 2007 study of welfare reform and public views toward the poor. By contrast, policy feedback effects on the political mobilization of government elites have been understudied, as Paul Pierson observes.

> Policy initiatives—which are, after all, the central undertakings of public officials—may provide resources and incentives affecting the capacities of government elites. Yet of all the dimensions of policy influence . . . those linking the resources and incentives generated by existing policies to the actions of government elites seem the least well established. (Pierson 1993, 603–4)

This book seeks to fill this void in the literature by investigating the feedback effects of one of the largest U.S. government programs of any kind on the political mobilization of state government elites.

MEDICAID: A SINGULAR CASE OF POLICY FEEDBACK

The central argument of this book is that following Medicaid's enactment, state leaders emerged as a supportive constituency, responding to the incentives built into the program in ways that have fueled the program's explosive growth over the past half-century. By offering generous open-ended matching grants to the states, along with broad discretion over eligibility and the scope of covered services, the program has created spoils that have motivated the governors to mobilize on behalf of programmatic expansion. Working both individually and as an organized interest group (the National Governors Association, one of the most powerful lobbying organizations in Washington), state leaders have sought to maximize federal financial assistance, with the byproduct of promoting the program's incremental growth. As is documented in this book, the governors have done so through a variety of channels, including lobbying Congress, negotiating with the White House, developing creative financing mechanisms to exploit Medicaid's open-ended financing structure, and applying for waivers to federal laws and regulations, among others. The infusion of funds and the delegation of new responsibilities have led to dramatic increases in state officials' administrative capability and technical expertise, which in turn has increased their access to Congress, the White House, and the news media—and thus their influence over federal Medicaid policy.

One of the defining characteristics of policy feedback is the reconfiguration of political dynamics in ways that hinder the adoption of previously feasible policy alternatives. Federal policymakers have, since Medicaid's very inception, tried on dozens of occasions to restructure the program's financing mechanism, but repeatedly failed to overcome state opposition. The governors have vehemently rejected numerous attempts to curtail federal assistance by capping Medicaid's open-ended matching grants. While some governors have, on occasion, expressed support for a Medicaid block grant—which would provide states with less funding, but more flexibility than the current arrangement—or a federal takeover of the program, federal-state negotiations over the terms of such reforms have routinely foundered due to the governors' financial concerns. As is argued in this book, the states' enormous financial stake in the status quo has proven to be an insurmountable obstacle to change.

Why has Medicaid had such important feedback effects on state leaders while other federal-state programs, such as cash assistance and highways, have not (as suggested by figs. 1 and 2)? The fact that public policies have the potential to set off a feedback process does not imply that they necessarily will. However, Medicaid clearly meets all three of Patashnik and Zelizer's (2010) criteria for policy feedback.

Medicaid meets the first criterion: policy design. When the program was created in 1965, its matching formula was considerably more generous than the formulas used to fund existing federal-state programs. For example, when Aid to Families with Dependent Children (AFDC) was created in 1935, it was funded with a 33 percent closed-ended matching grant.[15] The federal highway program offered a higher matching rate—between 75 and 80 percent for most states—but its grants are also closed ended. In fact, they are capped at such a low level that the federal government only pays about one-quarter of total highway spending, leading some scholars to argue that these matching grants effectively operate as block grants (Gamkhar 2003). Medicaid also offered more carrots and sticks to encourage state participation than previous federal-state health care programs for the poor—namely, medical vendor payments and the Kerr-Mills Program of Medical Assistance to the Aged—as is discussed in chapter 1.

Medicaid also meets the second criterion: timing. When the program was enacted in the mid-1960s, state capitals—like the federal government— were overwhelmingly dominated by liberals, and the political climate was characterized by heightened concern about poverty, inequality, and social justice (Stimson 1999). Medicaid's emphasis on alleviating suffering among the nation's most vulnerable populations was thus highly consistent with prevailing social norms. Had the program been enacted during the relatively conservative 1950s, it might have failed to establish such a secure toehold. Moreover, compared to cash assistance, health insurance was, and continues to be, more consistent with longstanding American social norms such as individualism and self-reliance. Americans are deeply ambivalent about government programs that give cash to the poor, but are generally much more supportive of health coverage for the same group—perhaps for paternalistic reasons, or because they view health care as a basic human right (Gilens 1999).

Finally, Medicaid was introduced at a time of greatly expanding institutional support at the state level. The mid-1960s witnessed a remarkable transformation in state governments due to the infusion of new federal grants-in-aid, the expansion of state tax authority, and the implementation of a variety of political and administrative reforms. Together, these changes attracted a new breed of more capable, experienced politicians to state capitals around the country. Thus, at the time of Medicaid's enactment, the states were particularly receptive to the new program's incentive structure.

More generally, when it comes to influencing federal policy, the governors have many institutional advantages that augment their capacity as a supportive constituency. Their status and legitimacy as high-ranking public officials and their direct electoral relationship with congressional members' constituencies makes them particularly influential on Capitol Hill. As implementers of federal policy, the governors can threaten noncooperation to gain leverage in changing the terms of their participation in federal-state programs.

However, as Patashnik and Zelizer note, policy feedback effects are weakened when the supportive constituency has multiple identities that are in tension with one another—as in the case of the governors, who identify not only as state leaders seeking federal financial assistance, but also as members of political parties. The two parties typically have very different positions on Medicaid policy, with Democrats preferring more expansive coverage than Republicans (Kousser 2002). Although partisan conflict threatens to undermine their cohesion and effectiveness as an interest group, the governors find it easier to agree on the need for additional federal funding than on any other issue (Posner 1998; Derthick 2001); indeed, as is demonstrated in later chapters, the governors' collective financial stake in protecting and augmenting federal Medicaid funds helps them overcome partisan and other internal cleavages, particularly during periods of resource scarcity, when fiscal considerations are especially salient.

In arguing that the governors have emerged as a supportive constituency, I am not claiming that Medicaid's growth is a reflection of their policy preferences. Despite the integral role they have played in promoting Medicaid's growth and protecting it against federal retrenchment, governors—particularly Republicans—routinely bemoan its expansion. Since the program's inception, state leaders have repeatedly complained to federal lawmakers that the state share of Medicaid spending is "out of control," "breaking our back," and "dragging us toward bankruptcy."[16] In fact, the governors have developed "a love-hate relationship" with Medicaid—they love the federal funding it brings in, but hate the mounting cost to the states (Grogan and Smith 2008, 204).

Rather, I argue that Medicaid's financial incentives have proven too powerful for even its biggest detractors to resist. For instance, in 2006, Governor Mitt Romney (R-Massachusetts)—a vocal critic of the "immensely expensive" Medicaid program—developed a comprehensive health care reform package that greatly expanded Medicaid eligibility, and relied on federal Medicaid funds for more than half its financing (discussed in chapter 8). Similarly, in 2010, Governor Rick Perry (R-Texas) declared that his state would opt out of the voluntary Medicaid program, only to retract the statement a month later when it turned out that the move would have cost his state's taxpayers billions of dollars, and would have decimated the state's health-care system (discussed in the conclusion). The often striking contrast between the governors' words and deeds underscores the irresistible incentives built into Medicaid's institutional arrangement, and suggests that Medicaid's growth is largely driven not by state policymakers' preferences but rather by the program's own institutional logic.

The governors' role in promoting Medicaid's growth over the past five decades highlights the irony of the states' legal challenge to the Affordable Care Act of 2010. In the lawsuit, 26 Republican governors and attorneys general argued that the mandatory expansion of Medicaid coverage was an "unprecedented encroachment on the sovereignty of the states," and the Supreme Court agreed in its June 2012 decision. Yet the Affordable Care Act was modeled on Governor Romney's health reform package, which in turn evolved from a series of creative financing mechanisms and "research and demonstration" waivers employed by Romney's predecessors in an attempt to extract the maximum federal funding from the Medicaid program (discussed in chapter 8). Moreover, although the Supreme Court decision makes the expansion of coverage optional, if history is any indication, most states will choose to expand coverage (as argued in the conclusion).

MANY ENGINES OF GROWTH

Of course, my claim is not that Medicaid's growth is entirely attributable to feedback effects arising from the program's federal-state cost-sharing structure. Rather than a comprehensive account of all of the factors that have shaped Medicaid's development, this book offers a crucial piece of the puzzle that has thus far been the subject of limited study. A host of factors has contributed to the program's incremental expansion, as has been documented by other scholars. These other expansionary forces—including health-care providers, nonprofit advocacy groups, public opinion, and federal government policy entrepreneurs—are complements to, rather than substitutes for, my argument, and in fact can help shed light on the motivations behind state leaders' efforts to expand and protect Medicaid.

First, health-care providers—the physicians, hospitals, nursing homes, public health clinics, community health centers, and other institutions that are reimbursed for their services by Medicaid—have exerted tremendous influence over the program's development (see for example Barrilleaux and Miller 1988; Sparer 1996; Olson 2010; Granneman and Pauly 2010). Providers have an enormous financial stake in Medicaid, which is a critical source of financial support, particularly for nursing homes and safety-net institutions. Although providers are primarily concerned with increasing provider reimbursement rates for existing Medicaid patients, they have also pushed for the expansion of covered services and, to a lesser extent, eligibility at various points in the program's history (Grogan 1994; Kronebusch 1997). Even though Medicaid's reimbursement rates are low compared to those of Medicare and private insurance, providers typically support eligibility expansions because the program covers low-income populations that would otherwise have difficulty paying for care (Sparer 2009). Also, since Medicare and most private insurers do not cover nursing-home services, the nursing-home lobby has been a particularly strong advocate of extending Medicaid eligibility (Grogan 1994).

Political pressure from providers can help explain state leaders' efforts to promote the program's growth and protect it against federal retrenchment. Providers are organized on a state basis and tend to be more influential in state politics than in national politics (Vladeck 1979; Palley 1997). In addition to exerting enormous influence over state Medicaid policy, providers thus use state leaders as a conduit through which to influence federal Medicaid policy. For instance, pressure from providers helped motivate the governors to lobby Congress to relax federal eligibility limits in the 1980s (chapter 4). As I explain in the conclusion, pressure from providers will also prevent most states from opting out of the Affordable Care Act's Medicaid expansion. State leaders are also acutely aware that by funneling federal money to health-care providers, Medicaid helps create jobs, purchases, and income associated with health-care service delivery, thereby augmenting state tax revenue. For instance, a Missouri study found that federal matching funds generated $5.82 billion in economic activity, supported 79,892 jobs, and increased income by $2.8 billion in 2004—generating $211 million in state tax revenue in 2004.[17]

Second, advocacy groups representing Medicaid beneficiaries have helped promote the program's growth (see for example Tanenbaum 1995; Sardell and Johnson 1998; Rosenbaum and Sonosky 2001; Palfrey 2006). For instance, the Children's Defense Fund, the American Academy of Pediatrics, and other child-advocacy organizations joined the governors in pressuring Congress to loosen federal eligibility rules in the 1980s, and to create the Children's Health Insurance Program—which gave the states the option of using the funds for Medicaid expansion—in 1997. Like providers, advocacy groups are often even more influential at the state level, where they lobby lawmakers to extend coverage beyond federal minimum standards (Sparer 1996; Berry and Arons 2003; Grogan and Gusmano 2007).

Third, public opinion is generally quite supportive of Medicaid. Despite the program's means-tested status and rapidly growing cost, only 13 percent of Americans favor major reductions in Medicaid spending, while 3 in 10 support minor reductions, and 53 percent want to see no reductions at all.[18] In part, Medicaid's popularity reflects the fact that it has increasingly become a program for not only the poor, but also the middle class, particularly when it comes to institutional care (Vladeck 2003; Grogan and Patashnik 2003a; Grogan and Patashnik 2003b; Grogan 2008). Although only 20 percent of survey respondents report having ever personally received Medicaid benefits, another 31 percent report having a friend or family member who has received Medicaid benefits—such as a parent in a nursing home—and many cite these personal connections as an important reason for their support. Medicaid's popularity may also reflect altruism or the possibility of needing Medicaid coverage in the future, as many respondents reported that they "like knowing that the Medicaid program exists as a safety net to protect low-income people who can't afford needed care." As political constructions of the growing Medicaid program have evolved from "stigmatized welfare" to "core social entitlement," federal and state leaders have become increasingly reluctant to cut the program (Grogan and Andrews 2011, 282).

Finally, federal government policy entrepreneurs—most notably Representative Henry Waxman (D-California)—have contributed to Medicaid's growth by championing the liberalization of federal laws and regulations governing eligibility, the scope of covered services, and provider reimbursement (Gilman 1998; Brown and Sparer 2003). Just as Medicaid's federal-state cost-sharing structure encourages state expansion, it also allows federal policy makers to accomplish health reform on the cheap—shifting the administrative burden and much of the cost to the states, and avoiding the tag of big government (Sparer, France, and Clinton 2011). Such incentives help explain why Medicaid expansion became a central pillar of the Affordable Care Act (Sparer 2009; Rosenbaum 2009).

In fact, Medicaid's federal-state cost-sharing structure often leads federal and state officials to "prompt and prod each other toward additional coverage expansions" (Sparer, France, and Clinton 2011). State activism can prompt federal activism, such as when Governor Romney's health care reform plan served as the template for the Affordable Care Act. Federal activism can also prompt state activism, such as when a series of federal eligibility expansions in the 1980s led the states to develop creative financing mechanisms to finance the program's mounting cost, thereby contributing to its further growth (chapter 5). Brown and Sparer (2003) have coined the phrase "catalytic federalism" to describe this phenomenon, while Nathan (2005) refers to it as "federal pull/state push."

OVERVIEW OF THE BOOK

Chapter 1 provides an account of Medicaid's political origins, arguing that a logic of expansion was embedded in the program's institutional structure, but not foreseen by its creator. When Wilbur Mills, the powerful and fiscally conservative chairman of the House Ways and Means Committee, first proposed the Medicaid program, it was widely hailed as an ingenious strategy for heading off subsequent pressure for expansion of coverage. However, due to Medicaid's unique policy design, timing, and state-level institutional support, this small safety net unexpectedly grew into one of the largest and costliest U.S. government programs of any kind. This chapter explores how Medicaid's policy design evolved from existing welfare medicine programs, and explains why experience with these programs led Mills—as well as other federal policy makers, interest groups, and the media—to underestimate Medicaid's potential.

Medicaid's unintended propensity for expansion was revealed immediately, as many state leaders moved quickly to design much broader programs than federal lawmakers had envisioned. Chapter 2 highlights the case of New York, where Governor Nelson Rockefeller attempted to make his state's Medicaid plan the "best in the nation" by extending eligibility to nearly half the state's population.[19] Federal policy makers subsequently grew alarmed that the "badly conceived and badly organized" program was generating "vast increases in government health expenditures."[20] Congress considered a wide range of amendments to the law in the program's first five years, including a cap on federal contributions in 1966, eligibility limits in 1967, reductions in federal matching rates for the medically needy in 1968, relaxation of coverage mandates in 1969, and reductions in federal funding for long-term care in 1970. Of these proposals, only the eligibility and coverage reforms succeeded; all three attempts to revise Medicaid's financing structure failed due to intense lobbying by the nation's governors. In a striking case of policy feedback, state leaders emerged as a supportive constituency for the new program, immediately constraining federal lawmakers' ability to reverse course.

The second half of chapter 2 documents the governors' mobilization as an interest group. Government action often stimulates interest-group formation, and the Great Society programs of the 1960s were no exception. The proliferation of federal grant programs—of which Medicaid quickly became the largest and most complex—meant that state officials suddenly had a compelling new incentive to organize and voice their interests in Washington. Moreover, the infusion of new funds and responsibilities increased the governors' resources for mobilization. Although the National Governors Association—originally known simply as the Governors' Conference—had existed since the beginning of the twentieth century, for its first six decades, the group had functioned primarily as a social club. It was not until the late 1960s that the governors established a permanent lobbying apparatus in Washington, organized standing committees, and began testifying before Congress on a regular basis. By the 1980s, the National Governors Association was widely considered one of the most influential lobbying organizations in Washington.

The Reagan administration made three major attempts at Medicaid retrenchment in the early 1980s and was defeated by the governors each time, as is documented in chapter 3. President Reagan first proposed to permanently cap Medicaid matching grants in 1981, but the governors successfully lobbied Congress to instead adopt a much smaller, temporary cut in the matching rate. Later that year, the administration considered converting the program's open-ended matching grants to block grants—offering the states more flexibility in exchange for less federal funding—but state leaders again rejected the idea. Realizing that the surest way to retrench the program was to remove it from state hands, the Reagan administration shifted gears in 1982, proposing a "swap" whereby the federal government would take full responsibility for Medicaid and, in exchange, the states would take full responsibility for cash assistance and food stamps. In an unprecedented move, the president invited the governors to participate in a high-profile series of negotiations at the White House. Although state leaders were eager to turn over Medicaid—the fastest-growing component of their budgets—to the federal government, they ultimately rejected the proposal when the administration revealed its plans to dramatically curtail Medicaid eligibility and benefits. However badly state leaders wanted out of Medicaid, the prospect of reduced federal support was even less appealing. The Reagan administration's failure to restructure and retrench Medicaid in the early 1980s is one of the most fascinating and unexpected paths not taken in the program's history.

Chapter 4 examines the critical role the nation's governors played in bringing about one of the most dramatic series of eligibility expansions in Medicaid's history. The recessions and budget cuts of the early 1980s contributed to increased poverty, a spike in the infant mortality rate, and a surge in uncompensated charity care costs at state hospitals. Many governors saw expanding Medicaid eligibility as a financially attractive solution to their mounting problems, realizing that if they could bring more of the uninsured into the program, the federal government would pick up half or more of the bill. In the mid-1980s the governors—led by Richard Riley (D-South Carolina) and several other Southern Democrats—repeatedly lobbied Congress to loosen federal eligibility rules to allow the states to enroll more infants and pregnant women in the program. Although most governors favored optional eligibility expansions, some preferred mandatory expansions to help them overcome political resistance from conservative state legislatures, as well as collective action problems arising from interstate competition. Congressional Democrats—taking advantage of the governors' increased receptiveness—passed a series of bills allowing or requiring the states to extend coverage to new groups. Early legislation targeting infants and pregnant women paved the way for later bills targeting older children, parents, seniors, and the disabled. As a result of these measures, enrollment rose by nearly 10 million people—an increase of roughly 50 percent.

Medicaid's federal-state cost-sharing arrangement presents numerous opportunities for cost shifting between levels of government; this was perhaps more evident in the late 1980s and early 1990s than at any other time in the program's history. As federal mandates proliferated and the national economy deteriorated, the governors grew increasingly desperate to relieve the mounting financial pressure on state budgets without scaling back coverage. Despite the national recession, most states avoided major Medicaid cutbacks—and some even extended eligibility and benefits—through the use of creative financing mechanisms, as is documented in chapter 5. Taking advantage of legal and regulatory loopholes, the states collected donations and taxes from medical providers and then used the funds to pay those same providers for Medicaid services, thereby qualifying for federal matching funds without putting up any additional state dollars. During this period, the National Governors Association played a critical role in representing the states' financial interests, providing legal and technical assistance on the structuring of creative financing mechanisms, and negotiating with the White House and lobbying Congress to keep the loopholes open as long as possible.

As the federal government began to set limits on the use of creative financing mechanisms in the early 1990s, state officials cast about for new ways to secure additional federal matching grants. An opportunity presented itself when Democrat (and former governor) Bill Clinton became president and—following months of intense negotiations with the National Governors Association—agreed to streamline the process by which states apply for research and demonstration waivers to federal Medicaid rules, making it easier for state officials to obtain additional federal funds for coverage expansions. The states rushed to apply for exemptions from federal regulations in order to cover otherwise ineligible populations or services, and in some cases—including Oregon and Tennessee—used federal funds to extend coverage to hundreds of thousands of uninsured individuals, as is documented in chapter 6.

In 1995, congressional Republicans drafted legislation that would have converted Medicaid's financing arrangement from an open-ended matching grant to a block grant. By offering the states increased programmatic flexibility, congressional leaders hoped to entice them into accepting explicit limits on federal funding. That conservative national leaders wanted to block grant Medicaid was nothing new; what was new was that an unprecedented number of governors supported the idea. As I argue in chapter 7, this turnaround was due to a unique set of political and economic factors that characterized the mid-1990s, including a large number of Republican governors, heightened party polarization, a recent spate of federal mandates, and a strong national economy. However, Democratic and some moderate Republican governors dragged their feet, fearing that without the federal government's open-ended financial commitment, the states would have insufficient resources to maintain current eligibility and benefit policies. Even conservative governors who wholeheartedly embraced the principle of a block grant found themselves engaged in a bitter formula fight over the distribution of funds. Ultimately, these internal divisions among the governors doomed the proposal's prospects in Washington. Despite unprecedented support for a Medicaid block grant at both levels of government, the governors' financial stake in the status quo once again shielded the program from retrenchment.

The central argument of this book is that Medicaid's federal-state cost-sharing arrangement has caused the program to persist and grow largely by its own institutional logic. Yet federalism—among other forms of institutional fragmentation—has also proven to be a formidable obstacle to the enactment of comprehensive health care reform in the United States (see for example Hacker 2002). Thus, this book's findings help to explain why recent efforts to solve the problem of the uninsured at both the state and federal levels rely heavily on the continued expansion of Medicaid. As I argue in chapter 8, incremental change and continued reliance on established institutions—not wholesale reform—has proven to be the path of least resistance.

The first half of chapter 8 examines Medicaid's central role in health care reform in Massachusetts, where Governor Mitt Romney's desire to avoid raising taxes led him to adopt a plan in 2006 that included a major expansion of Medicaid eligibility, and relied on federal Medicaid funds for more than half its financing. Four years later, federal policy makers' goal of a deficit-neutral health reform package led them to adopt the single largest eligibility expansion in Medicaid's history—extending coverage to an estimated 17 million additional people—in order to take advantage of state cost-sharing, as well as additional savings from the program's relatively low provider reimbursement rates and administrative costs, as is discussed in the second half of chapter 8. However, the governors proved once again to be an enormously influential force over federal Medicaid policy, convincing Congress to provide supplemental funding for newly eligible enrollees and convincing the Supreme Court that the expansion should be optional rather than mandatory.

This book's conclusion summarizes my central argument and explores its implications for the future of Medicaid. Despite Medicaid's rapid expansion over the past five decades, there are signs that its growth has begun to run into state-level fiscal and political constraints that may prove insurmountable. The recent combination of a severe national recession, an influx of Republican governors, and backlash against the Affordable Care Act has led to considerable speculation about the program's future. While theories of policy feedback can help explain persistence, they do not preclude dramatic change. Under the right circumstances, a countervailing set of forces can emerge that is sufficiently powerful to dislodge a long-lasting equilibrium (North 1990; Pierson 2000). This chapter concludes with an analysis of the political and economic factors that might converge to bring about a major change in Medicaid's trajectory, and the form that change might take.

CHAPTER I

The Birth of Medicaid: 1965

IN 1965, WILBUR MILLS, the powerful and fiscally conservative chairman of the House Ways and Means Committee, proposed a plan that was widely hailed as ingenious. The proposal, which Mills had secretly developed in collaboration with President Lyndon Johnson's administration over the course of a year, was to create two new health-care programs: Medicare for the elderly, and Medicaid for the poor. This plan had the virtue of combining elements of the proposals of Democrats, Republicans, and the powerful American Medical Association, making it politically unassailable from any angle. Creating a small safety net for the poor also had the advantage, in Mills's eyes, of heading off subsequent pressure for costly expansions of Medicare, which he feared would strain the Social Security system. Ironically, this small safety net grew so quickly that within one year observers were predicting that it would eventually "dwarf" Medicare.[1] Mills later referred to Medicaid as the most expensive mistake of his career (Zelizer 1998).

Wilbur Mills was not alone in underestimating Medicaid's potential. Federal policy makers, interest groups, and the media wrote off Medicaid as an incremental extension of small existing welfare medicine programs. Years of experience with these voluntary, state-administered programs (most notably the Kerr-Mills Program of Medical Assistance to the Aged)—under which state participation had been minimal due to lack of fiscal capacity and political commitment—led stakeholders to presume that Medicaid, too, would remain small. However, such predictions overlooked several expansionary seeds embedded in Kerr-Mills and Medicaid from the beginning, including not only the loosely defined eligibility standards and comprehensive scope of covered services that have been emphasized by other scholars (Stevens and Stevens 2003; Grogan and Patashnik 2003; Grogan 2006; Grogan and Smith 2008), but also the financial incentives created by open-ended matching grants. As I argue in this chapter and in chapter 2, these expansionary seeds only sprouted following Medicaid's enactment, when a confluence of factors—including incremental changes in policy design, increased institutional support, and the unique timing of the law's passage—prompted states to implement much more generous programs than anyone had anticipated.

MEDICAID'S POLITICAL ORIGINS

Medicaid's passage in 1965, and the program's unique institutional design, can only be fully understood in the context of the struggle to enact universal health insurance in the United States (Hacker 1998; Grogan and Patashnik 2003). Although nearly all industrialized nations adopted national health insurance programs in the twentieth century, efforts at such a reform repeatedly failed in America. Despite being introduced in Congress fourteen times throughout the 1940s and 1950s by Senator Robert Wagner (D-New York), Senator James Murray (D-Montana), and Representative John Dingell (D-Michigan), a payroll-tax-funded, compulsory, comprehensive national health-insurance program was never enacted. Its recurring failure is particularly striking given that Democrats controlled the presidency and both houses of Congress throughout most of this period and polls indicated that nearly three-quarters of Americans favored national health insurance (Harris 1969, 27).

Scholars have put forward a variety of theories to explain why the United States did not join other industrialized nations in adopting national health insurance in the twentieth century. Virtually all accounts point to the role of powerful special interest groups in impeding reform. Physicians—represented by the American Medical Association—and insurance companies resisted national health insurance as a threat to their financial interests, while employer groups and conservatives opposed the payroll taxes needed to finance coverage (Starr 1982; Quadragno 2005). These special interests were aided by the institutional fragmentation built into the American political system, as diffusion of power among multiple branches and levels of government creates numerous points of influence (Steinmo and Watts 1995; Hacker 2002). They were also aided by the United States' individualistic and antistatist political culture, which makes Americans "simultaneously supportive of significant reform and uneasy about expanding government involvement" (Jacobs 1993, 629). Moreover, there was no labor-sponsored initiative to counter the AMA since the rise of collectively bargained private health plans gave labor unions a vested interest in the private welfare state, effectively removing them from the struggle for national health insurance (Hacker 2002; Quadragno 2005).

In the late 1950s and 1960s, interest-group opposition led liberal reformers to scale back their ambitions by targeting two subsets of the population: the elderly, and welfare recipients. By limiting coverage to costly, difficult-to-insure groups, advocates hoped to minimize interest group opposition (Quadragno 2005). Targeting these groups also had potential public appeal. Impoverished mothers and children on welfare were widely seen as vulnerable, blameless victims, while the elderly were a politically active and sympathetic group who were twice as likely to need medical care and significantly less likely to hold private insurance than the rest of the population (Stevens and Stevens 2003).

One reform model—which ultimately became the template for Medicare—targeted the elderly, but retained the "social insurance" approach underlying national health insurance proposals, whereby health care would be universally available as a matter of right, regardless of need, as well as payroll-tax financing through the Social Security system. Advocates of national health insurance hoped this "foot in the door strategy" would establish "the precedent and practicality of public health insurance," paving the way for broader coverage over time (Gordon 2003, 24). Representative Aime Forand (D-Rhode Island) first introduced such a bill in 1957. In an effort to appease the AMA, Forand proposed to not only limit eligibility to the aged, but also to limit coverage to hospitalization, nursing-home, and in-hospital surgical care, omitting physician services. Despite these concessions, organized interests and conservatives vehemently opposed the bill for the same reasons they had opposed universal health insurance. Although the Forand Bill died in the House Ways and Means Committee, it reframed the debate by concentrating on the problems of the aged, setting off a "groundswell of grassroots support" among senior citizens that subsequently forced Medicare onto the national agenda (Starr 1982).

A second tactic, which ultimately paved the way for Medicaid, took a very different means-tested or "welfare medicine" approach, whereby government-financed health care is limited to only the neediest Americans—namely, recipients of public assistance, who were poor and met one of several categorical eligibility requirements (families with dependent children;

the elderly; the blind; and the disabled). This approach was more successful in minimizing interest-group opposition. As pressure for health reform mounted, physicians, insurers, employers, and conservatives came to see welfare medicine as the lesser of evils. As Stevens and Stevens note, "it was clear to the political realist that, if the movement for health insurance for the aged as part of the Social Security system were to be slowed down (if not stopped), there had to be a viable, or at least plausible, alternative" (2003, 28). Opponents of social insurance favored building on the American tradition of voluntary state administration of welfare programs, which dated back to the English Poor Laws (Sparer 1996). They took comfort in the belief that, given the states' proven lack of commitment and capacity to develop generous cash-assistance programs, state-administered welfare medicine would likely remain small and minimally intrusive as well (Moore and Smith 2005).

THE TWO WILBURS

The expansion of welfare medicine was spearheaded by two men named Wilbur: Wilbur Mills and Wilbur Cohen. Despite their close working relationship, the two Wilburs embodied the opposing sides of the philosophical divide over health reform. Like many opponents of the social-insurance approach, Mills saw welfare medicine as a preferable substitute. Like many advocates, Cohen saw it as a complement and potential stepping stone to broader coverage.

Wilbur Mills, a Harvard-trained lawyer and Democratic congressman from Arkansas, was routinely described as the most powerful man in Congress, and the second most powerful man in Washington after the president (Zelizer 1998). He served as chairman of the House Ways and Means Committee for a total of 18 years—longer than any other person in U.S. history.

Mills was a fiscal conservative who tended to define government programs in terms of their cost rather than human needs, and whose top policy objectives included low taxes and balanced budgets (Zelizer 1998). When it came to expanding access to health care, Mills feared that a Medicare program for elderly persons of all income levels funded by payroll taxes would threaten the actuarial soundness of the Social Security system. Social Security linked pension payments to an individual's wages during their working years; this was a predictable and controllable relationship, and Mills did not want to jeopardize it. He worried that health benefits would prove to be more expensive than anticipated, with "highly dangerous ramifications" for the cash benefits portion of Social Security (Patashnik and Zelizer 2001, 15). In particular, Mills warned that if Congress was forced to raise payroll taxes to cover the rising cost of health care, taxpayers and corporations would revolt against Social Security. These concerns were not unique to Mills—they resonated with many other members of Congress who, along with their constituents, had developed a vested interest in protecting the Social Security program, which was only beginning to emerge from the turbulence and uncertainty of the early years since its enactment in 1935 (Patashnik and Zelizer 2001).

Mills was also a highly skilled politician who was interested in advancing his own power within Congress. Biographer Julian Zelizer describes Mills as having chameleon- and sphinx-like characteristics. "As a chameleon, he absorbed the interests, the ideas, and the language of each faction . . . As a sphinx, Mills refused to commit himself to any particular proposal until the very end of deliberations." Mills also had an uncanny ability to gauge the political temperature. Fellow Congressman Joseph Barr remarked that he had "one of the keenest political ears in Congress" (Zelizer 1998, 218).

Mills was, by nature, a circumspect man with "a sense of caution that [led] him to use his influence only sparingly" so as not to dilute his power.[2] One of his defining characteristics as chairman was his refusal to report any bill out of committee unless it had an exceptionally high chance of passing. As Mills himself explained, "I was always determined that whatever came out of the committee passed, you know. It was a waste of time to spend a month or two in the committee developing something that you couldn't pass."[3] Social Security Commissioner Robert Ball recalls that Mills "was only defeated once on the House floor in all the time he was Chairman of the Ways and Means Committee . . . And he didn't like that. He always liked to win."[4]

Within the executive branch, a civil servant named Wilbur Cohen was widely considered the single most knowledgeable expert on the nation's social insurance and welfare programs. Cohen was the first member of the Social Security Administration, where he remained for 20 years. During this time, he helped Wagner, Dingell, Murray, and Forand draft—and repeatedly redraft—their health reform bills. In the 1960s, he went on to serve as assistant secretary, undersecretary, and ultimately, secretary of Health, Education and Welfare. Cohen came to be widely respected for his expertise: John F. Kennedy referred to him as "Mr. Social Security"; Lyndon Johnson praised him as the "planner, architect, builder and repairman on every major piece of social legislation" since 1935; and the *New York Times* called him "one of the country's foremost technicians in public welfare."[5]

Cohen was a progressive driven by the desire to extend Social Security to include more generous cash benefits, disability benefits and, especially, health insurance. He felt that until the Social Security system protected the elderly against the high cost of medical care—the single most important determinant of poverty in old age—the program would not be able to fulfill its fundamental goal.[6] Like many liberal advocates of the social insurance approach, he worried that a means-tested approach would be insufficient.

> I am convinced that, in the United States, a program that deals only with the poor will end up being a poor program. There is every evidence that this is true. Ever since the Elizabethan Poor Law of 1601, programs only for the poor have been lousy, no good, poor programs. And a program that is only for the poor—one that has nothing in it for the middle income and the upper income—is, in the long run, a program the American public won't support. This is why I think one must try to find a way to link the interests of all classes in these programs. (Cohen and Friedman 1972, 55)

However, Cohen was also a pragmatist and relentless incrementalist (Berkowitz 1995). *Time* magazine called him a "salami slicer" who was willing to "sacrifice cherished legislative objectives so long as he gets at least a small piece of what he wants . . . One slice does not amount to much, but eventually there is enough for a sandwich."[7] As such, Cohen fully embraced both the social insurance and welfare medicine approaches as potential stepping stones to universal coverage.

Cohen was a master of bipartisanship, cultivating close relationships with legislators on both sides of the aisle. Cohen's willingness to cooperate with Republicans and conservative Democrats occasionally prompted liberal members of Congress to accuse him of treachery or complain that he had "sold out" (Derthick 1979, 324). Yet Cohen's pragmatic approach was highly successful, as he repeatedly convinced Democrats and Republicans alike to support bills that created and expanded social-insurance programs.

Despite their obvious differences, Cohen and Mills developed a strong rapport. Recognizing that Mills's priorities differed from his own, Cohen would deliberately couch his arguments to Mills in financial and political terms, rather than speaking of people in need (Berkowitz 1996). Cohen came to admire Mills "extravagantly" for his brilliance and work ethic; Mills, in turn, came to trust and rely heavily on Cohen for his detailed technical expertise (Berkowitz 1995, 122). Since the Ways and Means Committee did not have much in the way of specialized staff at the time, Cohen came to serve as Mills's de facto staff, drafting numerous bills for him over the course of several decades.[8]

MEDICAL VENDOR PAYMENTS

Wilbur Cohen first got the idea for a program resembling Medicaid in 1942, when Rhode Island attempted to use federal public-assistance funds to pay for health services on behalf of welfare recipients (Moore and Smith 2005). The Social Security Administration determined that such payments were not permissible under the law at that time, which required states to pay public assistance funds directly to the welfare recipient rather than the recipient's doctor, landlord, or grocer.[9] However, as a growing number of states realized that the poor were using a large share of their public assistance funds to pay for private medical and institutional care, they began to lobby federal policy makers for the ability to directly reimburse providers (Grogan 2008). Cohen subsequently began working to draft an amendment that would permit states to use part of their federal welfare funds for medical vendor payments.

At the time, the United States had three main cash assistance programs: Old Age Assistance (OAA), Aid to the Blind (ATB), and Aid to Dependent Children (ADC)—later renamed Aid to Families with Dependent Children (AFDC)—which had been enacted as part of the Social Security Act of 1935 (a fourth program, Aid to the Permanently and Totally Disabled [APTD], was created in 1950). Prior to 1935, aid to the needy had been primarily a state and local responsibility—patterned on the English Poor Laws. The federal government only began to assume greater financial responsibility in response to the Great Depression, when state and local governments found themselves overwhelmed by demand for public assistance.

Under the 1935 law, the federal government provided capped matching grants to the states at a rate of 50 percent for OAA and ATB up to a maximum payment of $30 per person per month, and 33 percent for ADC up to a maximum of $18 per month for the first child, and $12 for additional children. These matching grants were designed to incentivize states to spend their own resources on expanding eligibility and benefits, which, in keeping with the tradition of decentralization, were largely left in state hands. Although a few responded to the incentives, most states—struggling to recover from the Great Depression and limited by constraints on their taxing authority and administrative capacity—adopted only meager programs (Perkins 1956).

Given the sad state of public assistance, the significance of Wilbur Cohen's proposal to allow states to use matching funds for direct payments to doctors and hospitals—lifting the prohibition against federally financed payments to elderly people living in public institutions—was largely overlooked. Congressional conservatives presumed that this extension of the tiny public-assistance programs would be low cost, and hoped it would undermine the movement for national health insurance. Liberals, too, failed to predict the eventual significance of medical vendor payments. Hoping that universal coverage was just around the corner, they saw welfare medicine as "a residual program that could be done away with" after the enactment of national health insurance (Grogan 2006, 206). Thus, without grasping the potential ramifications, Congress enacted medical vendor payments as part of the Social Security Amendments of 1950.

Shortly after passage, Cohen—ever the incrementalist—began working to expand the new system of medical vendor payments. Only a handful of states were implementing the new provision, and Cohen wanted to increase their incentives to do so. He was able to get provisions inserted into the Social Security Amendments of 1956 that augmented federal aid to the states by slightly increasing matching rates and lifting the caps on the amount of aid states could receive for public assistance and medical vendor payments (Schottland 1956). This paved the way for further liberalization in the Social Security Amendments of 1958, which introduced a progressive matching formula ranging from 50 percent for high-income states to 65 percent for low-income states to help ameliorate interstate differences in state capacity and need (Kramer 1959). Nonetheless, tight caps continued to apply to the amount of federal aid available for cash assistance and medical vendor payments. By 1960, 40 states were taking advantage of federal funding for medical vendor payments, but the total level of spending remained quite modest at $514 million.[10]

THE KERR-MILLS PROGRAM OF MEDICAL ASSISTANCE TO THE AGED

Upon taking his post as Ways and Means Committee chairman in 1957, Mills's keen political ear began to pick up the rumblings of growing support for expanded access to health care. First there was the aforementioned Forand Bill in 1957. Mills led the Ways and Means Committee in killing it, but a few years later Senator John F. Kennedy made a similar program, which came to be known as Medicare, the centerpiece of his 1960 presidential campaign platform. Surveys showed that a large and growing number of Americans supported such a program (Erskine 1975).

To head off pressure for a costly health-insurance program for elderly persons of all income levels, Mills offered a substitute measure to address the needs of poor senior citizens. Together with another conservative Southern Democrat, Senator Robert Kerr of Oklahoma, Mills sponsored a bill creating the Kerr-Mills Program of Medical Assistance to the Aged, an incremental extension of the existing medical vendor payment program. When Kerr and Mills asked Wilbur Cohen to draft the bill for them, Cohen was happy to oblige, seeing the new program as part of an incrementalist strategy. However, he had to repeatedly reassure liberal policy makers that he was "equally concerned about Medicare." As Cohen later explained, "at that time most people felt the Kerr-Mills was the substitute for Medicare. It was my position that you ought to have both of them."[11] Cohen worried that even if Medicare passed, there was still "the entire issue of what to do about people who were not covered by Medicare or, if they were covered by Medicare and their coverage was not sufficient to take care of everything."[12] As an advocate of universal coverage and a pragmatic incrementalist, Cohen saw the Kerr-Mills Program as potentially helpful in making up for Medicare's deficiencies.

Like medical vendor payments, Kerr-Mills provided federal matching grants in an amount that depended on the state's income, and left most of the initiative—including the decision of whether or not to participate—up to the states. However, Kerr-Mills included several new features designed to increase state participation. First, it extended eligibility by creating a new optional category of beneficiaries known as the "medically needy"—elderly persons whose incomes were not low enough to qualify them for public assistance, but whose resources were insufficient to meet the costs of necessary medical services. Second, in addition to listing a broad range of hospital, nursing home, physician, and other services that might be covered at the states' option, it required participating states to cover some institutional and some noninstitutional care as a condition of federal cost sharing. Third, it increased the top matching rate from 65 to 80 percent—disproportionately benefitting low-income southern states like those Kerr and Mills represented—and did not place a cap on the amount of federal aid states could receive. Although it went largely unnoticed at the time, the adoption of open-ended matching grants was unprecedented; federal funding for public-assistance programs had always been capped.

By building incrementally on medical vendor payments, the Kerr-Mills legislation "rocked no boats," which was the "essence of its political success" (Stevens and Stevens 2003, 28). However, liberals immediately expressed dissatisfaction with the legislation, worrying that a voluntary state-based program would be insufficient to meet the needs of the poor elderly due to the states' proven lack of capacity and commitment. Senator Patrick McNamara (D-Michigan) remarked that "it would be the miracle of the century if all of the states—or even a sizeable number—would be in a position to provide the matching funds to make the program more than just a plan on paper" (Marmor 1973, 36).

These fears turned out to be well-founded. Senator Kerr had predicted that 10 million recipients would benefit from the Kerr-Mills Program, but by 1965—five years after passage—fewer than 300,000 recipients were covered.[13] Nor were the benefits much more generous than those that had been available under medical vendor payments (Stevens and Stevens 2003). Although the majority of states chose to establish Kerr-Mills plans, the most active participation came from a handful of high-income states that had adopted the most substantial medical-vendor-payment programs prior to 1960. Thus, while the program's progressive matching formula had been designed to encourage the poorer states to participate, it was the richer states that were enticed by the prospect of additional federal funding to supplement and supplant existing state spending. Indeed, by 1965, five such states—California, Massachusetts, Minnesota, New York, and Pennsylvania— were receiving nearly two-thirds of the Kerr-Mills funds (Stevens and Stevens 2003). Mills argued that the program simply needed more time to take effect, defending his welfare medicine approach as "correct," while acknowledging that "as time develops" some "modifications" might be necessary (Zelizer 1998, 220).

Given the inadequacy of Kerr-Mills, pressure for expanded access to health care only intensified in the early 1960s. The civil rights movement drew public attention to the pressing needs of poor minority groups. Senior citizen groups became increasingly vocal in campaigning for a Social Security-based health-insurance program for elderly persons of all income levels. Medical costs continued to rise. In 1961, having won the presidential election on a campaign platform featuring compulsory health insurance for the elderly, President John F. Kennedy sent Congress a proposal that would extend Social Security to include hospital and nursing-home care. Unlike the Forand Bill, the proposal omitted surgery in a bid to appease the medical profession, which nonetheless registered strong disapproval (Marmor 1973).

When Representative Cecil King (D-California) and Senator Clinton Anderson (D-New Mexico) submitted the president's proposal in Congress, Wilbur Mills made sure it died in the Ways and Means Committee in 1961, and again in 1962, 1963, and 1964. The editorial page of the *New York Times* branded Mills the "One-Man Veto on Medicare," and lamented that "Mr. Mills prefers the restrictive approach to health care embodied in his own Kerr-Mills Act—a preference to which he clings despite the inadequacies demonstrated in the four years since that law's passage."[14] However, Mills defended his position as consistent with the will of his committee, and Congress as a whole. As one observer put it, his opposition to Medicare stemmed largely from his "great ability to count heads. He wasn't going to take on a crusade that was doomed to failure."[15] By most accounts, Medicare was at least three votes short on the Ways and Means Committee, and 23 votes short on the floor (Marmor 1973, Zelizer 1998). Acknowledging that a Medicare bill was unlikely to pass, Kennedy did not press the chairman about it.[16]

However, a window of opportunity opened following President Kennedy's assassination in November 1963. When Vice President Lyndon Johnson was sworn in, he vowed to fulfill his predecessor's pledge of a medical-care program for the elderly. In pursuing this objective, Johnson brought a genius for political strategy, an unparalleled tenacity, and 12 years of experience as "Master of the Senate" (Caro 2002). Calling Johnson "the smartest politician I ever knew," Senator Clinton Anderson noted that the new president "pushed heavily" for Medicare's enactment and that the president's efforts ultimately proved to be "very, very helpful on floor action."[17]

After the 1964 presidential election, Medicare seemed all but inevitable. The public's grief over Kennedy's assassination translated into a landslide victory for Johnson, which was widely interpreted as a popular mandate for Medicare since the program had been a central element of Johnson's campaign platform (Marmor 1973). This outpouring of support carried over to Congress: upon gaining 38 seats in the House, Democrats outnumbered Republicans two to one for the first time in more than three decades (the party already enjoyed a similar margin in the Senate). Among the Republicans' losses were three staunchly anti-Medicare members of the Ways and Means Committee.

The morning after the election, Chairman Mills resignedly told reporters that he would be receptive to a Medicare proposal in the upcoming legislative session; he later claimed in a speech that he "always thought there was great appeal" in a Social-Security-based health insurance program.[18] Asked why Mills's interviews and speeches suddenly began to sound increasingly pro-Medicare, one of his aides said "'Mene, Mene, Tekel' . . . a cryptic suggestion that Mr. Mills, like the Old Testament's King Belshazzar, saw the handwriting on the wall" foretelling the demise of his empire.[19] Years later, asked to describe his turnaround on Medicare, Mills explained, "the election of the President in 1964 had the major impact, made the major difference. He had espoused it in his campaign, you know, and here he was elected by a 2 to 1 vote, which was a pretty strong endorsement of it, I thought."[20] Realizing that he could no longer forestall Medicare, Mills shifted from opponent to manager (Marmor 1973).

THREE-LAYER CAKE

At the outset of the 89th Congress in January 1965, Representative King and Senator Anderson introduced H.R. 1 and S. 1, respectively—embodying the administration's proposal for a Social-Security-based system of hospital insurance for the elderly. Despite the changing political tides, fear of suffering additional defeats at the hands of the AMA had led the administration to omit physician services from the proposal. Continuing to embrace an incremental approach, the administration saw Medicare as only a beginning, hoping that additional services could be added later. However, the bill's supporters grew increasingly concerned that a large share of the elderly was under the mistaken impression that the bill did offer broad coverage including physician services, and would be disappointed when they learned otherwise (Marmor 1973).

An "alarmed, even panicky" American Medical Association—recognizing that its traditional arguments against Medicare were increasingly futile in the new political climate—turned to capitalizing on the misperceptions and mounting criticism surrounding Medicare.[21] As the Ways and Means Committee began to consider the King-Anderson Bill, the AMA launched a "last ditch fight against medical care for the aged under Social Security" and called an emergency meeting to discuss the possibility that a "stepped-up campaign to popularize the Kerr-Mills Act as a solution to the needs of the elderly would be enough to block Medicare in Congress."[22]

The AMA drafted a proposal for a program called Eldercare, which was essentially a "spruce-up" of Kerr-Mills, and solicited the help of Ways and Means Committee members Albert Herlong (D-FL) and Thomas Curtis (R-MO) in introducing the bill.[23] The AMA began running television and newspaper ads emphasizing the fact that, unlike Medicare, Eldercare would cover physician and surgical services, drugs, nursing-home fees, diagnostic and laboratory fees, and other outpatient services. The organization also funded a survey which revealed that 72 percent of respondents agreed that a government health plan should cover doctors' bills, and that 65 percent preferred a program that would pay an elderly person's medical bills only if he or she were in need of financial help over a universal program that would pay the medical expenses of everyone over the age of 65, regardless of their income (Marmor 1973).

However, the AMA's Eldercare proposal received little support from the left or the right. The AFL-CIO called the Eldercare proposal "Eldersnare," and accused the AMA of making empty promises since the proposal would make only cosmetic changes to the Kerr-Mills Program (Kooijmann 1999). Meanwhile, many congressional Republicans—fearing that their earlier partnership with the AMA in opposing health care for the elderly might have contributed to their party's losses in the 1964 election—wished to distance themselves from the proposal. However, they also wanted to prevent Democrats from creating a hugely popular program and taking all the credit (Marmor 1973). Also, since the AMA had spent millions of dollars advertising Medicare's inadequacy, they felt that any Republican proposal had to cover physician services.

Thus, in February 1965, the senior Republican on the Ways and Means Committee—Representative John Byrnes of Wisconsin—introduced an alternative to both Medicare and Eldercare. The Byrnes plan called for a voluntary health-insurance program that would be paid for out of a combination of general revenues and patient premiums, and would cover physician services as well as drugs. To distinguish his proposal from Medicare and Eldercare, Byrnes humorously referred to his bill as "Bettercare." As one participant recalls, the proposal was widely seen as a ploy to derail the Democrats' proposal, "something that the Republicans could point to and say, 'Well, our plan is much broader than yours . . . it's got all this good stuff in it that you don't have' . . . Byrnes never expected it pass."[24]

In considering the three proposals, Mills faced a dilemma. He continued to oppose the Social-Security-based Medicare program out of fear that the payroll tax needed to support such a program would grow "so high finally as to interfere with our capacity to compete in the world."[25] In particular, Mills was concerned that since the Medicare proposal did not cover physician services, it would leave the door open to public demands for liberalized benefits, forcing Congress to raise the payroll tax above an acceptable level. But neither did Mills want to fund health care for the elderly out of general federal revenues, as the Byrnes plan proposed, which he felt would "run the risk of bankrupting the Federal Treasury once and for all."[26] The Eldercare proposal to improve the Kerr-Mills Program appealed to Mills, both because that program's failure to catch on had become a source of personal embarrassment to the chairman, and because he continued to favor a means-tested, state-administered program. However, he recognized that Medicare supporters would not be satisfied with that approach alone.

Seemingly out of nowhere, Mills announced a solution that took nearly everyone by surprise. During an executive session of the Ways and Means Committee on March 2, 1965, as Mills listened to Representative Byrnes describe his Bettercare plan, the chairman suddenly seemed to have an epiphany—"you could see the light bulb flash on in his mind," reported one observer.

> Why not, Mr. Mills suddenly interjected, graft the Byrnes plan for doctor-bill insurance on top of the Social Security-Medicare plan for hospital benefits? Here at last was the dramatic Millsian splash, the antidote for the AMA ads, the way to prevent Congress from someday burdening the Social Security system with doctor bills.[27]

Mills went on to propose that the AMA's Eldercare program for the poor be grafted onto Medicare as well, enabling him to "turn their propaganda against them and say that he was doing what they were asking."[28] In short, Mills proposed to combine Medicare, Eldercare, and Bettercare—which had been presented as separate and mutually exclusive alternatives—into a "medi-elder-Byrnes bill." Wilbur Cohen exclaimed:

> The doctors couldn't complain, because they had been carping about Medicare's shortcomings and about its being compulsory. And the Republicans couldn't complain, because it was their own idea. In effect, Mills had taken the A.M.A.'s ammunition, put it in the Republicans' gun, and blown both of them off the map.[29]

Cohen predicted that this "combined package approach" made it "almost certain that nobody will vote against the bill when it comes on the floor of the House."[30] *Newsweek* referred to the strategy as a "Medicoup."[31]

The "medi-elder-Byrnes bill" was more than a political maneuver; Mills also hoped it would achieve his policy objectives. Recognizing that Medicare was inevitable, Mills sought to protect the program's fiscal integrity by surrounding it with other programs—funded through a combination of federal and state general revenues and patient premiums—to handle physician services and health care for the poor. Robert Myers, the chief actuary of the Social Security Administration, later recounted Mills's explanation of the logic behind the proposal.

> People have been led to believe they're getting a lot more than just hospital benefits. And instead of having continual pressure put on us, let's broaden the scope of the program and develop it the way we want under our own initiative, rather than under pressure from bureaucrats or the public.[32]

Mills himself later clarified in an interview that his plan was to "build a fence around the Medicare program" and forestall subsequent demands for liberalization that would burden the Social Security program and the economy (Marmor 1973, 69–70).

Most of the officials who were in the room when Mills dropped his bombshell were astonished. Fred Arner of the Congressional Research Service asked another onlooker, "He's kidding, isn't he?," while Representative Byrnes just sat there with his mouth open (Berkowitz 1995, 231; Zelizer 1998, 241). Another committee member recounted: "It was fantastic. It was Wilbur Mills at his best. His maneuvering was beautiful" (Zelizer 1998, 241).

"WE PLANNED THAT"

Wilbur Cohen claimed that Mills's three-prong approach had taken him by surprise as well, noting that "like everyone else in the room, I was stunned by Mills's strategy. It was the most brilliant legislative move I'd seen in thirty years." When Cohen sent the president a memo praising Mills's "ingenious" plan, media accounts suggested that the president, too, was "surprised and amused" by the news.[33] Numerous political histories of Medicare and Medicaid have repeated this version of events (see for example Marmor 1970; Stevens and Stevens 2003). Even Cohen's biographer, Edward Berkowitz, reported that Cohen was caught completely off guard by Mills's announcement (Berkowitz 1995).

We now know, however—through a series of interviews, memos, and recorded telephone conversations—that Cohen and Johnson had helped Mills develop the three-prong plan over the course of the previous year.[34] In an interview with historian Michael Gillette, Mills later admitted that his supposed bombshell had been anything but.

> GILLETTE: Wilbur Cohen described that process as the greatest legislative maneuver that he'd ever witnessed.
>
> MILLS: (Laughter) . . .
>
> GILLETTE: Cohen describes this almost with an element of amazement. Was it pieced together—?
>
> MILLS: No, it was planned.
>
> GILLETTE: It was? You'd been working on it for some time?
>
> MILLS: We planned that, yes. Oh, yes.[35]

Within weeks of President Kennedy's assassination—nearly a year before his landslide victory in the 1964 election—President Johnson began urging Wilbur Mills to report a Medicare bill out of his committee. He called Mills repeatedly, and took him out for meals. The president later joked that he courted Mills more assiduously than he had courted his own wife, Lady Bird (Blumenthal and Morone 2009, 178).

Johnson astutely realized that the only hope of enacting Medicare was to appeal to Mills's ego. Mills did not want Medicare to be the King-Anderson bill anymore; if it was going to pass at all, he wanted to rebrand it as the "Mills bill." Moreover, the chairman told the president that the bill would have to be "something that we could say was so different from the King bill itself that those of us who have repeatedly said we wouldn't vote for the King bill could vote for it," to which Johnson gamely replied: "That's exactly right. That's what you've got to do."[36] Johnson promised that if Mills would report out a bill, the White House would defer to him on the specifics and give him all the credit, telling him "you work it out" and "I'll come in and applaud you."[37] The president dispatched then-Assistant Secretary for Legislation of Health, Education, and Welfare Wilbur Cohen—who, Johnson knew, had both consummate technical expertise and a close working relationship with Mills—to "get him something . . . that he can call the Mills bill, that's what it amounts to, and you're smart enough to do that." Johnson instructed Cohen to "live with him if necessary."[38]

In January 1964—more than a year before Mills dropped his bombshell—Cohen proposed that Mills attach a "major revision and liberalization" of the Kerr-Mills Program to the Medicare legislation. Specifically, he proposed a "new title in the Social Security Act covering all public assistance vendor medical payments to needy persons (aged, blind, disabled, and children)" with an increased matching rate of up to 83 percent, a "flexible" eligibility test, and a "comprehensive" benefit package—in short, a program nearly identical to the Medicaid program that would be enacted a year later. Mills asked Cohen to provide supporting figures and language, and the Ways and Means Committee gave "extensive consideration" to a "major revision and liberalization" of Kerr-Mills throughout 1964.[39] Mills came to see this second prong as a key to his "face-saving operation," and potentially useful in "justifying a position for King-Anderson" after saying for years that he would never vote for it.[40]

When Mills told President Johnson in the summer of 1964 that he was considering Cohen's proposal to expand Kerr-Mills, the president pressed Mills to add a third prong: physician services. He told Mills: "I'd wait until you could get them all together because I think if you don't, why you just murder the other one [physician services], and I think the other is what's got sex appeal."[41] The cautious chairman told the president that Congress was likely to reject this three-prong approach, and that it was best to wait until after the upcoming election—hence the delay until the new Congress convened in 1965.[42]

Having promised to give Mills all the credit for the legislation, President Johnson and Secretary Cohen kept their involvement tightly under wraps. In fact, they were so secretive in their dealings with Mills that even Social Security Commissioner Robert Ball—who had sat with Cohen throughout the Ways and Means Committee's 1965 executive sessions on Medicare—continued to believe, even years later, that Cohen had been genuinely "astounded" by Mills's sudden announcement. Ball acknowledged that "there are people who think that isn't the whole story, that there was behind-the-scenes discussions of this—that it wasn't sprung on us," but maintained: "I really believe that it was a proposal that Mills pretty much put together quickly and tried out on us one afternoon."[43]

In fact, White House officials later acknowledged that Wilbur Cohen had worked tirelessly throughout 1964 to convince Mills to adopt the three-prong approach. When asked in an interview to describe what Cohen did to bring the legislation to fruition, presidential aide Larry O'Brien replied: "I don't know what he *didn't* do. I don't know as he slept at any time; he was a ball of fire who had the advantage of knowing the subject intimately [and] the ability to communicate with the Congress . . . He made one significant contribution to this struggle."[44] Presidential aide Douglas Cater confirmed that the "three-layer cake" had been Wilbur Cohen's idea, and that after it was implemented President Johnson had frequently told, with great pride, the story of how he and Cohen had "outfoxed the opposition on Medicare." According to the president's story, Cohen had said: "Well, all right. We'll buy all three of them." President Johnson asked, "Well, how much will it cost me?" Cohen said, "A billion dollars." And the president said, "Damn."[45]

"SLEEPER PROVISION"

On the afternoon of March 2, 1965, after Mills dropped his bombshell, there was a brief period of stunned silence. After that, Robert Ball reported, "There was no debate. The meeting just sort of broke up."[46] Chairman Mills turned to Wilbur Cohen and asked him to develop the details overnight of a proposal that would combine the three bills into one. Cohen was able to present a comprehensive proposal the next day by virtue of the fact that he and Mills already had been carefully considering it for more than a year.

The Ways and Means Committee reported the bill to the House floor on a straight party-line vote of 17 to 8 on March 23. True to his word, President Johnson saw to it that Representative King's original H.R. 1 bill was discarded and replaced with the committee's new bill—sponsored by Wilbur Mills— and waited until then to heap praise on the bill.[47] Just to be safe, the president called Cohen and instructed him to ask Mills, who was standing beside Cohen, "if it's alright for me to congratulate him . . . I don't want to jump the gun," to which Cohen replied: "Mr. Mills says go right ahead." Johnson then instructed Cohen to write a "statement that this is even a better bill than we had expected."[48]

President Johnson urged congressional leaders to push the legislation through Congress as quickly as possible. The president did not want the legislation to "lay around" stinking like a "dead cat," for fear that it would give opponents time to get organized against the bill. "For God's sakes, don't let dead cats stand on your porch . . . call that son of a bitch up before they can get their letters written."[49] At Johnson's urging, the bill moved through Congress with lightning speed. The House debated the bill on April 7 and 8 under a closed rule that limited amendments and restricted debate to 10 hours. On April 8, the House gave Mills a standing ovation before passing the bill by a margin of 313 to 115. The Senate Finance Committee reported the bill out on June 30; the Senate began debating the bill on July 6, and approved it with only minor changes by a vote of 68 to 21 on July 9. The Conference Committee to reconcile the two bills met from July 14 to 21, and filed the conference report on July 26. The House and Senate approved the report on July 27 and 28, respectively; President Johnson signed the bill into law as Public Law 89–97 on July 30.[50]

The legislation assigned new names to the three layers of the cake. Medicare Part A (Hospital Insurance) was modeled after the King-Anderson Bill; it would cover 60 days of hospitalization and related nursing care for the elderly, to be paid for through a dedicated payroll tax. Medicare Part B (Supplementary Medical Insurance) was modeled after the Byrnes Bill; it would provide the elderly with optional coverage of physician services, to be paid for through patient premiums and federal general revenues. Title XIX (later called Medicaid) was modeled on Eldercare; it would provide a broad array of medical services to certain categories of the poor, to be financed through federal and state general revenues.

Since Medicaid had been added to the Medicare legislation at the last minute, and the bill had been rushed through Congress, the provision largely flew under the radar. A legislative draftsman said that only half a day was devoted to consideration of Medicaid's provisions (Smith and Moore 2008, 21), while the *New York Times* reported that there had been "little floor debate" on the program.[51] In the 136-page final version of the law, Title XIX takes up a total of only nine pages.

Inattention to Medicaid largely reflected the belief that it was not a new program at all, but rather a minor extension of the tiny Kerr-Mills Program—a belief that was actively promoted by Wilbur Mills. Although Title XIX would replace Kerr-Mills with a new program, Mills—eager to both fix the Kerr-Mills Program and brand the legislation as his own—repeatedly referred to Title XIX as a "continuation of the Kerr-Mills program," "the revised Kerr-Mills program," or "the Kerr-Mills program . . . to make medical services for the needy more generally available."[52] Other members of Congress followed Mills's lead, referring to an improved, expanded, or more effective Kerr-Mills Program in committee reports and floor deliberations.

Nor did Title XIX receive much scrutiny from organized medicine throughout the legislative process. The American Medical Association saw Title XIX as a relatively unthreatening extension of a small, means-tested, state-administered program; indeed, this had been the organization's rationale for espousing Eldercare in the first place. Thus, as Congress began to draft legislation, the AMA focused most of its opposition on the seemingly more significant Medicare program.

President Johnson—who was primarily concerned with fulfilling Kennedy's pledge to enact a universal health-care program for the elderly—largely ignored the Medicaid provision as well; in fact, when he signed the Social Security Amendments of 1965, Johnson did not even mention Title XIX once in his remarks.[53] Most administration officials similarly paid little attention to Medicaid, seeing it as largely a state rather than federal concern—"up to the states to run as they pleased so long as no federal laws or restrictions were violated" (Smith and Moore 2008, 60).

The exception, of course, was Wilbur Cohen. Years later, Cohen noted that whereas the Medicare program had taken two decades to evolve and had been "fought in the front line trenches," Medicaid had been "largely overlooked . . . and thus it got the reputation of being a kind of sleeper provision." However, Cohen pointed out that "Those of us who were working on the development of legislation, like myself, of course, paid a good deal of attention to it because I was primarily responsible for the design of the Medicaid program."[54]

Congress added the Medicaid rider to the Medicare legislation with such great haste that historians later referred to the program's design as slapdash, casual, belated, ill-designed, and an afterthought (Friedman 1995; Stevens and Stevens 2003; Brown and Sparer 2003). Although Medicaid may have been an afterthought for most members of Congress, such claims overlook the fact that Wilbur Cohen—the nation's foremost expert on social-welfare programs—had been developing the program for more than a year.

POLICY FEEDBACK

Despite being widely written off as an incremental extension of a small pre-existing welfare program, Medicaid radically reshaped state leaders' incentives and resources in ways that immediately promoted rapid programmatic expansion. This surprising turn of events reflected Medicaid's unique policy design, timing, and institutional support—Patashnik and Zelizer's three conditions for policy feedback (2010).

Medicaid's policy design was modeled on the Kerr-Mills Program, which—despite eliciting minimal state participation—had tremendous latent potential for growth due to several expansionary provisions, including loosely defined eligibility standards and extensive benefits (Stevens and Stevens 2003; Grogan and Patashnik 2003; Grogan 2006; Grogan and Smith 2008) as well as open-ended matching grants. However, Medicaid's policy design was intentionally even more expansive than Kerr-Mills's. Wilbur Cohen later explained that in drafting the legislation, he had been "acutely aware of the inadequacies of the State medical assistance plans in the 1960's" (Cohen 1983, 10). Based on the Kerr-Mills experience, Cohen knew that any federal-state health-care program "would be operative only to the extent States undertake the financial responsibility to carry out the program."[55] Thus, he convinced Wilbur Mills that in order to correct the failures of the Kerr-Mills Program—and to create an effective fence around Medicare—it would be necessary to build into the new program a number of carrots and sticks to encourage greater state participation.

First, whereas the Kerr-Mills Act had limited eligibility to the low-income elderly, Medicaid required participating states to cover all persons receiving public assistance—including the aged, blind, disabled, and families with dependent children—and also gave states the option of covering medically needy persons in these same categories. The law thus permitted state officials to extend health coverage to a highly sympathetic and "deserving" group: children. Like Kerr-Mills, Medicaid allowed the states to define "medically needy" however they liked, setting no income ceiling on eligibility. In combination with the expansion of categorical eligibility, this opened the door to coverage of not only poor families with dependent children, but also those with moderate incomes as well.

Second, Medicaid required participating states to provide all beneficiaries with five mandatory services: (1) inpatient hospital care, (2) outpatient hospital care, (3) laboratory and x-ray tests, (4) physician services, and (5) skilled nursing-home services. Although many of these services had been authorized under Kerr-Mills, the only requirement under that program had been for the states to provide some institutional and some noninstitutional care—and few states had chosen to adopt comprehensive coverage. Mandatory coverage of nursing-home services was particularly consequential—especially since Medicare (and most private insurance) did not cover long-term care. The states could also elect to cover, and receive matching federal grants for, a long list of optional services including prescription drugs, dental care, eyeglasses, prosthetic devices, hearing aids, and physical therapy. Moreover, the legislation required a state that chose to cover one medically needy category—such as children—to provide the same benefits to other categories of the medically needy as well.

Third, the law included a maintenance-of-effort provision, specifying that states must expand eligibility and the scope of covered services as a condition of receiving federal funding, which is stated in section 1903 of the statute.

> The Secretary shall not make payments under the preceding provisions of this section to a State unless the State makes a satisfactory showing that it is making efforts in the direction of broadening the scope of the care and services made available under the plan and in the direction of liberalizing the eligibility requirements for medical assistance, with a view toward furnishing by July 1, 1975, comprehensive care and services to substantially all individuals who meet the plan's eligibility standards with respect to income and resources, including services to enable such individuals to attain or retain independence or self care.

This provision was designed in part to prevent state officials from using federal dollars to supplant, rather than supplement, current state spending. Wilbur Cohen noted that "there was no opposition to this ambiguous and general provision in 1965" (Cohen 1983).

Finally, although state participation in the new Medicaid program was voluntary, the law included several financial incentives to encourage all states to participate. Title XIX increased the average state's matching rate by five percentage points relative to Kerr-Mills (Cohen and Ball 1965). States with national average income received a federal match of 55 percent instead of 50 percent, while those with the lowest incomes received 83 percent, in contrast to 80 percent under Kerr-Mills. This new formula was the most generous in the history of public-assistance programs in the United States. Moreover, the law permitted states that established Medicaid plans to apply this more liberal matching formula to AFDC and other cash-assistance programs, which were still funded with capped matching grants at that time (Smith and Moore 2008). As an additional inducement, states that did not establish Medicaid programs by 1970 would lose their Kerr-Mills funding.

By providing unprecedentedly generous financial incentives and giving the states broad discretion over eligibility and benefits, Title XIX paid scant attention to cost containment. This might seem surprising in light of the fiscal conservatism of its sponsor, Wilbur Mills; however, Moore and Smith remark:

> The legislation seems to have been acceptable to those who worried about costs because it was based on a presumption—not unreasonable given the history of Kerr-Mills—that States would be slow and careful about taking up this option, would set eligibility standards and income and assets tests close to those for public assistance recipients, and would, therefore, limit both State and Federal financial outlays. (Moore and Smith 2005, 49)

This assumption turned out to be incorrect, however, due to the unique timing of Medicaid's enactment and the sudden expansion of state-level institutional support.

First, the timing of the program's introduction in 1965 was highly conducive to expansion. Following the 1964 election, state capitals—like the federal government—were overwhelmingly dominated by liberals. The public, too, was more receptive to government intervention. After a period of relative conservatism during the 1950s and early 1960s, the late 1960s were characterized by a new political climate of concern about poverty, inequality, and social justice (Stimson 1999). Also, whereas Kerr-Mills had been introduced during the national recession of 1960–61, the economy was booming by the mid-1960s, and states were flush with resources.

Second, Medicaid was introduced at a time of greatly expanding institutional support at the state level. The 1960s witnessed a remarkable transformation in state governments due to the infusion of federal funding—for Medicaid as well as numerous other federal-state programs; the adoption of income and sales taxes by many states; the implementation of a variety of political and administrative reforms; and numerous other policies designed to increase state capacity, as is documented in chapter 2. Together, these reforms attracted a new breed of politician to state capitals around the country. Almost overnight, the "political pipsqueaks" who had run state governments earlier in the century were replaced with state leaders who were "capable, creative, forward-looking, and experienced" (Sabato 1983, 1).

In short, the expansionary features embedded in the Kerr-Mills Program and extended in Title XIX reflected the mistaken assumption that states would continue to lack the fiscal capacity and political commitment to adopt generous coverage. At the time of Medicaid's introduction, however, the states were suddenly exceptionally receptive to the new program's incentive structure.

CONCLUSION

For Wilbur Cohen, the progressive architect of the Medicaid program, Title XIX of the Social Security Amendments of 1965 was the culmination of a dream—and more than two decades of hard work—to expand health coverage for vulnerable populations. For Wilbur Mills, the legislation's fiscally conservative sponsor, Medicaid reflected a political compromise that quickly turned into a nightmare, as the program's institutional design turned out to be considerably more expansive than the Ways and Means Chairman had ever intended or believed possible. In fact, less than a year after the program's inception, Mills was already frantically trying to rewrite the law.

CHAPTER 2

The Sleeping Giant Awakens: 1966–80

THE INITIAL ESTIMATES OF Medicaid's cost proved to be "absurdly low."[1] Congress had failed to anticipate the extent to which the states would take advantage of the program's financial incentives to adopt generous coverage. By 1969, just three years after Medicaid's inception, a federal report stated that the "badly conceived and badly organized" program had generated "vast increases in government health expenditures" and contributed to "crippling inflation in medical costs."[2] Federal lawmakers began drafting legislation to redesign the program almost immediately after the program went into effect. As one senator put it, "Congress never expected any such eventuality. Now being embarrassed by the fact that their open-ended invitation was too generous, they have to set some limits."[3]

Medicaid's early vulnerability, and the governors' efforts to combat federal retrenchment, is one of the largely untold sagas in the program's history. In Medicaid's first five years, federal policy makers considered a wide range of amendments to the law including a cap on federal contributions in 1966, eligibility limits in 1967, reductions in federal matching rates for the medically needy in 1968, relaxation of coverage mandates in 1969, and reductions in federal funding for long-term care in 1970. Of these proposals, only the eligibility and coverage reforms succeeded; all three attempts to revise Medicaid's financing structure failed due to intense lobbying by the nation's governors. In a striking case of policy feedback, state leaders emerged as a supportive constituency for the new program, immediately constraining federal lawmakers' ability to reverse course.

Medicaid's enactment contributed significantly to the governors' mobilization as an interest group. Initially, Governor Nelson Rockefeller of New York, who had developed the most ambitious Medicaid plan in the nation, battled the federal cutbacks virtually singlehandedly. Over time, however, state leaders joined forces to protect their collective financial stake in the program with increased strength and organization; indeed, it was largely in response to the introduction of Medicaid, among other federal-state programs, that the governors established a full-time lobbying apparatus in Washington, and began issuing policy statements and testifying before Congress to an unprecedented extent. The governors' transformation into an organized, influential interest group marked a critical turning point in American federalism, with enormous implications for the future trajectory of U.S. health policy.

NEW YORK'S CONTROVERSIAL MEDICAID PLAN

When federal Medicaid funding became available for the first time in January 1966, large, liberal, high-income states that had developed relatively expansive Kerr-Mills plans—such as New York, California, and Massachusetts—were among the first in line. Eager to start taking advantage of the new funding available under Medicaid, these states "rudely jostled their way toward the Title XIX trough, to the increasing consternation of legislators and administrators in Washington" (Stevens and Stevens 2003, 81).

Governor Nelson Rockefeller of New York took a particularly keen interest in the new Medicaid law. Although Rockefeller was a Republican, he was also a liberal; indeed, in his day, left-leaning members of the Republican Party were known as "Rockefeller Republicans." According to biographer Joseph Persico, if there was one policy area in which the governor was "indisputably" liberal, it was health care, which Rockefeller considered a basic human right (Persico 1982, 224). In his earlier role as undersecretary of the U.S. Department of Health, Education, and Welfare (HEW), Rockefeller had helped Wilbur Cohen create the medical-vendor-payment program, which had paved the way for Kerr-Mills and Medicaid (Moore and Smith 2005). As governor of New York, he boasted that he had developed "the largest and most liberal program of medical assistance under the Kerr-Mills Bill, utilizing more than twenty-five percent of all the money spent for this program in the United States."[4]

Governor Rockefeller had adopted a generous Kerr-Mills plan in 1960 despite his concern that its federal-state cost-sharing structure would create a "serious financial drain on the States." For years, Rockefeller had expressed a strong preference for a Social Security-based national health-insurance program in which "a definite percentage of the cost is borne by those who ultimately receive the benefits," so as to create "a built-in safeguard against the constant pressure for irresponsible and extravagant additions to the scheme which is politically difficult to resist."[5] However, when such a program failed to materialize, Rockefeller made do with Kerr-Mills, even though he believed it was "basically unsound fiscally."[6] Several years later, when Congress modeled Medicaid on Kerr-Mills, Rockefeller declared the new program "a unique opportunity for New York State to build upon its record of leadership," despite similar reservations about its financing mechanism.[7] In the absence of a national health-insurance program, he saw Medicaid as an alternative, albeit imperfect, stepping stone to universal coverage (Grogan 2008).

In early 1966, Governor Rockefeller announced his intention to implement a Medicaid plan so generous that 45 percent of the state's population—or eight million people—would be eligible for coverage. Title XIX allowed the states to define "medically needy" however they liked, and Rockefeller defined it as a family of four with an income of $6,000 or less, which was close to the median household income at that time. Under his proposal, fully 70 percent of the state's Medicaid spending would go to the relatively well-to-do medically needy, while only 30 percent would go to recipients of cash assistance (Grogan and Smith 2008).

Rockefeller's proposed eligibility standard was considerably higher than the ceilings under consideration elsewhere. A handful of states, such as California and Pennsylvania, proposed a $4,000 standard, but most states' limits were between $2,500 and $3,600 (Greenfield 1968). New York's income limit was also orders of magnitude larger than anything Congress had anticipated. In fact, the estimated federal cost of New York's program—$217 million—was more than HEW Department estimates had initially suggested the program would cost for all 50 states combined,[8] prompting Senator Jacob Javits (R-New York) to exclaim: "My God, Nelson, at the rate you're going, New York State will use up all the Medicaid money that Congress appropriated for the whole country" (Persico 1982, 224). But the governor defended his generous plan as "in keeping with New York's economic leadership, living costs, and humanitarian social outlook"[9] and pointed out that it would "enable New York State to receive the maximum federal aid under Title XIX."[10]

Governor Rockefeller urged the state assembly to vote quickly on his proposal, noting that if New York enacted a plan before April 1, the federal government would provide retroactive aid for the first quarter of 1966.[11] By creating a sense of urgency over the potential loss of federal funds, Rockefeller was able to spur the bill through the legislature in less than two months, after the briefest of hearings and virtually no floor debate. The bill passed both chambers by wide margins: 64 to 1 in the Senate, and 132 to 21 in the assembly.[12] The governor applauded the legislature's speedy action on "the most significant social legislation in three decades" and asserted that New York's Medicaid program would be "the best in the nation."[13]

Suddenly, the news media was full of stories about how New York had unlocked Medicaid's potential. The *Wall Street Journal* reported that New York had "turned a spotlight on Medicaid by showing just how generous a state can make its Title 19 programs."[14] The *New York Times* noted that "it was not until New York State established the plans for its program . . . that most persons realized Medicaid would eventually be a far greater and more significant program than Medicare."[15]

The state assembly had enacted Rockefeller's Medicaid plan with such great haste—the media characterized the process as "rush-hour lawmaking"— that many lawmakers failed to fully comprehend the bill they had voted for.[16] As one advocate put it, "it's a damn good thing because they never would have voted for it if they had."[17] Upon returning home to their districts, lawmakers from conservative parts of the state faced a "storm of protest" and "mass hysteria" over the alleged "socialization of medicine."[18] One Republican legislator from Erie County who had voted for the bill subsequently led an unsuccessful campaign to repeal the entire act.[19]

Medical providers and insurers, concerned about the financial implications of large-scale government intervention in the health-care market, also registered their disapproval. The Association of New York State Physicians and Dentists sent a letter to dozens of members of key congressional committees calling New York's plan a "careless, almost wanton, distortion of the worthwhile purpose intended by Congress," and recommending that Congress establish stricter limits on eligibility and a ceiling on federal contributions.[20] Together with the Aetna and Travelers Insurance companies, the association also sent a 27-page memorandum to HEW Undersecretary Wilbur Cohen, urging him to reject New York's Medicaid plan as "inconsistent with the purpose and standards of the Federal statute," "inviting the over-utilization of limited health facilities," and benefitting "those who are not in financial need."[21]

The irony of organized medicine's protests was obvious. The New York plan implemented a federal law that had been enacted with strong support from the American Medical Association in the hopes of scuttling Medicare. The medical profession had long expressed a preference for welfare medicine programs like Medicaid over universal programs like Medicare on the premise that the former's relatively small size posed little threat—as was discussed in chapter 1. However, Medicaid was turning out to be far bigger than anyone had predicted.

The uproar over Rockefeller's proposal extended to the nation's capital. When New York officials presented their plan in Washington, the House Ways and Means Committee and Senate Finance Committee summoned HEW Undersecretary Wilbur Cohen, and demanded to know how a state could do such a thing. The answer was simple: the law Congress had passed encouraged states to adopt expansive plans, and unless Congress rewrote the law, HEW had no grounds for withholding approval.[22] Thus, only six months after Medicaid went into effect, congressional leaders hurriedly set out to rewrite the law so as to restrict the scope of New York's plan and prevent other states from following suit.

SOCIAL SECURITY AMENDMENTS OF 1967

Not surprisingly, Wilbur Mills—the Medicaid program's fiscally conservative architect—was among the first federal legislators to attempt to rewrite the law. Realizing that he had miscalculated in creating Medicaid as a check on the growth of public health-care spending, and embarrassed by media coverage of the "great goof" Congress had made in designing the law, Mills began to see the program as an "intolerable blot" on the Ways and Means Committee's proud record.[23] Moreover, he did not want to break his promise to the American Medical Association that he would watch over the new program to see that it did not get out of hand (Smith and Moore 2008).

Chairman Mills led the Ways and Means Committee in considering several alternative approaches to curbing Medicaid spending in the summer of 1966. Recognizing that Medicaid's open-ended matching grants were enticing states to adopt generous plans, Mills first proposed to place a ceiling on federal Medicaid contributions to each state. One such formula would have limited federal Medicaid spending to $12 per capita per year—thereby capping New York's annual allocation at its estimated first-year cost of $217 million—which was expected to soar to $700 million within a few years under the original law. The committee also considered imposing tighter in-

come limits on eligibility to prevent states from adopting expansive definitions of the medically needy. The proposed income standard for New York
was rumored to be $4,150 for a family of four—considerably less than Gover-
nor Rockefeller's $6,000 limit (Stevens and Stevens 2003).

Mills's plan to obstruct New York's Medicaid plan was a potentially embarrassing development for Rockefeller, particularly as the governor campaigned for reelection on a platform that touted the program as one of his
most important achievements. Thus, as Mills began to draft a Medicaid bill,
Rockefeller called on Representative Eugene Keogh (D-New York), a senior
member of the Ways and Means Committee, to block the bill from making it
out of committee. Despite belonging to different political parties, Rockefeller and Keogh shared the desire to expand access to health care and to promote their state's financial interests, and formed a "firm, if unaccustomed"
alliance.[24]

Like Wilbur Mills, most members of the Ways and Means Committee
worried that Medicaid's unintended growth reflected poorly on their legislative craftsmanship, and initially seemed predisposed to rewrite the law.
However, when Keogh notified the representatives of several large states
with ambitious Medicaid plans, including California and Massachusetts, of
the committee's plans to curtail their states' funding, they joined him in
warning the committee against any legislative changes. Suddenly, the committee's near-unanimous support for Medicaid reform disintegrated as its
members realized there was no way to curb federal spending without squash-
ing the plans of several powerful states. As one committee member admitted,
"We got cold feet." As another put it, "We're like the man who casually invited his country cousin to come have dinner someday and then has the guy
arrive on his doorstep with his whole damn family. You'd like to slam the
door in his face but how the hell can you do it?" After the proposal died in
committee, media reports marveled that despite much "huffing and puff-
ing," the powerful Ways and Means Committee was "helpless to prevent
states from grabbing all the goodies in the surprise package."[25]

Mills was unwilling to concede defeat, however. Realizing that any large,
visible cut in federal aid would elicit resistance from powerful state leaders,
he took a different approach. Instead of capping federal matching grants, he
sought to clarify the definition of medically needy, specifying that the federal government would not provide any matching funds for able-bodied
adults under 65 who were not on welfare. This measure was significantly less
severe than the first, and would have cost New York an estimated $50 million

instead of $500 million in lost federal funding per year.[26] Over Representative Keogh's protests, the Ways and Means Committee reported this relatively mild bill to the House floor in October 1966.

As the Senate began to consider parallel action, Rockefeller again lobbied the New York delegation to kill the measure. The governor convinced Senate Finance Committee member Jacob Javits (R-New York) to demand that the committee delay consideration of the bill until Rockefeller had a chance to testify. Javits's effort to stall the legislation came as a surprise, as the senator had irked Governor Rockefeller only a few months earlier by speaking of the urgent need to set "reasonable limits" on federal Medicaid commitments.[27] Some speculated that Javits's reversal was related to the fact that he had since become the governor's campaign manager.[28] As a result of the delay, the Democratic leadership announced that no action would be taken on Medicaid until the following year. Many observers registered shock that legislative action that had enjoyed widespread congressional support, and had seemed like a virtual certainty earlier in the year, had somehow failed to materialize.[29]

Determined to revise the Medicaid law, Mills resumed his efforts in 1967. As a growing number of states submitted ambitious Medicaid plans, pressure to rewrite the law mounted. In an effort to find a middle ground, the Johnson administration put forward a proposal of its own. Wilbur Cohen, eager to avoid imposing federal limits on the definition of medical indigence, proposed to instead tie the means-test level for Medicaid to the cash assistance standard in each state, thereby retaining state control over eligibility (Stevens and Stevens 2003). Under the administration's proposal, the federal government would only help pay for Medicaid coverage for recipients with incomes under 150 percent of the state's standard to qualify for welfare payments. Mills drafted a bill that made this limit slightly more restrictive, calling for the standard to decline in stages from 150 percent in 1968 to 133 percent by 1970. This tightening of eligibility rules would affect not only New York, but also 14 of the 35 states that had enacted Medicaid programs by this time.[30]

The compromise measure enjoyed widespread support in Congress. During Senate Finance Committee hearings, Senator Albert Gore Sr. (D-Tennessee) argued forcefully for limiting the definition of medically needy, questioning "the justice of taxing a person in Nebraska who has earnings of $4,000 a year to pay the medical expenses of a citizen in New York who earns $6,000 a year."[31] The Senate finance committee report on the bill noted:

The tendency of some States to identify as eligible for medical assistance under title XIX large numbers of persons who could reasonably be expected to
pay some, or all, of their medical expenses has not only significantly increased the amount of Federal funds flowing into this program currently but
has developed future cost projections of a level totally inconsistent with the
expectations of the Congress when it enacted title XIX in 1965.[32]

Governor Rockefeller fought the measure both personally and through
his state's congressional delegation. In congressional testimony, he protested that his Medicaid plan was merely an attempt to comply with Title
XIX's maintenance-of-effort provision, which specified that states could
only qualify for increased aid if they expanded eligibility, so as not to merely
replace existing state funding with federal funding.

To improve our existing program and thereby qualify for the funds from the
Federal Government, we raised our standard for eligibility . . . we already had
high standards and we went higher in order to fulfill the intent of the Federal
law as written by the Congress—then there was a tremendous reaction in the
Congress . . . This was not our fault. We complied with the law in order to get
the maximum funds.[33]

At Rockefeller's urging, Representative Jacob Gilbert (D-New York) told his
colleagues that his and other states had acted in "good faith" in establishing
Medicaid programs in accordance with federal law, that the program's rising
costs were a sign of success rather than failure, and that his home state would
suffer greatly if the law was amended.[34]

Rockefeller was outnumbered, however. Congress passed the bill, and
President Johnson signed it into law as part of the Social Security Amendments of 1967. The legislation proved to be a fairly effective curb on the program's growth. The prospect of diminished federal aid prompted New York
lawmakers to reduce the income eligibility cap for a family of four from
$6,000 to $5,000 by 1969, resulting in the elimination of one million individuals from the Medicaid rolls (Sparer 1996, 81).

Nonetheless, New York's program—and, to a lesser extent, those of several other states—continued to be significantly more generous than Congress had intended. Although the Social Security Amendments of 1967 had
imposed limits on one of the "expansionary seeds embedded in Medicaid's
beginnings"—namely, medical indigence—two others remained: compre-

hensive benefits and open-ended matching grants (Grogan and Smith 2008, 228). Thus, Congress resumed efforts to revise Medicaid's financing mechanism.

CONGRESS TARGETS MATCHING RATES

Almost immediately upon Medicaid's implementation, it became obvious to federal and state lawmakers alike that generous open-ended matching grants were fueling the program's rapid growth. An exchange between Senator (and former governor) Clifford Hansen (R-Wyoming) and Governor Hulett Smith (D-West Virginia) during a hearing of the Senate Subcommittee on Intergovernmental Relations in February 1967 illustrates this growing awareness.

> SENATOR HANSEN: Would you agree with me that sometimes because— well, each state gets its share of dollars, that we provide matching funds for Federal programs that may not be as important sometimes as our other areas of need in the State and yet we pretty well get pushed into a position where we have to put in so many dollars to match Federal dollars?
>
> GOVERNOR SMITH: This is ever-occurring. With the passage of a program somebody says, well, here is something we have got to take advantage of . . . this question has come up, particularly in regard to Title XIX . . . I think every governor wants to use the total funds available to him to the best advantage of his State . . . [I]n the various programs— the matching ratio changes as far as the Federal government or the State government—you find the greatest heat is put on because this is 75 percent Federal aid 25 percent State and everybody is all for that one whereas if it is 50–50, it kind of slides back and if it is 30–70 it slides back further. You find the great drive and thrust of everybody to be—to take advantage of that one where it might not be the most important thing in that particular State . . .
>
> SENATOR HANSEN: . . . I think you call attention to a weakness in this system, in that we do not always go into these programs on the basis of what is of greatest need to the State, but rather on the basis of what will bring about the greatest infusion of Federal dollars into the Treasury of the state . . . Would you agree?
>
> GOVERNOR SMITH: I agree with that.[35]

Senate Finance Committee Chairman Russell Long (D-Louisiana) was particularly concerned about the incentives created by generous matching grants. Senator Long, a fiscal conservative, a close friend of Wilbur Mills, and one of the most powerful members of Congress, proposed to reduce matching rates from 50–83 percent to 25–69 percent for the medically needy. This amendment was directed at states such as New York, where, in Long's words, "middle-income people were being made eligible as medical indigents . . . if the states want to be more liberal than we intended to be, let them put up a higher percentage of money to be liberal with."[36]

Governor Rockefeller again urged New York's congressional delegation to block the bill, which he called "very disturbing" in a letter to Senators Javits and Robert F. Kennedy (D-New York).[37] A few days later, Javits carried Rockefeller's message to the Senate, arguing that it was "discriminatory to cut the federal share of costs of benefits for the medically indigent who were not eligible for or did not choose to accept public assistance."[38] Rockefeller also sent President Johnson a telegram, cosigned by New York City mayor John Lindsay, imploring him "to do everything possible" to kill the measure, which he alleged would have a "serious impact on many destitute children, their families, and the medically needy of this state."[39] The governor also testified before Congress, noting that "it is very difficult . . . to have Federal legislation passed and then have the legislation changed. The States must then backtrack and that is not easy."[40]

This time, Rockefeller's was not the only state official's voice heard in Washington. He was joined by Massachusetts's Republican governor, John Volpe, who sent a telegram to key members of Congress complaining that his state stood to lose $30 million per year if the measure passed. Volpe argued that cutting the federal matching rate would deal a "telling blow" to state finances, not only in his state, but also around the country.[41]

Despite the efforts of Governors Rockefeller and Volpe, the Senate Finance Committee passed the measure in September 1968, sending "shock waves" throughout the Johnson administration and state capitals alike. Wilbur Cohen called the reduction "absolutely unrealistic," noting that many states would be forced to cut eligibility and services, and predicted that governors would join him in "vigorously opposing" the amendment;[42] indeed, Governor Rockefeller lambasted federal lawmakers for failing to honor their commitments to "the needy sick who cannot pay for the health care they require and to states who accepted, in good faith, Federal approval of their Medicaid programs." He denounced the bill, which would cost New York an estimated $130 million per year, as a "planned act of reneging" that would be even more damaging than the Social Security Amendments of 1967.[43]

Once again, Governor Rockefeller's most potent weapon was his influence with his state's congressional delegation. In October 1968, Senators Javits and Charles Goodell (R-New York) used a filibuster to kill the measure—speaking at length against the Medicaid cutbacks, and lining up other senators to speak and offer amendments. Senator Long was forced to withdraw the provision, announcing: "I have been defeated by a successful filibuster." When Long vowed to resume his efforts to curtail federal Medicaid contributions the following year, Javits warned that he and Governor Rockefeller would continue to work together to block the legislation.[44]

One year later, Republican President Richard Nixon, having won the 1968 election on a campaign platform of reining in federal spending, put forward a new proposal to curb Medicaid's growth. Recognizing that enacting a broad reduction in matching rates had proven politically difficult and that institutional care was the largest and fastest-growing component of Medicaid spending, Nixon proposed to reduce federal matching funds for nursing homes and mental institutions. He defended his proposal on the grounds that the program's original purpose was to provide medical treatment rather than "custodial care."[45]

The president's proposal was met with sternly worded disapproval from a chorus of governors. As the Senate Finance Committee began considering the measure, Governor Norbert Tiemann (R-Nebraska) wired committee member Carl Curtis (R-Nebraska), complaining that the bill would cost their state nearly $3 million per year.[46] Governor William Cahill (R-New Jersey) submitted testimony that his state's losses would be nearly $17 million per year.[47] And Governor Marvin Mandel (D-Maryland) warned that cutting federal funding for nursing homes and other long-term care facilities would be "an act of bad faith by the federal government." Mandel argued that the states did not have the money to pay a larger share of health costs, and faulted the federal government for "grossly" underestimating the cost of Medicaid prior to enactment.[48] Under pressure from their states' leaders, congressional support dwindled, and the measure died.

RELAXING MANDATES

With the repeated failure of efforts to redesign Medicaid's financing structure, it was becoming clear that the nation's governors would be a formidable obstacle to any reductions in federal Medicaid contributions; indeed, state leaders were expressing a growing irritation with the federal government's efforts to rewrite the law. As one state official put it, "The federal government publicizes the program. It is ballyhooed nationwide. The states are pulled into the program, and then the Federal Government starts changing the ground rules [and] the states are left holding the bag."[49]

Congress subsequently switched tactics—proposing instead to relax the program's mandates so as to enable states to scale back coverage, thereby cutting both federal and state costs. The governors were generally more receptive to this approach, since it increased their flexibility without reducing federal cost sharing. Giving states greater discretion thus presented Congress with a more politically feasible path to retrenchment.

In fact, as Medicaid began to eat up a rapidly growing share of state budgets in the late 1960s, several governors had begun calling for such reforms. California's Republican governor, Ronald Reagan, complained that his state's Medicaid costs were rising at a rate of 50 percent per year, and that "something must be done before this ill-conceived program bankrupts the state" (Stevens and Stevens 2003, 112). Even Nelson Rockefeller—struggling to find the money to pay for New York's increasingly costly program, and facing mounting criticism from his state's taxpayers—acknowledged that he might have been "wrong in the beginning by going so enthusiastically for Medicaid."[50] He repeatedly urged the federal government to adopt national health insurance, and scale back Medicaid to a mere "second line of defense." He reiterated his long-standing concern that "taking the money out of the general treasury" to pay for Medicaid was "a far less responsible approach" than the payroll taxes and patient copayments that funded the Medicare program. He noted that unlike Medicare, Medicaid contained "no self-restraining force to curb abuse and excessive expansion."[51]

One of the states hit hardest by Medicaid was New Mexico. Although its program was not particularly generous—"bare-bones" compared to those of New York and California—the state legislature did not anticipate how rapidly costs would rise, and when the money ran out, refused to appropriate more funds (Stevens and Stevens 2003, 158). As a result, the state was forced to temporarily drop out of the program for nine days in May 1969, resulting in the eviction of thousands of nursing-home residents. Republican Governor David Cargo declared a state of emergency in order to free up the state funds needed to start up the program again, and began to seek relief from federal lawmakers.

Governor Cargo found a receptive audience in Senator Clinton Anderson (D-New Mexico). Although Senator Anderson had long supported the expansion of health coverage—and had even cosponsored the King-Anderson Bill, which had evolved into the Medicare program—he had grown increasingly concerned about the financial condition of his home state, which had been "driven to the wall by the fantastic costs" of Medicaid and was "paying too much for too many kinds of care for too many people."[52]

In May 1969, Senator Anderson proposed a bill to repeal two provisions of the Medicaid law. The first was the maintenance-of-effort provision prohibiting states from receiving federal assistance if they reduced their own spending on medical services for the poor. The second was the mandate that states provide "comprehensive care" to all individuals who met the plan's eligibility standards by July 1, 1975—which, as Anderson put it, amounted to "mandated bankruptcy no later than 1975."[53] In introducing his bill in Congress, he noted that it would "relieve my state of New Mexico of virtually unbearable fiscal pressure."[54]

In a poll of the nation's governors, nearly all favored the proposed changes (Stevens and Stevens 2003). Most members of the Senate Finance Committee also supported the amendments, stating in a June 1969 report that they were "greatly concerned over the sharp, accelerated, and unanticipated increases in the costs of Medicaid," and sought "to relieve what is for many states a serious burden and for some an intolerable one."[55] Many Senate liberals opposed the cuts, however, warning that the amendments would have a "seriously regressive effect on the goals of the Medicaid program."[56] Senator Javits—sympathizing with the liberal senators' desire to protect the program but acknowledging the pressure to address mounting cost concerns—helped secure passage of a compromise bill. States were permitted to drop some services, such as optometric services and dental care, but could not cut the five mandatory services or reduce overall spending below current levels. Instead of eliminating the deadline for establishing a comprehensive program, the legislation extended the deadline from 1975 to 1977. Javits argued that this compromise was a "balance between efforts to attain the national goals of the Medicaid program and the need to meet the acute financial distress being faced by several states."[57]

Anderson's amendments were later enacted as part of the Social Security Amendments of 1972, however. Under pressure from a diverse coalition of twenty organizations including the AFL-CIO, Common Cause, and the National Welfare Rights Organization, and dissatisfied by the existing patchwork of welfare programs, Congress created Supplemental Security Income (SSI), a national cash-assistance program to replace federal grants-in-aid programs for the blind, aged, and disabled. Since states were required to provide medical assistance to all cash assistance recipients, and since the SSI program's liberalized federal eligibility standard was expected to double enrollment, state leaders denounced the burden the law would impose on state budgets. Under pressure from the governors—and looking for ways to contain its own share of costs—Congress added several provisions to ease mandates on the states. The final legislation eliminated the maintenance-of-effort requirement, allowing states to reduce expenditures on Medicaid from one year to the next, as well as the 1977 deadline for comprehensive care. The law also specified that states were not required to provide medical assistance to the aged, blind, or disabled if such assistance was not required as of January 1, 1972, unless the state deemed such persons medically needy. "In plain language, this was a loophole created for states that did not wish to be tied to the SSI definitions or levels of income eligibility but might still wish to cover the medically indigent" (Smith and Moore 2008, 104).

Such efforts to relax mandates were a significant departure from previous efforts at cost containment. Unlike federal lawmakers' failed attempts to cap or cut federal matching rates, the elimination of the maintenance-of-effort and comprehensive care mandates aimed to reduce costs without scaling back the federal share of the program's costs. Powerful states with generous Medicaid programs could continue to offer a comprehensive benefit package without losing federal funds. This shift from cutting aid to loosening mandates reflected the growing influence of the governors in the federal-policy arena.

GOVERNORS PROPOSE NATIONAL HEALTH REFORM

An even more dramatic display of the governors' growing strength occurred in September 1969, as state leaders switched from responding to federal action to initiating action of their own. Mounting concerns about rising Medicaid costs led the governors to adopt a policy statement calling on the federal government to replace the federal-state program with a national health-insurance program. Under their proposal, all workers would be required to purchase health insurance from private insurance companies, financed out of employer and employee contributions, and the federal government would subsidize insurance for those below the poverty level. By shifting health-care costs to employers, employees, and the federal government, the governors' proposal would relieve the states of the growing financial burden imposed by Medicaid.

Governor Rockefeller presented this proposal at the annual gathering of the governors—then known as the National Governors' Conference—in September 1969. Rockefeller reminded his colleagues that "the cost of Medicaid, for those of you who have experimented with it under Title 19, can be prohibitive . . . it would not be possible under such a system to give the kind of protection that is essential in this country." He urged the governors to join him in recommending that the federal government adopt a national universal health-insurance program "as the primary method of keeping rising health costs from preventing all people from receiving the medical care they need."[58] The governors, eager to alleviate their states' mounting Medicaid costs, adopted Rockefeller's policy statement with only a handful of dissenting votes. The dissenters—Ronald Reagan (R-California) and Stanley Hathaway (R-Wyoming)—unsuccessfully proposed an amendment—submitted on behalf of the American Medical Association—to make the system voluntary, rather than compulsory.

The governors' virtually united front on health care represented a notable departure from past experience. Social policy had traditionally divided the governors along ideological and geographical lines, particularly during the civil rights era, with liberal Northerners promoting antipoverty programs and conservative Southerners questioning the need for such programs. But as Medicaid began squeezing state budgets, the governors increasingly found themselves ignoring regional differences as they sought financial relief. Indeed, at the 1969 meeting, Governor George Romney (R-Michigan) noted that prior to Medicaid's enactment "the Conference almost split up . . . over partisan politics and partisan views. Since then, fortunately, the Governors' Conference is increasingly recognizing the paramount importance of the problems that Governors face regardless of party."[59] Governor Buford Ellington (D-Tennessee) concurred that the meeting had been transformed almost overnight from a forum for "partisan and sectional squabbles" to a platform for "discussion of substantive issue."[60]

The governors' collective endorsement of a national social-policy initiative signified a newfound solidarity arising from the financial pressure created by the Medicaid program. The move also foreshadowed the increasingly prominent role that governors would play in setting the national health-policy agenda. After the governors voted to adopt his policy statement, Governor Rockefeller declared:

> The governors have moved ahead of the Washington scene in their perception of the needs and problems we face as a nation. It seems to me we have done more to grapple with national issues and take positions than any conference I have ever attended [and will] assume a more important role in the formulation of national policies.[61]

After attending the governors' annual meeting, President Nixon took a "sudden and serious interest" in their reform proposal. Nixon had opposed national health insurance during his presidential campaign the previous year, but the governors' proposal led him to reconsider the reform as a cost-cutting measure, since it would entail turning over a large share of costs to the private sector. He directed HEW secretary Robert Finch to lead a task force in examining the potential costs and benefits of replacing Medicaid with a "Medicare program for all ages," citing the governors' policy statement as the driving catalyst.[62]

The Task Force on Medicaid and Related Programs issued its report in June 1970. The report warned that Medicaid was not sustainable in its current form, noting that "the Federal-State grant structure on which it is based cannot, for the long run, stand the massive stresses of paying for quality services," and singling out long-term care as an especially large burden on the states. The task force concluded that "Medicaid should be converted to a program with a uniform minimal level of health benefits financed 100 percent by Federal funds," and that federal-state matching should be retained only for benefits and individuals not covered under the minimum plan, offered at the states' discretion.[63]

The Republican president developed a more limited proposal than the one recommended by his task force, however. Declaring that Medicaid was "plagued with serious faults," and that the program had "defrauded the taxpayer," President Nixon proposed to replace it with a new voluntary national health-insurance plan for families with incomes under $5,620. To minimize the burden on the taxpayer, Nixon's plan would require beneficiaries to pay a share of the cost themselves, based on a sliding scale that varied with the recipient's income. The federal government would pay the full cost for families with incomes under $1,600.[64]

Nixon's proposal was met with skepticism from congressional conservatives and liberals alike. Conservatives rejected it as the opening wedge for full-scale national health insurance financed by the federal government—echoing concerns that had been raised about Medicare several years earlier—while liberals rejected it as grossly inadequate. Senator Ted Kennedy—a leading contender for the Democratic presidential nomination—slammed Nixon's proposal as "poorhouse medicine," and countered with his own costlier, more ambitious proposal, which would fold all existing public and private health plans into a single compulsory, universal program.[65]

The reemergence of universal health insurance on the U.S. policy agenda subsumed Medicaid into a much larger and more intractable debate that dragged on throughout the 1970s without resolution. And as medical cost inflation skyrocketed, the question of federal versus state responsibility for funding health care for the poor took a back seat to issues such as health maintenance organizations and cost-containment measures. Nonetheless, the governors' proposal marked a significant turning point in intergovernmental relations, with major implications for national health policy.

THE RISE OF THE GOVERNORS

The governors' policy statement on health care reform reflected a broader trend toward greater organization, cohesion, and initiative among state officials in voicing their collective interests in Washington. This trend was unfolding in the background throughout the late 1960s as the federal government and the states clashed over Medicaid. The rise of the governors can be traced to three main sources: the sudden proliferation of federal grants and mandates—most notably those related to Medicaid, state-level institutional changes that transformed the nature of the governorship, and the evolution of the national party system.

The 1960s and 1970s witnessed an explosion of federal grants and mandates. In 1955, federal grants had constituted only 12 percent of state and local budgets; by 1978, that figure had nearly tripled to 32 percent.[66] Much of this growth stemmed from President Johnson's Great Society programs—including not only Medicaid, but also a number of smaller education, transportation, and antipoverty programs. The Great Society extended the reach of the federal government to an unprecedented degree, infusing state coffers with federal aid, but also imposing on state and local officials a staggering number of new mandates. Of all the federal-state programs that emerged during this period, Medicaid quickly rose to the top in prominence. Within a few years, the governors were warning that "Medicaid has become the most rapidly escalating cost of state budgets" and identifying the program as "an item of highest priority" for the states.[67]

Scholars of federalism have put forward a variety of theories about the ramifications of programs like Medicaid for intergovernmental relations. Although cooperation has long been central to American federalism (Elazar 1962; Grodzins 1966), some early scholars argued that the proliferation of intergovernmental programs caused a shift from "dual federalism"—in which the federal and state spheres had operated relatively autonomously—to "cooperative federalism," whereby the states acted as friendly servants carrying out federal policies (Corwin 1950; Davis 1978). By emphasizing the states' transition from autonomy to subservience, such theories suggest that the proliferation of intergovernmental programs has weakened the states.

More recent scholarship has posited that intergovernmental programs have, in fact, exacerbated the conflict, disagreement, and tension inherent in intergovernmental relations (Rosenthal and Hoefler 1989; Kincaid 1990). Stephens and Wikstrom note that "in a rather ironic sense, the federal grants-in-aid system designed to promote cooperation between the federal government, the states, and localities has been the cause, or instigator, of political and intergovernmental controversy and conflict" (2007, 69). The states' ability to use their power as implementers of federal policy to resist, challenge, and dissent suggests that increased reliance on the states may have actually augmented their influence (Bulman-Pozen and Gerken 2009).

Consistent with this view, several scholars have observed that as federal and state governments have become progressively intertwined, intergovernmental relations have become increasingly characterized by bargaining under conditions of partial conflict (Wright 1978; Derthick 1987; O'Toole 2007). These theories suggest that as the federal-state partnership has become more complex and contentious, state officials have sought to negotiate the terms of that partnership to their collective advantage. As grants and mandates multiplied, the stakes grew—strengthening the governors' incentives to seek ways to augment their bargaining capacity.

A second and closely related factor that led to the growing prominence of the governors in Washington in the late 1960s was the changing nature of the governorship itself. For generations, the states and their leaders had been the subject of widespread criticism and ridicule. In 1949, Robert S. Allen described the states as the "tawdriest, most incompetent and most stultifying unit of the nation's political structure" (Allen 1949). In 1962, James Reston wrote that "the governors of the states, taken as a whole, are a poor lot," adding that "the state capitals are over their heads in problems and up to their knees in midgets," singling out Nelson Rockefeller as one of a few notable exceptions.[68]

The reasons were largely institutional, and reflected a longstanding suspicion of concentrated executive power that dated back to colonial times. Traditionally, many governors had served two-year terms, while others were limited to a single four-year term in office. They had few formal powers, tiny staffs, and small budgets—in fact, until the 1960s, many states had neither an income tax, nor a sales tax. Since governorship offered few advantages, it tended to attract "good time Charlies" who were primarily interested in the social and ceremonial aspects of office rather than matters of substance (Sabato 1983); as Governor Rockefeller put it, "great men are not drawn to small office" (Rockefeller 1967, 209).

Following the enactment of Medicaid and other federal-state programs in the 1960s, state officials had a rapidly expanding set of duties and resources. Some of the resulting impetus for change came from within, as state officials struggled to meet the new demands of office and began to modernize state administrative structures. Pressure for change also came from the federal government, with an eye toward seeing its programs executed competently. Citizens, too, expected more of their state officials, as postwar prosperity increased the demand for government services. Citizens' expectations of their governors only intensified in the 1970s, as the Vietnam War and Watergate led to disillusionment with federal government, and a relative trust in state and local government (Teaford 2002).

Together, these pressures unleashed a series of state reforms extending term lengths, loosening term limits, giving the governors additional administrative powers, expanding staffing, and creating state budget offices. A growing number of states adopted income and sales taxes or raised existing tax rates—greatly increasing state resources—and many states switched from biennial to annual legislative sessions to more effectively allocate those resources. These reforms, in turn, attracted a "new breed" of experienced, competent, ambitious politicians to state capitals (Sabato 1983, 2).

David Broder summarized the governors' transformation in a 1974 *Washington Post* article titled "The Rise of the Governors."

> For most of the past two generations, the American governors have been piti-
> able figures. Penniless, powerless, prone to defeat . . . they were—with a few
> notable exceptions—richly entitled to the contempt they received from the
> public and the press.

However, Broder noted, the late 1960s and early 1970s saw an "astonishing
rise in the status of the state executives"—due in large part to the "bootstrap
efforts most of the states have made to reclaim their leadership role in domestic affairs" through "courage in raising taxes, in modernizing state con-
stitutions and administrative structures, in improving state services." As a
result of these reforms, Broder remarked that there had never before been a
more capable group of 50 governors in office.[69]

A third factor that contributed to the growing organization of the governors was the overhaul of the national party system that occurred in the late
1960s. Historically, the governors had—together with other state and local
officials—helped select presidential and congressional candidates by choos-
ing the delegates who would vote on candidates at the national party convention. Under this system, state leaders would choose the nominee who
would help them the most in their own reelection campaigns. Once selected,
the national candidate was dependent on state and local leaders to support
his or her candidacy, and to deliver a good turnout on Election Day. Although citizens in many states voted for candidates in primaries, the primary vote was virtually worthless because the results did not bind state and
local officials' selection of delegates (Crotty 1983).

A dramatic turn of events in 1968 brought an abrupt end to this system.
President Lyndon Johnson, facing a growing storm of protest over the Vietnam War, civil-rights related political unrest, and challenges from several
strong Democratic contenders, announced that he would not run for reelection. Instead, he rallied state and local officials into supporting his vice president, Hubert Humphrey. When Humphrey won the Democratic Party
nomination—despite his unpopularity with voters and failure to enter a
single state primary race—the other candidates' supporters were outraged.
To heal the divisions that had erupted within the party, the Democratic National Committee established a Commission on Party Structure and Delegate Selection. The commission recommended a number of reforms, including open delegate selection procedures, so that party leaders could no longer
hand-pick convention delegates behind closed doors. These reforms were
ultimately adopted by both parties.

Subsequently, state party organizations came to play a much smaller role in the candidate selection process. Candidates for national office began shifting their focus away from garnering support from state and local officials, and toward building campaigns designed to help them win primary elections. As politicians increasingly appealed directly to voters, the news media displaced state and local officials as the main link between candidates and the electorate. In addition, a "cluster of powerful centripetalist competitors" including pollsters, political consultants, and political action committees began to carry out many of the functions that the decentralized party system had previously performed (Walker 1991, 108).

The growing independence of national political candidates from state party organizations left the governors feeling like just another interest group—and not a particularly well-organized one (Kincaid 1990). Suddenly, they had to find new ways to establish a collective identity and new mechanisms for influencing national policy. As Haider notes, the new party system meant that "banding together to deal with their federal constituency" had become a "political necessity" (1974, 11). Meanwhile, the individualization of the political system also meant that members of Congress could not rely as heavily on their party organizations, and needed to make it on their own by bringing home the bacon to their districts—fueling the aforementioned growth of federal grants to the states (Conlan 2006).

THE GOVERNORS GET ORGANIZED

In the mid-1960s, the governors began to descend on Washington. Between 1964 and 1969, nearly half of all governors set up a state liaison office in the nation's capital. More significantly, the governors established a collective national voice by opening a permanent office in Washington in 1967.

The establishment of a full-time lobbying apparatus in Washington was a major turning point in the governors' history. The National Governors' Conference (NGC) had existed since 1908, when President Theodore Roosevelt invited the governors to the White House to help him pressure Congress to enact his natural resource conservation program (Haider 1974). The governors subsequently organized an annual conference—originally known simply as the Governors' Conference. The location of the meeting rotated around the nation, as governors took turns hosting their colleagues. For decades, the NGC operated primarily as a social club. The governors' annual meetings were "occasions for elaborate entertainment," and placed "a marked emphasis on social affairs."[70] As one governor put it, the NGC's "basic significance was as a place where governors could meet each other . . . Not too much serious business came out of the Conference" (Sabato 1983, 171).

To the extent that the governors addressed substantive matters during their annual meetings, they focused primarily on the technical aspects of running state government, and on interstate affairs; indeed, until the mid-1960s, the governors expressed remarkably little concern with what was going on in Washington. On the rare occasions when they did, they had trouble reaching a consensus and often issued tentative, "half-hearted" policy resolutions (Sabato 1983, 171). These recommendations were reached through an "unsystematic process," with decisions made "on an ad hoc basis and with insufficient study."[71] Their effectiveness was further undermined by the fact that typically only about half the governors even showed up to the conference to vote on resolutions (Haider 1974). Not surprisingly, the governors "scored few if any victories and nearly all defeats," were at most "mildly obstructive on federal-state matters," and "generally proved ineffectual as a national political interest group" (Haider 1974, 22).

All that changed in the mid-1960s, when the federal government began to intervene in state affairs to an unprecedented degree with the creation of new federal-state programs like Medicaid. Federal policy was suddenly high stakes for the governors, and they became increasingly concerned about their lack of organization and influence in Washington. As one governor recalled, "We simply weren't going anywhere under the then existing structure" (Haider 1974, 23). The governors' desire to organize themselves more effectively also reflected the increased competence and motivation of the new breed of governors entering office during this period: "The lackluster conference was a product of its membership; therefore, as the governors grew more capable and directed, this development was reflected in their organization" (Sabato 1983, 172).

In December 1966, the governors voted unanimously to establish an office in Washington. Governor John Love (R-Colorado), who led the movement, explained the need for a full-time lobbying apparatus: "Congress passes legislation creating new programs and the administrators promulgate rules for their operation without any effective consultation with the Governors, and yet we wind up with the responsibility for administering these programs." According to Love, the governors also acted out of frustration with their own members of Congress, who they perceived as representing personal and national interests above state interests. "Ideally, the Senators and Representatives should be state-oriented, and many of them are, but the system just hasn't worked well enough to sufficiently represent the views of the states."[72]

The governors opened their Washington office—funded by annual appropriations from the individual states—in March 1967, with the goal to "improve the effectiveness of the states, and particularly the governors, in dealing with problems arising out of federal-state relations." Almost overnight, the organization was transformed from a loosely organized social club to an influential interest group. As Haider observes, "Few governors seemed to grasp fully the significance of what they had done. In effect, they had put behind them the nonfederal functions and purposes of the organization so characteristic of the past. They had created a full-time governors' lobby in Washington" (Haider 1974, 27).

To increase their influence in Washington, the governors overhauled their leadership and internal organization. They replaced the "political pipsqueaks and goodtime Charlies they used to endow with the empty honor of the governors' conference chairmanship" with their best and brightest.[73] They also replaced their ad hoc committee structure with permanent standing committees focused on specific policy areas such as human resources (including health), natural resources, and commerce—mirroring the organization of congressional committees. This new system nurtured policy experts among committee chairmen and vice chairmen, providing a useful resource for communication and consultation with federal policy makers.

Beginning in 1968, the governors began gathering for a second annual meeting in midwinter in Washington—inviting presidents, cabinet members, congressional leaders, and other top federal officials to attend. The winter meeting enhanced the governors' ability to lobby federal policy makers on behalf of their preferred policies. Virtually all governors began attending the winter meeting, as well as the annual meeting in September.

The pace of the governors' activities in Washington accelerated rapidly in the late 1960s. They began to issue more policy statements, informing federal officials of the states' collective opinions on national policy matters, and testified more frequently before Congress—often in response to proposed changes in the Medicaid law. As NGC chairman John Volpe noted at the organization's midyear conference in 1968:

> The governors presented more oral testimony in Washington in the past
> twelve months than they had in the previous ten years . . . It is through the
> National Governors' Conference . . . that we governors have been able to reas-
> sert the need for our own pivotal role in domestic policies and programs of
> this nation. (Haider 1974, 30)

Throughout the 1970s, the governors grew progressively more organized.
In 1974, they created a think tank called the NGC Center for Policy Research
and Analysis to "liberate them from the pattern of always reacting to congressional and presidential initiatives, and enable the governors to propose
their own programs for national consideration."[74] In 1975, the NGC created
a Hall of the States—located only steps away from the U.S. Capitol—bringing
together the headquarters of state officials and lobbying groups that previously had been scattered around Washington, in order to improve communication and coordination (Sabato 1983, 174). Additionally, in 1977, the governors voted to change the name of their organization from the National
Governors' Conference to the National Governors Association (NGA) to reflect the transformation from an annual meeting to a full-time lobbying organization. In introducing the measure, Governor Reubin Askew (D-Florida)
remarked upon this transformation.

> There have been many governors over the years who have felt that the name
> of the organization ought to be changed because it implies a conference, a
> meeting, and not an ongoing organization. We now have a physical presence
> in Washington, we've got a substantial staff, we're working all the time.[75]

To be sure, the governors were not the only intergovernmental lobbying
group to organize during this time. Other groups included the National
Conference of State Legislatures, the National Association of Counties, and
the U.S. Conference of Mayors. But as the embodiment of the states, the governors were by far the most prominent and influential among these groups
(Haider 1974; Cammisa 1995).

STRENGTHS AND WEAKNESSES

As a bargaining agent for the interests of state governments, the National
Governors Association has several unique strengths. Due to the governors'

status and legitimacy as high-ranking public officials, they enjoy considerable access to federal government officials, as well as the news media. The governors' direct electoral relationship with congressional members' constituencies makes them particularly influential in Congress, and, above all, in the Senate—organized as it is along state lines (Haider 1974). As administrators of an expanding set of federal-state programs, governors have hands-on expertise that has made them a valuable resource to federal policy makers. Also, as the implementers of federal policy, governors can threaten noncooperation to gain leverage in changing the terms of their participation in federal programs (Posner 1998).

Indeed, the NGA received unprecedented access to federal officials almost immediately after setting up shop in Washington. President Nixon attended the governors' 1969 conference—at which they proposed replacing Medicaid with a national health-insurance program—bringing with him nearly a dozen other top administration officials. This "outpouring of Washington officials" was widely interpreted as an indication of the governors' growing influence and the president's desire to strengthen ties with state officials.[76]

Nonetheless, the governors often struggled to influence federal policy as they first began to get organized. One observer noted in 1970:

> The Governors are spending more time, much better organized, in serious debate than they did at their meetings a few years ago. But it would be inaccurate to claim that the Governors had found the way to underscore their policy statements with the very real political and governmental influence they enjoy back in their capitals.[77]

Indeed, the governors had—and continue to have—a number of notable weaknesses as an interest group. When it comes to influencing federal policy, the governors have a limited number of tools in their arsenal, such as issuing policy statements, testifying before Congress, and communicating with individual lawmakers. Nor do the governors possess many of the resources that typically characterize powerful lobbying organizations, such as extensive financial resources, or effective mechanisms for sanctioning uncooperative members.

The governors also face a number of challenges arising from their identities as elected officials, partisans, and representatives of diverse constituencies. First, since the NGA is comprised of elected officials, each with his or her own personal ambitions and policy agendas—or "fifty prima donnas" as Haider puts it (1974, 24)—achieving the internal consensus needed to effectively formulate and communicate a single set of policy recommendations to the federal government can be difficult. Moreover, high membership turnover and geographical dispersion tend to inhibit the social bonds that promote cooperation.

Second, the governors' cohesion as an interest group is undermined by partisan cleavages, as the NGA's members are typically split fairly evenly between the two parties. When it comes to Medicaid, for example, Democratic governors typically favor more expansive coverage than Republican governors (Kousser 2002). Cognizant of this challenge, the governors have collectively adopted an organizational structure designed to promote bipartisanship. The NGA's Articles of Incorporation require that the chairmanship rotate annually between the two parties; that the chair and vice chair be from different parties; and that the nine-member executive committee consist of four members of the chair's party, and five members of the vice chair's party. Moreover, a vote of two-thirds of the governors in attendance is required to pass a formal policy resolution in order to help prevent the majority party from steamrolling the minority party.[78]

Regional cleavages pose a third challenge. For instance, distributional fights over Medicaid funds often break down along geographical lines, since the progressive matching formula redistributes resources from wealthier Northern states to poorer Southern states.[79] In order to "siphon off" factional concerns that threaten to undermine consensus within the NGA, subsets of governors have organized themselves into separate associations along regional lines (the Midwestern, Southern, and Western Governors Associations, and New England Governors' Conference), as well as party lines (the Republican and Democratic Governors Associations) (Haider 1974, 25).

CONCLUSION

The governors' growing influence over federal policy in the late 1960s was indisputable. The federal-state struggle over Medicaid during this period provides ample evidence of their remarkable political transformation. In Medicaid's vulnerable first few years, Governor Nelson Rockefeller of New York worked tirelessly, in collaboration with his state's congressional delegation, to fight federal retrenchment. Over time, his efforts were reinforced by other governors such as John Volpe of Massachusetts, Marvin Mandel of Maryland, and William Cahill of New Jersey. Remarkably, this handful of governors managed to repeatedly prevent the House, Senate, and president from revising the program's federal-state financing structure.

Following Medicaid's enactment, the governors briskly organized into what would soon become one of the most influential interest groups in Washington. Through communication with federal policy makers, congressional testimony, and policy statements, they began to assert their collective financial interests with increased frequency and strength. It was not long before the governors found themselves at the White House, negotiating the terms of a potential overhaul of the Medicaid program—as discussed in chapter 3.

CHAPTER 3

Retrenchment and Repudiation in the Reagan Era

THE REAGAN ADMINISTRATION made three major attempts at Medicaid retrenchment in the early 1980s, but was blocked by the governors on all three occasions. The White House first proposed to permanently cap Medicaid matching grants in 1981, but state leaders successfully lobbied Congress to instead adopt a much smaller, temporary cut in federal matching rates. The administration next proposed converting the program's open-ended matching grants to block grants—offering the states more flexibility in exchange for less funding—but abandoned the idea when the governors declared themselves "violently opposed."[1] Realizing that the surest way to retrench the program was to remove it from state hands, the Reagan administration shifted gears in 1982, proposing a "swap," whereby the federal government would assume full responsibility for Medicaid if the states would accept full responsibility for two other programs: Aid to Families with Dependent Children, and food stamps. However, following an unprecedented series of high-profile negotiations with the White House, the governors rejected the proposal when the administration revealed its plans to dramatically curtail Medicaid eligibility and benefits.

The Reagan administration's failure to restructure and retrench Medicaid in the early 1980s is one of the most fascinating and unexpected paths not taken in the program's history. In fact, the odds seemed stacked against Medicaid in the Reagan era. The Republican president, still in his honeymoon period, had won a landslide victory on a platform of limiting the growth of government. He faced a friendly, Republican-controlled Senate, a weak, disorganized Democratic majority in the House, and an electorate eager for spending and tax cuts. State officials were also open to change, having recently called on federal policy makers to realign federal and state responsibilities—and specifically to take over the rapidly growing Medicaid program. However, in negotiating the details of a federal takeover, the Reagan administration's budget-cutting agenda came into direct conflict with the states' financial prerogatives. A scaled-back national Medicaid program would have forced states to make a politically difficult choice: alienate voters by raising taxes to maintain service levels, or alienate the powerful health-care industry by allowing coverage to erode and the uninsured rate to rise (Thompson and Fossett 2008). However badly governors wanted out of Medicaid, the prospect of reduced federal support was even less appealing—particularly at a time of back-to-back recessions, budget shortfalls, and rapid medical-cost inflation. In short, Medicaid's federal cost-sharing structure had turned state officials into stakeholders in the status quo.

THE REAGAN REVOLUTION

In November 1980, Ronald Reagan won a decisive victory over incumbent Jimmy Carter on a platform of cutting spending and taxes, balancing the federal budget, and devolving power to state and local governments. Upon assuming the presidency, Reagan told a reporter that he hoped his legacy would be to "restore to local and State government functions that are properly theirs."[2] As governor of California, Reagan had bristled at the growing intrusion of the federal government in state affairs, and had been a particularly vocal critic of Medicaid, comparing the program's rapid cost growth to "a cancer eating at our vitals."[3] Reagan was also an outspoken opponent of national health insurance, having recorded an album for the American Medical Association in 1961 called *Ronald Reagan Speaks out against Socialized Medicine,* in which he warned that government intervention in the health-care market threatened the sanctity of the doctor-patient relationship.

Thus, it came as no surprise that when Reagan presented his first budget to Congress in February 1981, Medicaid was near the top of his hit list. In his remarks, the president singled out Medicaid's "unlimited matching payments"—and the states' resulting incentive to adopt generous policies—as the primary driver of the program's rapid growth. Reagan argued that capping federal Medicaid payments, so that states would bear full responsibility for every dollar of spending above the cap, would "attack waste" while protecting those with "true need."[4] Specifically, he proposed a 5 percent cap on the growth of federal Medicaid contributions for 1982; thereafter, federal contributions would be capped at the inflation rate. Since federal

Medicaid spending had been growing at a rate of 15 to 20 percent per year, this measure would result in considerable federal savings: $1 billion in the first year, and as much as $5 billion per year by 1985.[5] To sweeten the deal, the White House proposed to loosen federal eligibility and benefit standards to allow states to scale back their programs and reduce their own share of costs.

In addition to the Medicaid cap, the Reagan administration's first budget included two other proposals that would cut federal aid to the states in return for increased flexibility. First, the White House proposed to replace nearly 90 small categorical grants with 7 more flexible block grants, trimming support for these programs by 20 to 25 percent. Second, Reagan called for an eventual sorting out of responsibilities, whereby each level of government would take full responsibility for a broad set of government functions. Although the president was initially vague about which programs he thought belonged at which level of government, his advisors soon revealed that the administration was eager to turn over responsibility for Medicaid, Aid to Families with Dependent Children (AFDC), and food stamps— "programs which encourage profligacy"—to the states.[6] Thus, the proposed Medicaid cap was simply an interim measure; ultimately the Reagan administration hoped the states would take over full responsibility for the program.

Reagan's stated motive for his federalism initiatives was economic recovery. At the time he took office, the country was experiencing a bout of stagflation—high inflation combined with high unemployment—due to expansionary monetary policies and a series of oil price shocks in the 1970s, exacerbated by a mild recession in the first half of 1980. Framing the troubled economy as a "calamity of tremendous proportions"[7] caused primarily by the "uncontrolled growth of government spending,"[8] the president argued that the only solution was to slash public spending: "only if our Government grows less will our economy grow more."[9]

Although many Americans welcomed Reagan's proposals as a bold move to remedy the troubled economy, economic forecasters were dubious that his measures would have the promised effect, causing the stock market to dip following Reagan's budget presentation (Wilentz 2008). For their part, the governors—a majority of whom were Democrats—feared the president's budget was merely a Trojan Horse for cutting aid to the states, and saw his emphasis on economic recovery as an attempt to dramatize the need for budget cuts.[10] Many Democrats and some Republicans in Congress shared the governors' concerns, and warned state leaders to read "devolution" as a synonym for "retrenchment."[11]

Reagan initially denied that his goal was to dismantle the welfare state, but later admitted in his memoir that he considered Lyndon Johnson's Great Society programs a waste of money and an encroachment on Americans' freedoms. "The liberals had had their turn at bat in the 1960s and they had struck out," Reagan wrote, and now that it was his turn, he planned to undo Johnson's work (Reagan 1990, 198–99). David Stockman—the fiscally conservative director of the Office of Management and Budget, and a driving force behind Reagan's budget-cutting agenda—confirmed that the president's first budget was "a frontal assault on the American welfare state" designed to scrap "forty years' worth of promises, subventions, entitlements, and safety nets issued by the federal government to every component and stratum of American society." The administration was braced for "risky and mortal political combat with all the mass constituencies of Washington's largesse" including "state and local officials" (Stockman 1986, 9).

AN UNEASY PARTNERSHIP

One week after Reagan announced his budget, the governors gathered in Washington for their winter meeting. The president and several top aides and cabinet members spent an unprecedented three days with the governors. The purpose, according to Richard Williamson, Reagan's assistant for intergovernmental affairs, was to convey the administration's commitment to federalism and interest in developing a partnership with state leaders.[12]

The governors had mixed feelings about the president's first budget. On the one hand, they welcomed the conversion of small categorical grants to block grants and were willing to accept some funding cuts in exchange for increased flexibility since the financial stakes were relatively low. They also supported the idea of sorting out responsibilities for larger programs. In fact, in 1980, the NGA had adopted a policy resolution calling on the president and Congress to consider a new "division of labor" among the federal government and the states.[13] Thus, NGA chairman George Busbee (D-Georgia) told the president that the governors gladly accepted his invitation to consider a realignment of responsibilities.[14] On the other hand, Reagan's specific proposals for redistributing responsibilities were inconsistent with the NGA's official position that the federal government should administer and finance programs for the poor, while the states should specialize in funding education, local transportation, and public safety.[15]

The governors were not alone in this view; many economists and political scientists have put forward a variety of arguments for central administration and financing of redistributive programs. First, Wallace Oates notes that "poverty is, in a fundamental sense, a national problem" (1982, 476). Since the poor are unevenly distributed across the country, "on purely equity grounds, one can contend that a 'fair' resolution of the poverty problem requires central-government participation" so as to ensure a uniform level of benefits and to spread the burden evenly among the nation's nonpoor citizens. Second, safety-net programs for the poor serve as "automatic stabilizers" for the national economy—since more people receive benefits when the economy weakens—and there is general agreement that the responsibility for macroeconomic stabilization rests with the central government (Oates 1982). Third, "serious constraints" limit the states' ability to adopt redistributive policies since "the high degree of mobility within national borders implies that one jurisdiction cannot tax a certain group significantly more heavily than elsewhere without creating incentives to move" (Oates 1982, 475). Thus, the federal government's ability to pool resources with little danger of capital flight makes it the "most competent agent of redistribution" (Peterson 1995, 27). By contrast, the states are often said to have a comparative advantage in the "productivity agenda," including education and infrastructure (Rivlin 1992).

For these reasons, the Advisory Commission on Intergovernmental Relations (ACIR)—a bipartisan group consisting of federal, state, and local officials, as well as private citizens—issued a series of reports in the 1960s, 1970s, and 1980s calling for federal assumption of social-welfare functions, including health care for the poor. The ACIR argued that "just as the national government has necessarily assumed paramount responsibility for managing the economy in the aggregate, it also should accept responsibility for meeting the basic human needs of those whom the economy has failed," and noted that "only national financing can assure that an adequate standard of benefits exists throughout the nation."[16]

Congressional Democrats also tended to share the governors' view. The 1980 Democratic Party platform called for "serious reform" of the federalist system, referring to the nation's programs for the poor as "inequitable and archaic," and warning that the states "find themselves in deepening fiscal difficulty."[17] Some Democratic members, such as Senator Daniel Patrick Moynihan of New York, advocated increasing the minimum federal matching rate from 50 percent to 90 percent so as to assign primary responsibility for financing Medicaid (as well as AFDC) to the federal government.[18]

Even some Reagan administration officials admitted that the governors' argument had merit. During the NGA meetings, Governor Lamar Alexander (R-Tennessee) pointedly asked Robert Carleson—special assistant to the president for policy development—if the governors' position was not "perfectly in accord" with Reagan's desire to sort out federal and state responsibilities. Carleson acknowledged that "there's no doubt the federal government is the most efficient instrument" of redistribution, but argued that programs for the poor should only provide temporary relief for those most in need, and that the states were best able to determine the extent and duration of need.[19] The Reagan administration's determination to turn over the costly Medicaid program to the states led some governors to grumble that the White House's approach to federalism was driven by "pure expediency."[20]

To be sure, the governors themselves were clearly motivated by financial self-interest, as well as philosophical concerns about the proper distribution of responsibility. In their 1980 policy position on Medicaid, the governors made their complaints known.

> The design and administration of the program have produced a system which is bankrupting the states . . . Medicaid has become the most rapidly escalating cost of state budgets . . . The spiraling cost of this program must be controlled, but without holding the poor hostage to forces beyond their control.[21]

As the *New York Times* editorial page opined, "The governors' position, though guided by self-interest, keeps the needs of poor people clearly in view."[22]

In addition to disagreeing with Reagan's long-term plans for sorting out responsibilities, the governors vehemently opposed his more immediate plans for a Medicaid cap, which they saw as a blatant attempt to shift costs to the states. They feared that the cap would require them to increase their own financial contributions to the program at a time when two-thirds of the states were already struggling with significant Medicaid-related financial difficulties as a result of the recession.[23] Estimating that the cap would decrease federal Medicaid assistance to New York by 20 percent, Governor Hugh Carey warned that "The state has no money to fill the void." The Democratic governor called the president's proposal "obnoxious," and said that he would accept the cap "over my prostrate body."[24] Even NGA chairman George Busbee—a fiscal conservative who was eager to negotiate with the Reagan administration on other aspects of the budget proposal—called the Medicaid cap "completely unacceptable."[25] In the economic context of the early 1980s, the president's offer of more flexibility over Medicaid in exchange for less money was simply not attractive to the governors.

The governors thought it was particularly unfair that they should have to take on a bigger share of Medicaid costs given that national economic policy had contributed to the recession, which in turn caused state revenues to decline and demand for programs like Medicaid to rise. Moreover, they felt that national health policy—including the larger Medicare program's reimbursement policies—had contributed to medical cost inflation, and that the federal government was therefore in a better position than the states to slow cost growth. Pointing out in a letter to the White House that "States purchase medical services from a large and complex medical delivery system, and Medicaid programs constitute only about one-tenth of that market,"[26] the governors expressed doubt that the additional flexibility Reagan was offering the states would be of much help with cost containment.

Despite the governors' mixed feelings about Reagan's budget, Chairman Busbee urged them to adopt a conciliatory tone in their policy resolution. Busbee advised the governors to take comfort in the fact that the president was "not fixed in concrete on a lot of things" and seemed genuinely open to their input.[27] He encouraged his colleagues to embrace, in bipartisan fashion, the president's offer of a new partnership—convinced that presenting a united front would augment the governors' ability to shape national policy (Williamson 1983). Although some governors—particularly Republicans—seemed to share Busbee's optimism, many Democratic governors registered concern. Governor Jerry Brown (D-California) warned his colleagues that Reagan's budget would simply shift financial burdens from the federal government to the states, referring to Reagan's proposals as "a shell game" and "a red flag," and warning that "coming from my own state, I have some experience of my predecessor, Mr. Reagan . . . there is a tendency to shift and not to cut."[28]

Busbee prevailed, and the governors endorsed a resolution stating that the states were prepared to accept funding cuts in a wide range of small federal grant programs in exchange for greater flexibility. However, the resolution warned that "the federal budget reductions must not result in imposing an unfair and disproportionate burden on the poor, disadvantaged, and the handicapped."[29] The resolution also specified that the federal government should eventually move toward primary responsibility for Medicaid and AFDC.

Despite the openness expressed in their resolution, many governors left the NGA meetings with a sense of trepidation, particularly when it came to the Medicaid cap. Several governors began to make phone calls and write letters to sympathetic members of Congress, who would soon begin hearings on the president's budget. Governor Carey expressed optimism that the Democrat-controlled House of Representatives would be particularly receptive to the governors' concerns, declaring: "I see the beginning of a coalition."[30]

BATTLE ON CAPITOL HILL

Shortly after the governors' meeting, the two congressional committees with jurisdiction over Medicaid—the House Commerce Committee and the Senate Finance Committee—began to consider the president's proposals, and governors and NGA officials began to lobby extensively on Capitol Hill. In testimony before the health subcommittee of the House Commerce Committee, NGA executive director Steve Farber noted that of all of the elements of Reagan's budget, the proposal that was of greatest concern to the governors was the Medicaid cap, which he called a "retreat from what the Governors strongly believe is a fundamental part of a sorting out process and is primarily a Federal responsibility."[31] Governor James Hunt (D-North Carolina), testifying before the same committee, echoed the governors' "very serious concerns" with the administration's proposal to cap Medicaid.

> Every Governor in this country, all 50, would like to be here this morning . . . There is not a single issue facing Governors . . . that is of greater concern and is putting us into a greater financial bind than this issue . . . the immediate effect of such a move will be to shift costs to the States . . . and we simply cannot absorb cuts of this magnitude.[32]

The governors had a friendly audience in subcommittee chairman Henry Waxman—a liberal Democrat from California, and champion of the Medicaid program. Waxman agreed with the governors that "a cap simply shifts costs to the states . . . It does not cap the aging process. It does not change people's basic need for medical care." Recognizing that budget cuts were inevitable in the current political and economic climate, Waxman preferred a more moderate approach that retained the federal government's commitment to "carry its share of the burden."[33] Waxman later explained in an interview that he was "just trying to hold onto the Medicaid program being an entitlement without any caps or limits on it at the federal level because that would have been such a fundamental change that would have made it impossible for states to pick up the slack."[34]

Waxman developed a proposal that retained Medicaid's open-ended financing structure, but made a series of relatively small, temporary cuts in the federal matching rate: 3 percent in fiscal year 1982, 2 percent in fiscal year 1983, and 1 percent in fiscal year 1984. He also included a provision allowing states to avoid all or some portion of the cuts if they had high unemployment rates, and adopted certain cost-containment measures. The estimated loss to the states was a total of $1 billion over three years—considerably less than the Reagan administration's permanent cuts (Smith and Moore 2008).

Despite being controlled by Republicans, the Senate Finance Committee also developed a more moderate alternative to the Reagan administration's proposal—in part because the Senate's organization along state lines predisposes its members to accommodate federal programs to state interests (Haider 1974). Chairman Robert Dole (R-Kansas) spoke of the large number of "governors in this country worried about Medicaid," and pledged to "work out some accommodation."[35] Several committee members, including John Chafee (R-Rhode Island) and David Boren (D-Oklahoma), were former governors themselves, and were thus particularly sympathetic. As a committee staffer explained in an interview: "there was no question that the presence of former governors had an impact on our deliberations, members who knew very clearly what it would be like to essentially have an economy go south on them and not have any flexibility and who counted on these federal funds."[36]

The Senate Finance Committee proposed to place a cap of 9 percent on the growth of federal Medicaid contributions—considerably looser than that proposed by the Reagan administration.[37] However, at Senator Dole's urging, the committee also proposed lowering the bottom matching rate from 50 percent to 40 percent to generate additional savings. The bill would cost the states $1-2 billion per year in lost funding—the majority of which would be sustained by seven states with high per capita incomes—only one of which was represented on the Senate Finance Committee; the senator from that state, Bill Bradley (D-New Jersey), voted against the bill.[38]

As the Reagan administration scrambled to win congressional support for its Medicaid cap, it became increasingly clear that Congress was unlikely to acquiesce without the governors' stamp of approval. President Reagan met with NGA chairman George Busbee to seek his cooperation, and when

Busbee refused to budge, the president frantically called his staff together for a last-minute meeting to discuss options for overcoming the governors' opposition, causing a half-hour delay in a speech he was supposed to deliver.[39]

Meanwhile, Chairman Busbee led governors of both parties in a flurry of lobbying activity on Capitol Hill. Governor James Hunt (D-North Carolina) told Senator Jesse Helms (R-North Carolina) of his "deep concern" at the prospect of a Medicaid cap, warning that their state would have to cut back on much-needed health services for poor children to make up for the loss of federal aid.[40] Similarly, Governor Bill Milliken (R-Michigan) warned the Michigan delegation to the House of Representatives that "unduly large reductions in the federal government's share of costs would have grave consequences" for their state.[41]

The Democrat-controlled House became the central battleground for the clash over Reagan's budget. Although Representative Waxman's small, temporary Medicaid cuts initially appeared likely to emerge from the Commerce Committee with bipartisan support, the committee deadlocked after ranking Republican member Edward Madigan reluctantly withdrew his support under pressure from David Stockman (Smith and Moore 2008). The impasse presented a window of opportunity for Reagan's conservative allies in the House, as Representative Jim Broyhill (R-North Carolina) proposed an amendment that would replace Waxman's proposal with the Reagan administration's Medicaid cap. Although the idea was unpopular with most House Democrats, it won the support of 44 conservative Southern Democrats known as "Boll Weevils" who had banded together as an influential swing group (Iglehart 1981).

However, the "Gypsy Moths"—moderate to liberal northeastern Republicans—opposed the amendment. Representative Bill Green of New York assembled a coalition of 20 Republicans from states for which the Medicaid cap would have required extensive cuts, and demanded that the administration loosen the cap. Desperate to win their votes, the White House bent over backward trying to accommodate their requests. David Stockman described this predicament in *The Triumph of Politics.*

> We were tacking on adjustments to the Broyhill amendment faster than could be recorded. It was a mess. Bill Green of New York wanted the Medicaid cap raised—first by 1 percent, then by 2 percent, then by 3 percent . . . I gave it all to him, thereby eliminating all but an insignificant portion of the savings. (Stockman 1986, 239)

However, at the urging of their states' governors, the Gypsy Moths later announced that even this looser cap was unacceptable, and many vowed to vote against a cap of any size.[42]

Mounting congressional opposition to the Medicaid cap posed a serious problem for the White House, particularly since the administration had chosen to use a relatively new and little-used procedure known as reconciliation—which combines dozens of measures into an enormous omnibus bill and limits the debate to 20 hours—to push its budget priorities through Congress. Administration officials hoped that fast-tracking the president's budget and forcing an up-or-down vote would increase the odds of getting everything they wanted. It was a risky strategy, however, since the president's entire budget could go up in flames if any part of the bill garnered sufficient opposition.

Shortly before the House vote, Republican leaders counted up the likely votes and realized that the Broyhill amendment might fail—dealing an embarrassing blow to the president, and potentially jeopardizing the budget as a whole. As Stockman explained, "the GOP-Boll Weevil leaders finally succumbed to battle fatigue. Without even checking with the White House, they huddled briefly on the floor and decided to dump the Broyhill amendment entirely—and with it the Medicaid cap" (Stockman 1986, 242). By default, Waxman's relatively mild Medicaid cuts prevailed in the final House bill.

After the Senate passed its bill, the two chambers convened the largest, most unwieldy conference in congressional history—consisting of 69 Senators and nearly 200 House members, or roughly half of Congress—to work out the differences between the two budget bills.[43] Medicaid was the major sticking point, and threatened to derail the entire conference. Despite Senate Republicans' efforts to get their 9 percent cap into the final bill, Representative Waxman dug in his heels, warning "there is no way in the world I would ever agree to sign onto a conference report that capped the Medicaid program," and that "the whole thing could come tumbling down if they pushed too hard."[44]

In an eleventh-hour compromise, the committee agreed not to cap Medicaid payments—thus retaining the program's open-ended federal matching contribution—but rather to cut the matching rate by more than the House bill had called for: 3 percent in 1982, 4 percent in 1983, and 4.5 percent in 1984.[45] The conference committee scaled back the magnitude of these cuts for some states—such as those with high unemployment rates, or those that adopted cost-containment measures, as in the House bill.

The law also included a number of provisions that increased the states' flexibility to reduce Medicaid benefits, eligibility, and provider payments so as to lower both federal and state costs. Prior to 1981, if a state chose to cover the medically needy, federal regulations required the state to cover all individuals within that income range, and provide them all with the same services; the new law relaxed this provision. The law also gave the states more flexibility in setting provider payment rates, allowed them to substitute home-care services for costlier nursing-home care, and made children aged 18–21 an optional, rather than mandatory, group. Importantly, however, the law did not drop federal assistance for any mandatory or optional services (Bovbjerg and Holahan 1982).[46]

When it came to federal grant programs other than Medicaid, the budget passed by Congress was closer to the Reagan administration's initial proposals. Congress cut federal grant programs by $6.6 billion for 1982, relative to 1981 levels, representing a reduction of 13 percent in real terms. The cuts disproportionately affected programs related to social services, education, training, and employment. Sixty-two programs were terminated altogether, and another 77 were consolidated into 9 block grants. Aid to Families with Dependent Children was cut by $2 billion, or 14 percent (Conlan 1998).

When the president signed the Omnibus Budget Reconciliation Act of 1981 (OBRA 1981) into law on August 13, 1981, many observers hailed it as a decisive victory for the Reagan administration. But budget director David Stockman called it "nothing of the sort," singling out the Medicaid cap as the most significant defeat in the president's first budget battle (Stockman 1986, 243). Moreover, despite the administration's stated goal of balancing the budget, the legislation the president ultimately signed included $280 billion in tax cuts, and only $130 billion in spending cuts over three years. If Reagan was to come anywhere close to fulfilling his campaign pledge, it was obvious he would have to "unload the great bulk of present federal responsibilities, other than defense and Social Security, onto someone else—and the governors are first in the likely receiving line."[47]

THE GOVERNORS' COUNTERREVOLUTION

The NGA's annual meeting in August 1981 provided the governors with an opportunity to reflect on the recently enacted budget, and, like the Reagan administration, they had mixed feelings about it. As Joe McLaughlin, spokesman for the National Governors Association, put it, "We got far less than what we wanted but probably far more than what most people thought we'd get."[48] However, when it came to Medicaid, the governors were overjoyed. Chairman Busbee told his colleagues: "I think we can all agree that we were the major factor in defeating the Medicaid cap." In a moment of levity, Governor Scott Matheson (D-Utah) presented Busbee with a hat as a symbol of the governors' appreciation of his efforts, explaining that "George deserves a little extra credit because he is the one who went up on the Hill and basically insured that we would have a Medicaid program without a cap. I am here to award you a Medicaid cap without a cap," to which Busbee jokingly replied: "The chair rules that totally in order."[49]

The governors did not waste much time celebrating, however. As they prepared to negotiate the sorting out of responsibilities with the White House, many governors—particularly Democrats—began taking a more critical tone, despite pressure within the NGA to mute their criticisms for the sake of the negotiations.[50] In a *Washington Post* op-ed titled "The Governors Will Fight," Governor Bruce Babbitt (D-Arizona) warned that if Reagan again tried to "abdicate federal responsibility" and "dump" Medicaid on the states, this time the governors would not be "sitting on the bench" but rather "on the field, ready to fight for a federal system of logically divided program responsibilities."[51] Even Governor Busbee, who had previously expressed trust in and eagerness to negotiate with Reagan, began to bemoan the administration's desire to "save a buck by passing the buck," and to decry its philosophy of federalism as guided by:

> one sole criterion—what makes it easiest to balance the federal budget. From the point of view of budgetary tunnel vision, federalism becomes an easy matter. Pick out the most expensive, the most difficult to manage, the most politically controversial federal programs and hand them back to the states and localities with a heartfelt sigh of relief.[52]

The change in the governors' tone was so striking that some observers began to speak of a gubernatorial counterrevolution to the Reagan revolution.[53]

A handful of Republican governors, including incoming NGA chairman Richard Snelling (R-Vermont) and Lamar Alexander (R-Tennessee), convinced their wary colleagues that negotiating with the White House was the governors' best hope for shifting greater responsibility for Medicaid—"our most expensive and rapidly growing program"—to the federal government.[54]

Snelling led the governors in passing a resolution stating that they were prepared to negotiate a phase-out of federal aid for education, transportation, and law enforcement if the federal government would assume greater responsibility for Medicaid and AFDC. The resolution reiterated the governors' "strong belief that the so-called 'safety-net' programs . . . have been, are, and should continue to be primarily a federal responsibility. We will continue to resist . . . any effort to shift Medicaid or Aid to Families with Dependent Children in any way."[55] But as they looked ahead to the next round of negotiations, many remained uneasy. In his parting remarks as NGA chairman, George Busbee warned: "More and more, I'm convinced the major effort will be made in the very near future to transfer responsibility for income maintenance programs to the states."[56]

Governor Busbee's fears were realized the very next day, when Robert Carleson leaked news that the White House, in its determination to balance the federal budget, was seriously considering cutting federal funding for Medicaid and AFDC. Reagan's economic team continued to believe that open-ended matching grants put insufficient pressure on states to restrain the growth of eligibility and benefits, streamline administration, and reduce waste, since the federal government paid between half and three-fourths of the states' costs, no matter how high. They hoped to convert funding for both programs to more restrictive block grants, making the states responsible for 100 percent of spending above a fixed federal contribution.

The governors were outraged. A spokesman for the NGA announced that an "overwhelming majority" of governors of both parties "violently opposed" the idea of block-granting Medicaid and AFDC.[57] In response to their strong reaction, President Reagan sent a letter to all 50 governors, pledging not to make fundamental changes to federal-state welfare programs without consulting them.[58]

As White House officials mulled a block grant proposal throughout the fall of 1981, intergovernmental affairs advisor Richard Williamson urged the administration to drop the idea. In a memo to Reagan's economic team, Williamson warned that state officials were "near revolution as a result of our most recent round of budget cuts," and that the "key element of political trust" had been "exhausted."[59] Much to the White House's annoyance, NGA chairman Richard Snelling had launched an all-out public relations offensive, stating that he was "shocked to the core" by some of Reagan's federalism proposals, and warning that his policies would lead to an "economic Bay of Pigs."[60] Snelling also wrote a letter to the president reaffirming the governors' strong opposition to any reduction in Medicaid grants, and suggested that federal budget cuts instead target other programs—such as national defense and Social Security.[61] White House officials grew increasingly irritated with Snelling's outspoken, critical style. As Williamson put it in a memo to the president, "Governor Snelling is bright and articulate, but fair men would say he is somewhat difficult to deal with."[62]

The governors were not the only ones opposed to further cuts to the social safety net; opposition was also mounting in Congress. Many Democrats and moderate Republicans did not want to enact any additional cuts in social programs until there were bigger cuts in other areas, such as defense. Underscoring the governors' influence within Congress, Richard Williamson urged President Reagan not to antagonize them: "If they are united in their opposition to the Administration's program when it is presented on the Hill, we will, in all probability, lose."[63] Reluctant to proceed without the governors' support, the Reagan administration decided not to continue down this path. Instead, the White House suddenly took a very different federalism approach, much to the governors' surprise.

THE NEW FEDERALISM NEGOTIATIONS

In January 1982, when Reagan unveiled his budget proposals in the State of the Union address, he announced the federal government's plans for Medicaid.

> Starting in fiscal 1984, the Federal Government will assume full responsibility for the cost of the rapidly growing Medicaid program to go along with its existing responsibility for Medicare. As part of a financially equal swap, the States will simultaneously take full responsibility for Aid to Families with Dependent Children and food stamps.[64]

Reagan subsequently clarified that this "swap" would actually benefit the states since surrendering Medicaid would save them an estimated $19.1 billion in the first year, while the additional cost to the states of taking over AFDC and food stamps was projected at only $16.5 billion. Moreover, Reagan argued that since Medicaid costs were increasing several times faster than the other programs' costs, the federal government would be relieving the states of a growing financial burden.[65]

A second component of Reagan's proposal—the so-called turnback—involved phasing out 44 education, transportation, community development, and social service grant programs worth a total of $30.2 billion. To compensate the states for the lost funds, Reagan proposed to establish a temporary "grassroots trust fund," which the states could use as they saw fit. States that stood to lose under the swap would receive more money from the trust fund, while those that would profit from the swap would receive less. Beginning in fiscal year 1987, the trust fund would be phased out over four years.

Reagan emphasized that his proposal was merely a starting point for negotiations, noting that the full details would have to be worked out through "close consultation" with the governors.[66] Reagan had learned the hard way the previous year that he could not accomplish his federalism agenda without state leaders' cooperation. Indeed, the ranking Republican on the House Ways and Means Committee pointed out that the prospects for Reagan's swap and turnback were bleak without the governors' strong endorsement: "If the states want it, they can probably have it, but if the administration can't convince the states it's a good deal, it will not pass."[67]

The governors were, of course, very receptive to the idea of relinquishing responsibility for Medicaid, expressing relief that the president finally seemed prepared to move halfway toward their long-standing goal of federalization of federal-state programs for the poor. However, many governors worried—given the administration's stated objective to reduce federal spending, as well as its recent attempts to permanently cap and block-grant Medicaid—that after taking over the program, the White House would seek to slash eligibility and benefits. Moreover, the prospect of taking over the federal-state AFDC program and the federal food-stamps program was a nonstarter for most governors. Governor Hugh Carey (D-New York) complained that the administration was "dumping" these programs on the states, while Governor Bill Clements (R-Texas) said of the food-stamps program: "I ain't going to buy a pig in a poke."[68]

Other stakeholders also registered concern at the prospect of turning over AFDC and food stamps to the states. House Speaker Tip O'Neill (D-Mass.) spoke for many congressional Democrats when he called the proposal "little more than a disguised attempt to balance the budget on the backs of states,"[69] and part of an "overall retrenchment on social policy."[70] Many congressional Republicans, concerned about how the president's growing unpopularity would affect their prospects in the upcoming midterm elections,

saw Reagan's emphasis on federalism as a diversion from more pressing problems that required his attention, such as the faltering economy and ballooning national deficit (Conlan 1998). The press questioned the logic behind
federalizing only the Medicaid program, asking "Do poor people get equally
sick in different places but not equally hungry?"[71] Advocates for the poor
worried about the implications of devolution for vulnerable populations,
and providers and insurers worried that a federalized Medicaid program
would "bypass the state-based hospital lobbies and enable national officials
interested primarily in cost-cutting to set the rules."[72]

Undeterred, the president launched an unprecedented series of meetings
with state and local officials which came to be known as the "new federalism
negotiations" (Williamson 1983). Throughout the spring and summer of
1982, Reagan and his key advisors on intergovernmental, policy, and economic affairs—Williamson, Carleson, Stockman, and counselor to the president for policy Edwin Meese, among others—met repeatedly with the governors' negotiating team: Governors Snelling, Busbee, Matheson, Babbitt,
Alexander, and James Thompson (R-Illinois), as well as state legislators, state
budget directors, mayors, and county officials. As Williamson later wrote,
"Never before had a president commenced such thorough and complete
consultations with state and local officials designed to reach a consensus on
realigning governmental responsibilities" (Williamson 1983, 11). But, of all
the state and local officials who participated, Williamson considered the
governors to be "the key group on the New Federalism initiative," noting
that "if an acceptable compromise can be worked out between the Administration and NGA, passage of the initiative in Congress is far more likely."[73]

At the outset, the president reassured the governors by outlining several
guiding principles for the negotiations, among them: (1) the federalism initiative is not a vehicle for budgetary savings; (2) it includes a dollar-for-dollar
exchange of programs along with the revenue sources to pay for them; (3)
there should be no winners or losers among the states; and (4) state and local
officials should be able to count on stability and certainty in federal funds.
At the same time, however, the White House warned: (5) "The federal government is overloaded, having assumed far more responsibility than it can
efficiently or effectively manage."[74]

Despite his reassurances, the president's initial silence on the administration's plans for federal aid programs in the upcoming fiscal year made
the governors nervous. The swap and turnback, which had featured so
prominently in Reagan's State of the Union address, would not begin until

1984; the administration's intentions for 1983 remained unclear. Governor Thompson noted that "the '83 budget is absolutely critical if this whole thing is to make sense. A lot depends on how much we're hit in the '83 budget."[75]

The governors soon got their answer, and it was not welcome news. In February, the president outlined $10 billion in proposed cuts to federal grant programs for fiscal year 1983, including a three-percentage-point reduction in the Medicaid matching rate for all medically needy beneficiaries, and for all optional services. Reagan justified the cuts as necessary to "eliminate the fat that has grown in the program," and limit coverage to "those who really need it."[76] The budget proposal also included nearly $4 billion in cuts to AFDC and food stamps, purportedly to make the swap arithmetic come out evenly.

The governors—already struggling to cope with the deteriorating economy and OBRA 1981 cuts—were outraged, and warned that unless Reagan dropped the cuts the new federalism initiative was dead. The administration immediately withdrew the proposal, and Reagan again reassured the governors that his federalism initiative was not a federal budget-cutting device, acknowledging that "realistically, that is the only way this program will have your support and will have a chance of being passed by Congress."[77] But the damage had been done: the proposed budget cuts revived the governors' fears that the swap was simply a veiled attempt to shift costs to the states. Richard Williamson later noted that the timing of the proposal, just as the negotiations were getting off the ground, "severely poisoned the well for federalism reform" (Williamson 1983, 31).

At the end of the NGA's winter meeting, the governors issued a policy resolution supporting only half of the swap. Although the governors were "in full accord with the president's proposal for a federal assumption of Medicaid," they rejected the state takeover of AFDC and food stamps as "not consistent with existing policy positions of the National Governors Association." They suggested that the latter be "temporarily set aside as we build a program based on existing areas of mutual agreement."[78] After reiterating his belief that AFDC and food stamps belonged in state hands, Reagan pronounced that the governors' response had opened the door to useful negotiations. The president's mild reaction reflected his relief that the governors had not walked away from the negotiating table, dooming the swap's prospects in Congress.[79]

The Reagan administration subsequently made two significant concessions to the governors. First, when the governors refused to budge from the NGA's long-standing policy position on income maintenance programs, the administration agreed to retain full responsibility for the federal food-stamps program. Second, when the governors' negotiating team tentatively agreed to this proposal on the condition that the federal government establish a "safety net supplemental assistance fund" to protect states against future periods of high unemployment, Reagan's advisors agreed to consider the possibility—seeing it as politically helpful for the negotiations, but ultimately unlikely to secure congressional passage given the ballooning federal deficit and the fact that the swap already included a grassroots trust fund.[80] Once these matters were tentatively settled, the big remaining question was what the federalized Medicaid program would look like.

FIVE OPTIONS FOR A FEDERAL MEDICAID PROGRAM

Throughout the spring and summer of 1982, the Reagan administration mulled over options for a federal takeover of the Medicaid program. A series of White House memos from this period reveals that, for Reagan's economic team, a major goal for the reform was to control costs by eliminating the expansionary incentives generated by open-ended matching grants. As Don Moran of OMB explained in a memo to Richard S. Williamson:

> The major driving element in Medicaid costs is the expansion of eligibility and benefits. This has resulted from the fact that, while States have the great majority of control over these two variables, the financial risk for the outcome of these decisions has been split, due to the matching grant relationship, between the Federal government and the States. The result has always been that the easiest form of short-term cost control has not been cost control at all, but rather the ability of the Federal government and the States to push costs off onto each other. The cardinal lesson to be learned from this is that control over benefits and eligibility should remain in the hands of the party bearing the financial risk.[81]

Although the most obvious way to address the state incentive problem would be for the federal government to take over full control and full financial risk, this conflicted with the Reagan administration's goal to rein in federal spending on social-welfare programs. Thus, White House officials faced the daunting task of trying to design a Medicaid program that realigned states' incentives at the lowest possible federal cost, and yet had a chance of winning the support of state officials. Moreover, the new program had to live up to Reagan's rather unrealistic promise of "no winners and losers among the states."

A few days after the governors' conference, secretary of health and human services Richard Schweiker sent a memo to policy advisor Edwin Meese outlining five options for restructuring the Medicaid program. The first three options consisted of complete federalization—that is, a fully federally administered program with uniform eligibility, benefit, and reimbursement policies—but differed in scope. Option 1 consisted of a broad Medicaid program with a "relatively high eligibility level," and coverage of most optional benefits currently being offered by the states. Option 2 consisted of federalization of a more limited program, covering only AFDC and SSI recipients, and providing only the mandatory benefit package. Option 3 consisted of federalization of an even more limited "core" program with continuation of federal-state cost-sharing for additional coverage beyond the core, although the memo did not define what the core might include. Options 4 and 5 consisted of federal assumption of only the financing role. Option 4 consisted of federal assumption of 100 percent of Medicaid costs, with eligibility based on the state's cash-assistance standards, and benefits based on the state's currently offered package. Option 5 consisted of a block grant; the federal government would provide the states with a predetermined amount of money, and the states would have the freedom to choose their own eligibility and benefit policies.

Schweiker's memo outlined each option's advantages and disadvantages for each level of government, noting that federal and state interests were, not surprisingly, diametrically opposed. Option 1 would be most attractive to the states, but "extremely expensive" for the federal government, effectively doubling federal spending on Medicaid. Options 2 and 3 would be less expensive for the federal government, but less attractive to the states. Since all three options would implement a uniform set of eligibility and benefit policies, all three would create winners and losers among the states—not to mention Medicaid beneficiaries. The redistributive effects would be potentially enormous due to the wide state-level variation in eligibility and benefits. In 1980, Medicaid eligibility levels ranged from $1,680 in Texas to $6,828 in Oregon, 34 states had a medically needy program, about half the states covered optional services such as eyeglasses and physical therapy, and hospital benefits varied from 10 days to unlimited coverage.[82]

Option 4 would allow the states to continue to tailor their Medicaid programs, thereby mitigating the winners-and-losers problem; however, it would perpetuate differences among states. Schweiker also pointed out that increasing the federal financing role while retaining state administrative and policy-making authority might decrease the states' incentive to constrain costs. Moreover, if states took over full responsibility for AFDC as part of the swap, they could use their increased control over that program's eligibility standards to increase the number of Medicaid enrollees at the federal government's expense. Option 5 was the most attractive for the federal government since it would impose a firm dollar limit the federal contribution, and give states an incentive to control costs. However, since states would be liable for any costs beyond the block—and since state leaders had rejected a similar proposal the year before—Schweiker surmised that the governors were "quite likely to resist this proposal."

Reagan's economic advisors initially opposed the first four options as too costly. Moreover, in a memo to Edwin Meese, Robert Carleson argued that options 1, 2, and 3 could have "disastrous" long-run implications because "federalizing Medicaid, drawing it closer to Medicare, would give complete control of the programs to the Federal government making it easier for a subsequent Administration to effect National Health Insurance." He also worried that since federalization would sever the link between Medicaid eligibility and a state's AFDC standard, it might lead to pressure for a more generous—and thus expensive—national Medicaid eligibility standard. Fortunately, Carleson noted, the president had only committed to paying "the cost" of Medicaid, and had avoided any reference to "federalizing" the program.[83]

Reagan's economic advisors worried that option 4—100 percent federal financing of existing state eligibility and benefit policies—would exacerbate the incentive problem underlying the existing financing mechanism. As Carleson put it, "simply to retain the present system with the Federal government assuming the full cost would result in a raid on the Treasury, because States determine eligibility and service levels." Thus, Carleson felt that the best approach was option 5, which he characterized as "containing costs through the federal appropriation process by granting to each State a finite amount of money sufficient to cover the agreed upon 'full costs' of the current program as projected."[84]

However, the economic team acknowledged that state leaders, having vehemently rejected a Medicaid block grant the previous year, were unlikely to agree to option 5. Although Moran called the block grant approach "the fastest, easiest, and most certain way of meeting the President's commitment to taking over the cost of the Medicaid program," he conceded that this option "may not satisfy the NGA."[85] Thus, Reagan's economic team settled for their second-favorite model: option 3—federalization of a "core" program with federal-state cost sharing for coverage beyond the core.

SWAP SHELVED

As the White House deliberated, the governors nervously awaited news of the president's Medicaid proposal. They were especially eager to ascertain whether the federalized Medicaid program would cover not only categorically eligible welfare recipients, but also the medically needy. Adequate coverage of long-term care was another major concern.

Not surprisingly, the administration—eager to cut costs—decided that the federalized Medicaid program would not cover the medically needy. Robert Carleson worried that "in addition to cost implications, attempting to nationalize this amorphous group would be a nightmare, both legislatively and administratively."[86] Don Moran raised another concern: to the extent that a medically needy program "might induce self-employed individuals, or low-wage employers, to reduce or eliminate private coverage, the bill could mount quite rapidly."[87] Nor did Reagan's economic advisors wish to cover costly long-term care—let alone most optional services such as eyeglasses and dental care—in the core package of services to be funded entirely by the federal government.

Instead, the economic team envisioned a national Medicaid program that would offer a "bare minimum" package of routine-care benefits—inpatient and outpatient hospital services, physician services, laboratory services, out-of-hospital prescription drugs, and skilled nursing-home-facility coverage of up to 100 days—for only AFDC and SSI recipients.[88] They would offer the governors an $8.4 billion block grant for long-term care—enough to cover 100 percent of projected 1984 costs—putting the onus on the states to control costs thereafter.[89] The block grant would cover only the cost of institutionalization; thus, nursing-home residents who did not qualify for SSI would lose acute-care coverage. The White

House presented these coverage reductions as "fiscal necessities unrelated to the federalism objective."[90]

State leaders were extremely unhappy with the administration's Medicaid plan, seeing it as both inadequate and a deviation from the "no winners and no losers" pledge. Under the proposal, at least one-third of the states would have to either reduce coverage, or spend their own funds to maintain service levels at a total cost of $14 billion per year. States with relatively generous Medicaid programs—such as New York and California—would be hit particularly hard. One New York State official estimated that the Reagan administration's proposal could cost the state as much as $2 billion per year, and would result in a "fiscal crisis."[91] Even for the so-called winners—states with less generous programs, such as Mississippi and Texas—the upside of increased coverage of acute care would be largely offset by the downside of greater responsibility for long-term care.

NGA chairman Richard Snelling wrote a letter to the president, imploring him to revise the Medicaid plan. He explained that the governors were "deeply concerned" that the proposal would "force the states to choose between inadequate benefit levels and unacceptably high levels of state and local taxation." He urged Reagan to cover the medically needy in order to "make possible broad based state support for the final proposal and . . . mute many of the concerns and criticisms of those who will otherwise strongly oppose the plan."[92] Eager to get an acceptable proposal from the White House in time for a vote at the NGA's annual meeting in August, Snelling grew increasingly agitated as the summer wore on without word from the White House. One week before the meeting, he reminded the president that "if [the swap] is to succeed in Congress, and in the public view, we are essential allies," and cautioned that "the momentum and unity among the Governors behind your federalism initiative is in serious jeopardy."[93]

When it became clear that the governors would not accept the administration's bare minimum Medicaid package, Reagan's economic team lost interest in the swap. Unable to use the new federalism negotiations as a vehicle for federal spending cuts in a rapidly deteriorating economic climate, Don Moran and Robert Carleson began to obstruct the talks' progress. Richard Williamson lamented that "certain administration officials . . . dragged their feet and hindered efforts to produce a federalized Medicaid package" out of "an obsession over short-term budget considerations" (Williamson 1983, 31). In the end, Reagan's economic advisors prevailed as the president proved unwilling to sacrifice his budget goals for the sake of his federalism agenda

(Conlan 1986). The president called each member of the governors' negotiating team on the eve of the NGA meetings to apologize for suspending the negotiations.

Budget and economic considerations also impeded the governors' willingness to negotiate. In addition to having "fortified suspicions that the president had agreed to federalize Medicaid merely to gain the control he needed to reduce the program," the economic climate hardened the governors' own bargaining position (Conlan 1998, 190). As Richard Williamson observed, the states' fiscal woes stemming from the 1982 recession prompted the governors to "shift from philosophical concerns and structural issues to matters of fiscal security" (Williamson 1983, 11). Perhaps in a more favorable economic climate, the governors would have been more open to accepting less money in exchange for fewer responsibilities, but in the context of large and growing budget shortfalls, financial prerogatives dominated and they preferred to deal with "the devil they knew" (Farber 1983, 36).

The upcoming elections also caused many state leaders to harden their positions on the swap. In 1982, 36 of the 50 governors were up for reelection, and as November approached, the NGA's bipartisan unity grew strained. Many governors wanted to avoid supporting any controversial policy initiatives that might diminish their reelection chances (Williamson 1983). Moreover, election-year politics led many Democratic governors to seek opportunities to portray Reagan's domestic agenda as a coldhearted attack on vulnerable Americans.[94]

Yet even under different economic and political circumstances, it is unclear that federal and state officials could have reached an agreement on the details of a swap. As health-policy analysts Alan Weil and Louis Rossiter observe, shared fiscal responsibility makes it intrinsically difficult for the two levels of government to extract themselves from Medicaid.

> The argument for the swap is that shared fiscal responsibility is a recipe for cost shifting and inefficiency, and indeed there is evidence to support this view. Yet . . . neither level of government wants to take on a larger current or expected future fiscal burden. Neither level of government is sufficiently confident that, given full responsibility for a population, it will be able to meet the needs of that population at lower cost. (Weil and Rossiter 2007, 114)

Despite their common desire to set Medicaid on a different path, federal and state leaders proved unable to find a mutually agreeable exit strategy.

CONCLUSION

In the years that followed the new federalism negotiations, the Reagan ad-ministration made several additional attempts to cut federal Medicaid spending—all unsuccessful. In the spring of 1984, as the expiration date of the OBRA 1981 Medicaid cuts approached, the president proposed extending the measure for another three years. The governors responded with a flurry of congressional testimony, letters, phone calls, and media appearances. As one senator put it, "what we are hearing from our Governors . . . is, in effect, a loud scream."[95] After Congress rejected the extended cuts, Reagan resur-rected his 1981 proposal to cap the growth of Medicaid grants at the rate of inflation, provoking another round of gubernatorial lobbying. When the measure died in Congress, Governor Thomas Kean (R-New Jersey) congratu-lated his colleagues on their "complete victory," calling it "a wonderful ex-ample of how this organization can work together to achieve an end."[96] The Reagan administration's attempts to cap federal Medicaid grants in 1986, 1987, and 1988 met a similar fate.

Medicaid's virtual imperviousness to retrenchment throughout the two terms of the Reagan administration was nothing short of remarkable. As one of the largest and fastest-growing components of the federal budget, the pro-gram was a major target for fiscal hawks in the White House, as well as the Republican-controlled Senate, and yet—with the exception of the tempo-rary OBRA 1981 cuts—Medicaid emerged from the Reagan years virtually un-scathed, largely due to state leaders' entrenched interest in preserving the status quo. As Representative Waxman later explained in an interview, the Reagan administration repeatedly found that efforts to cut Medicaid elicited "a lot of political problems . . . with the governors and the states."[97] In fact, the governors not only succeeded in protecting the program against re-trenchment throughout this conservative era in American politics, they also successfully championed one of the largest series of eligibility expansions in Medicaid's history—documented in chapter 4.

CHAPTER 4

Options and Mandates in the 1980s

THROUGHOUT U.S. HISTORY, when the pendulum of national social policy has swung toward conservatism, the states have been a source of activism, innovation, and expansion (Nathan 2005). The 1980s were no exception, as the Reagan administration's restrictive social policies prompted state leaders to lobby Congress to loosen federal eligibility rules to allow them to enroll more infants and pregnant women in Medicaid (Johnston 1997). Although many governors favored optional eligibility expansions, some—particularly Southern Democrats—lobbied for mandatory expansions to help them overcome political resistance from conservative state legislatures, as well as collective action problems arising from interstate competition.[1]

Congressional Democrats, taking advantage of the governors' increased receptiveness, as well as a relatively new budget technique known as reconciliation, enacted a series of measures allowing or requiring the states to extend coverage to new groups. Early legislation targeting infants and pregnant women paved the way for later bills targeting older children, parents, seniors, and the disabled. As a result, enrollment rose by nearly 10 million people, or roughly 50 percent. Thus, in an ironic twist—despite the Reagan administration's attempts to use devolution as a tool for retrenchment, as documented in chapter 3—"catalytic federalism" promoted an enormous expansion of Medicaid coverage in the 1980s.

"PROTECTORS OF THE SOCIAL SAFETY NET"

Reagan's 1981 budget cuts—including a three-year reduction in federal matching grants for Medicaid as well as cuts in numerous other state-administered welfare programs—went into effect just as the national economy entered a pronounced recession. Unemployment soared, millions of workers lost employer-sponsored health insurance, and the need for Medicaid and other social-safety-net programs grew dramatically. Yet, in response to reduced federal aid and shrinking state revenues, most states began to implement cost-containment measures including scaling back Medicaid eligibility; reducing the amount, scope, and duration of covered services; and cutting already-low provider reimbursement rates, diminishing the number of doctors willing to treat Medicaid patients (Rowland, Lyons, and Edwards 1988).

The effect of federal and state budget cuts and the economic downturn on coverage rates was striking. The share of America's poor covered by Medicaid dropped from 63 percent in 1976 to approximately 50 percent by 1985 (Engel 2006, 184). The share of poor children covered fell from 90 percent to 70 percent, despite the fact that 22 percent of children were living in poverty—the highest rate in two decades (Cohen 1990). The timing of the budget cuts seemed cruel, heightening sympathy for the downtrodden.

Of particular concern was the fact that the nation's infant mortality rate—already high compared to other industrialized nations—had begun to reverse its steady decline. In 1984, the *New York Times* reported that there were parts of the United States in which a baby had less chance of surviving to his first birthday than a baby born in Trinidad, Guyana, or the Soviet Union.[2] The infant mortality problem was particularly pronounced in the South, with its large numbers of poor, uninsured, predominantly African American, single mothers, and its traditionally limited Medicaid programs. The factor most commonly associated with infant mortality was low birth weight, which in turn was highly correlated with inadequate prenatal and neonatal care.[3]

Once the economy began to improve in 1984, these concerns prompted many state leaders—particularly in Southern states—to begin to reverse the earlier Medicaid cuts. Thirty states expanded their Medicaid programs to include at least one additional optional service between 1984 and 1987. Several states including Arkansas and West Virginia set up special funds to expand health care for the indigent, while others including South Carolina, Georgia, Texas, and Florida established medically needy programs for the first time.[4] As Governor Richard Riley of South Carolina proudly put it in a letter to the editor of the *Washington Post*, "Southern states have historically had more limited Medicaid programs, [but we] are now attempting to develop innovative, cost-effective and progressive programs to address the unmet needs of our poor children."[5]

The leadership of Southern governors reflected not only the region's dire infant mortality problem, but also the emergence of a new brand of governors: young, ambitious, progressive, popular, highly educated politicians who personified the decade's version of "New South" politics.[6] This group of governors—primarily Democrats, plus a handful of moderate Republicans—included not only Richard Riley (D-South Carolina), but also Bill Clinton (D-Arkansas), Lamar Alexander (R-Tennessee), Mark White (D-Texas), and Bob Graham (D-Florida), among others.

The governors' heightened interest in expanding Medicaid also reflected the unusually large number of Democratic governors in office at the time. Dissatisfied with the Reagan administration's first two years, voters gave the Democratic Party a net gain of eight governorships in the 1982 and 1983 elections—in addition to increasing the Democrats' margin in the House of Representatives—bringing the total number to 35 out of 50 governors in 1984. As a result, gubernatorial activism extended beyond the South. For instance, upon taking office, Michigan's new Democratic governor, James Blanchard, pledged to "make prenatal care a right of citizenship in our State."[7] According to one Michigan official, state leaders "wanted to be trailblazers in Medicaid . . . We were looking for opportunities where we could move forward and be out front and be one of the early innovators."[8]

It is perhaps not surprising that, at a time of conservatism in social policy making at the national level, the nation's relatively liberal governors took on the role of social policy entrepreneurs. As James Martin, legislative counsel to the National Governors Association, put it, federal retrenchment had led the nation's governors to take on the role of "protectors of the social safety net."[9] A *New York Times* editorial, "The Governors and Poor Children," observed that state leaders were "stepping into the breach" left by the Reagan administration's policies in an effort to "assure a fair chance for every child."[10]

In addition to their progressive ideology, powerful financial incentives also motivated state leaders to expand Medicaid eligibility for infants and pregnant women. For one thing, a growing body of medical research suggested that investing in preventive prenatal and neonatal care would save the states money by reducing the astronomical costs of not only neonatal intensive care, but also disability, mental retardation, and other health, learning, and behavioral problems later in life.[11] Moreover, the recession, budget cuts, growing number of uninsured, and rising demand for health services meant that state hospitals were increasingly racking up large costs of uncompensated care.[12] Between 1980 and 1987, the amount of uncompensated care nearly tripled from $3.5 billion to almost $9 billion, and public hospitals bore most of the burden (Fraser 1991, 304). State officials were eager to shift a portion of these costs to the federal government by expanding Medicaid.

A final factor that drove states to voluntarily expand Medicaid coverage was pressure from the health-care industry. In many states, interest groups representing hospitals, nursing homes, and other providers pushed state leaders to make up for the loss of federal funding and rising cost of uncompensated care. For example, lobbying by the medical profession was a "crucial factor" in Mississippi's decision to adopt a medically needy program in 1984 (Nathan, Doolittle, and Associates 1987, 218). A study of discretionary Medicaid spending in 46 states in the 1980s confirms that the medical lobby played an important role in promoting the expansion of coverage (Kousser 2002). In the political tug-of-war over scarce state resources, the "well-organized and politically strong" associations representing medical providers gave Medicaid a major advantage over other programs targeted by Reagan's budget cuts, such as Aid to Families with Dependent Children (Nathan, Doolittle, and Associates 1983, 201).

STATES SEEK FEDERAL HELP

The governors soon began to encounter obstacles to expanding Medicaid coverage, however. One of the biggest hurdles was the longstanding link between Medicaid eligibility and a state's standard for Aid to Families with Dependent Children (Rowland, Lyons, and Edwards 1988). In order to receive federal matching funds to expand Medicaid to more categorically eligible infants and pregnant women, a state also had to expand eligibility for AFDC. However, many states had allowed their AFDC standards to be heavily eroded by inflation. Between 1975 and 1984, the average income eligibility threshold plunged from 75 percent to 47 percent of the federal poverty level (FPL) (Hill 1990, 76). AFDC standards were so low in the early 1980s that two-thirds of poor women and children did not qualify for cash assistance.[13] Eligibility standards were particularly low in the Southern states. For example, standards were around 20 percent of FPL in Alabama, Texas, and South Carolina, compared to more than 80 percent in Alaska, California, and Wisconsin (table 4).

This decline in state funding for AFDC was largely a product of recessions and reductions in federal aid. However, it also reflected changes in public attitudes toward welfare. Compared to the relative liberalism of the 1960s, Americans held considerably more conservative views beginning in the mid-1970s. The percentage of Americans who reported believing that the United States spends too much on welfare jumped from the low 40s in the early 1970s to the low 60s later in the decade (Shapiro and Young 1989). Political scientists have traced this pattern to a variety of factors including the sluggish economy (Shapiro and Young 1989), the news media's "racialization" of welfare and poverty (Gilens 1999), and the rhetorical attacks of political elites, such as Reagan's famous depiction of welfare beneficiaries as "Cadillac-driving welfare queens."[14]

Despite serving a similar population, Medicaid was—and continues to

TABLE 4. Medicaid/AFDC Eligibility Standards as a Percentage of the Federal Poverty Level, 1984

Alabama	17%	**National Average**	**47%**
South Carolina	20%	Iowa	47%
Texas	20%	New Jersey	47%
Tennessee	23%	Montana	48%
New Mexico	24%	Kansas	49%
Georgia	27%	Maine	49%
Arkansas	29%	Massachusetts	50%
Florida	31%	Oregon	50%
Nevada	31%	Pennsylvania	52%
Idaho	34%	Oklahoma	53%
Missouri	34%	Michigan	56%
North Carolina	34%	West Virginia	56%
Kentucky	36%	Nebraska	59%
Louisiana	36%	North Dakota	60%
Indiana	37%	Washington	60%
Mississippi	37%	Hawaii	62%
Delaware	38%	Utah	63%
Ohio	39%	Minnesota	66%
Wyoming	40%	New York	68%
South Dakota	41%	Rhode Island	68%
Illinois	42%	Vermont	70%
Virginia	42%	Connecticut	71%
Maryland	44%	Wisconsin	81%
Colorado	46%	Alaska	88%
New Hampshire	46%	California	91%

Source: Data from Rowland, Lyons, and Edwards 1988.

be—considerably more popular than cash assistance. Whereas Americans have long been skeptical of programs that give cash to the poor, in keeping with American social norms such as individualism and self-reliance, they tend to have fewer misgivings about providing health care to the poor—either for paternalistic reasons or because they view health care as a basic human right. This distinction is particularly striking when it comes to beliefs about the "deservingness" of Medicaid versus AFDC beneficiaries—despite considerable overlap between the two populations. In a 1986 survey, respondents were significantly more likely to say that, compared to Medicaid enrollees, AFDC recipients do not really need the benefits, do not use their benefits wisely, do not want to be independent, and are eligible through some fault of their own (Cook and Barrett 1992).

Due to declining support for cash assistance, the link between AFDC and Medicaid eligibility made it increasingly difficult for states to expand health coverage for the poor in the 1980s. A state could, with a little creativity, expand Medicaid eligibility standards for AFDC beneficiaries without appropriating new funds for AFDC. Since the federal government set no minimum welfare benefit, a state could hold down the cost of Medicaid expansion by setting an extremely low AFDC payment. As one gubernatorial aide explained, beneficiaries "would receive a very tiny AFDC check—but they got Medicaid coverage."[15]

States could only get so creative, however, because the definition of medically needy was also linked to AFDC eligibility standards. The Social Security Amendments of 1967 had established a limit whereby the federal government would not help the states pay for health care for individuals with incomes above 133 percent of the standard to qualify for cash assistance in that state, as discussed in chapter 2. Thus, many states' medically needy standards declined in the 1980s along with their AFDC standards. Moreover, federal rules limited states' discretion over the scope of benefits. For instance, if a state wanted to receive federal matching grants to help pay for nutritional counseling or prenatal vitamins, it had to apply for a waiver from the Health Care Financing Administration.[16]

In addition to federal legal limits, many governors encountered a second set of obstacles to Medicaid expansion within their own states. In some cases—particularly in conservative corners of the South—governors who wanted to expand coverage faced "bruising, uphill battles with state lawmakers" reluctant to appropriate the necessary funds.[17] Many state leaders also encountered collective action problems stemming from intergovernmental competition (Posner 1998). If one state voluntarily made its Medicaid program more generous than its neighbors', it risked scaring away businesses and wealthy taxpayers. Thus, some governors hoped that federal action to raise Medicaid standards across the board would provide "political cover" if state lawmakers objected or taxpayers threatened to "vote with their feet" (Conlan 1991, 57).

In the mid-1980s, governors increasingly began to ask Congress to help them expand Medicaid eligibility. At the forefront of this movement was Governor Richard Riley of South Carolina. A moderate Democrat and former naval officer with a quiet, self-effacing style, Riley was so popular that citizens amended the state constitution to permit him to run for reelection. Riley cared passionately about health care—and, particularly, the prevention of disabilities—having suffered from an excruciatingly painful spinal condition known as spondylitis as a young man. According to his wife, Ann, "suffering that much and not letting it get the best of him . . . made him a stronger person . . . He has a wonderful power of concentration. He can just do what has to be done."[18]

In 1984, Governor Riley spearheaded the creation of the Southern Regional Task Force on Infant Mortality with the goal of publicizing the infant mortality problem, and compelling Congress to allocate more resources to address the problem. This task force was a joint undertaking of the Southern Governors Association—of which Riley was chairman—and a regional legislative group called the Southern Legislative Conference, and included several members of Congress, governors' wives (including Hillary Rodham Clinton), state Medicaid commissioners, and the leaders of health care and child advocacy groups such as the American Hospital Association and the Children's Defense Fund.

The task force's decision to focus on maternal and infant health was largely a response to rising infant mortality rates, but it was also a politically astute calculation. Governors Riley, Clinton, Alexander, and others were interested in expanding health care access to all poor Americans, but they realized that a broad increase in eligibility would be a hard sell due to complicated racial politics and anti-welfare sentiments, so they decided to focus on a widely attractive and less divisive subset of the poor (Smith and Moore 2008). Moreover, Riley and his colleagues hoped that limiting their focus to infants and pregnant women would appeal to even the most fiscally conservative state and federal policy makers. First, there was a growing awareness that investing in prenatal and neonatal care was cost-effective. Second, they hoped that enlisting a "limiting principle" would help alleviate cost concerns, particularly given that the principle was based on a "utilitarian calculus of eligibility—that is, deservingness of, in proportion to the measurable usefulness of, health care services" (Tanenbaum 1995, 945). Emphasizing infants and pregnant women thus enabled Southern governors to play a delicate two-level game, bargaining with federal policy makers over liberalizing Medicaid while maintaining electoral viability in their home states.

HENRY WAXMAN, POLICY ENTREPRENEUR

Meanwhile, Congress was gradually growing more amenable to the idea of expanding Medicaid. Following the 1982 elections, Democrats had solidified their control of the House, and while the Senate remained in Republican hands, Reagan's declining popularity, the recession, and a growing sense of sympathy for the poor led many Republican Senators to take a more moderate stance. Moreover, members of Congress were increasingly hearing from the governors of their home states that the poor had inadequate access to health care, and that the federal government needed to do more.

One member of Congress—Representative Henry Waxman (D-California)—was particularly interested in expanding health care for the poor. A liberal Democrat and longtime champion of national health insurance, Waxman chaired the Commerce Committee's Subcommittee on Health and the Environment, which had jurisdiction over the Medicaid program. Before serving in Congress, Waxman had served as chairman of the health committee in the California State Assembly during Ronald Reagan's tenure as governor, and was thus accustomed to playing the role of Reagan's dramatic foil when it came to health policy.

According to John Kingdon's 1984 "policy streams" theory, new policies emerge when a policy entrepreneur recognizes a window of opportunity to couple the "problem stream" (a public issue in need of attention), the "politics stream" (a favorable political climate), and the "policy stream" (a proposal for change). When it came to Medicaid in the 1980s, Henry Waxman played the role of policy entrepreneur, ushering in a series of major changes in federal law over the course of seven years (Gilman 1998). Recognizing that the Reagan budget cuts had, ironically, "developed an enormous amount of support for the Medicaid program," and that many state and federal policy makers subsequently had become "quite horrified" by America's growing infant mortality problem, Waxman resurrected an unsuccessful Carter administration proposal called the Child Health Assurance Program (CHAP).[19] The goal was to relax some of the family-structure-related limits on Medicaid eligibility to address the needs of poor pregnant women and children who did not fit the traditional "categorically needy" definition of families with dependent children. Specifically, the program would extend Medicaid coverage to women who were pregnant for the first time—and therefore did not have the children necessary to qualify for AFDC—as well as poor children in two-parent families.

Waxman's success—despite the measure's earlier failure as well as initial opposition from the White House and many members of Congress—was largely attributable to Richard Riley's mobilization of the Southern governors, who worked hard to win the support of reluctant legislators from the region (Brown 1990). As Waxman recalls, "the Southern governors were tremendously helpful in pushing for this. A big part of their economy in some of these states was health care under the Medicaid program. And this was a large amount of federal dollars that they could use to cover people."[20]

Ultimately, Congress passed a variation on Waxman's proposal as part of the Deficit Reduction Act of 1984 (DEFRA 1984) over the objections of fiscally conservative lawmakers like Representative Bill Frenzel (R-Minnesota), who complained that inserting spending increases into a bill designed to cut deficits was "outrageous and scandalous."[21] The legislation authorized nearly $300 million in new federal matching grants per year, and required the states to provide Medicaid coverage to several groups meeting AFDC income and resource requirements: (1) first-time pregnant women; (2) pregnant women in two-parent families with an unemployed parent (AFDC-UP); and (3) children up to age five in two-parent families, to be phased in gradually according to birth date.[22]

States moved quickly in response to the legislation, in many cases complying with the new mandates ahead of the deadline Congress had set or going further than Congress had required. For instance, in October 1984, Texas expanded its Medicaid program to cover all pregnant women regardless of marital status, and all children up to age 18 in families with incomes up to the state's AFDC standard; Mississippi adopted a similar program a few months later. Virginia expanded Medicaid eligibility to all pregnant women up to 133 percent of the state's AFDC standard; South Carolina and Georgia did the same, and also covered all children through age 18 up to 133 percent of the AFDC standard.[23]

The states' eager response prompted Waxman to pursue another incremental expansion the following year. A provision of the Consolidated Omnibus Budget Reconciliation Act of 1985 (COBRA 1985) required the states to cover all pregnant women meeting state AFDC income and resource standards, regardless of family structure or employment status. It also gave states the option of immediately extending coverage to all qualifying children up

TABLE 5. Time Line of Major Medicaid Options and Mandates: 1984–90

Deficit Reduction Act of 1984	*Mandate:* Children up to age 5 (born after 9/30/1983) meeting state AFDC income and resource standards, regardless of family structure; pregnant women who would qualify for AFDC or AFDC-UP (unemployed parent) after the child is born, regardless of whether the state has an AFDC-UP program.
Consolidated Omnibus Budget Reconciliation Act of 1985	*Mandate:* Pregnant women meeting state AFDC income and resource standards, regardless of family structure.
Omnibus Budget Reconciliation Act of 1986	*Option:* Pregnant women, infants, and children up to age 5 (born after 9/30/1983) up to 100% of the federal poverty level (FPL); payment of Medicare premiums and cost-sharing for elderly and disabled beneficiaries up to 100% of FPL.
Omnibus Budget Reconciliation Act of 1987	*Option:* Pregnant women and infants up to 185% of FPL; children up to age 8 (born after 9/30/1983) up to 100% of FPL. *Mandate:* Children up to age 8 (born after 9/30/1983) meeting state AFDC income and resource standards.
Family Support Act of 1988	*Mandate:* 12 months' transitional medical assistance to families leaving AFDC due to earnings from work; all AFDC families with an unemployed parent (AFDC-UP).
Medicare Catastrophic Coverage Act of 1988	*Mandate:* Pregnant women and infants up to 100% of FPL; payment of Medicare premiums and cost-sharing for elderly and disabled beneficiaries up to 100% of FPL.
Omnibus Budget Reconciliation Act of 1989	*Mandate:* Pregnant women and children up to age 6 up to 133% of FPL; expanded EPSDT coverage for Medicaid-eligible children up to age 21.
Omnibus Budget Reconciliation Act of 1990	*Mandate:* Children up to age 18 (born after 9/30/1983) up to 100% of FPL; payment of Medicare premiums and cost-sharing for elderly and disabled beneficiaries up to 120% of FPL.

Source: Data from Kaiser Family Foundation; Government Accountability Office; Coughlin, Ku, and Holahan 1994.

to the age of five instead of phasing them in gradually. (See table 5 for a time-line of federal options and mandates.)

Waxman's success was attributable to not only the governors' support, but also the relatively new budget reconciliation process, which he used to push the measure through Congress and prevent a presidential veto. Recon-ciliation, which combines dozens of measures into an enormous omnibus bill and then limits debate, is designed to force committees to meet the spend-ing limits contained in the budget resolution. President Reagan had been us-ing reconciliation to cut the budget since 1981 (as discussed in chapter 3), but Waxman and his staff realized that the same procedure could be used to pro-mote their agenda as well.[24] Tucking a Medicaid expansion into a fast-tracked omnibus bill greatly increased the odds of passage, relative to proposing a stand-alone measure. Opponents might grumble, but they were unlikely to reject the entire bill as long as the expansion was fairly modest in scope. Wax-man would go on to use this technique repeatedly throughout the late 1980s.

"A FISCAL IMPERATIVE"

Despite the 1984 and 1985 liberalizations of federal eligibility rules, Gover-nor Riley was not satisfied. In an effort to spur Congress to further relax fed-eral eligibility limits, his Southern Regional Task Force on Infant Mortality issued a series of reports throughout 1985. The first, *A Fiscal Imperative: Prena-tal and Infant Care,* emphasized the potential cost savings from investing in maternal and infant care, arguing that "prenatal and infant health care pays for itself over and over. In contrast to the human and financial costs of infant problems associated with inadequate maternity care, outpatient prenatal and infant health care is quite inexpensive."[25] The report drew on research from a variety of sources, including a study by the American Academy of Pe-diatrics showing that every dollar spent on prenatal care ultimately saves two to ten dollars on care later in life. The report also urged the states to do their part, pointing out the financial advantages of making "full and creative use" of federal Medicaid funding. "Because federal monies match state in-vestments . . . savings from expenditures in prevention can be maximized."[26] Moreover, the report noted that expanding Medicaid would greatly reduce the cost of treating the uninsured in state and local—as well as private—hospitals, noting that three-fifths of hospitals' bad debts were attributable to the uninsured—and the largest category of uncollected costs was for maternity-related care.

The task force's second report, *An Investment in the Future: Legislative Strategies for Maternal and Infant Health,* described the actions many states had taken to expand access to health care and urged more states to follow suit. Like the first report, it focused on the financial advantages of exploiting Medicaid's federal-state cost-sharing arrangement.

> Expanding Medicaid is one of the most cost-effective ways to provide more women with adequate prenatal care [because] the Federal Government pays from 50 to 77 percent of Medicaid costs. In the South, this means that states pay an average of only 36.8 percent of their total Medicaid benefit expansion.[27]

The report encouraged the states to expand Medicaid in three ways: by extending eligibility to cover more people, broadening the range of services offered, and increasing provider reimbursement rates.

The Task Force's last report, *Final Report: For the Children of Tomorrow,* called on Congress to make federal Medicaid eligibility rules more flexible. Noting that "the cost of providing state match for AFDC and Medicaid has been a financial obstacle for many Southern states which wish to provide health care for poor working families," the report urged Congress to allow states to extend Medicaid eligibility to poor families with incomes above the state's AFDC standard of need without also being required to provide AFDC payments to those families.[28] The report also recommended that Congress amend the Medicaid law to provide comprehensive coverage for all pregnant women and infants below the federal poverty level.

The Southern Governors Association and the Southern Legislative Conference immediately endorsed the task force's report, and at the NGA's February 1986 meeting, Governor Riley asked his colleagues to do the same. To make the case, Riley cited a long list of research findings, including an Oregon study showing that for the cost of treating five high-risk babies, it would be possible to provide prenatal care to 149 women, as well as a Missouri study that found that women who received prenatal care had a prematurity rate that was 50 percent lower than that of women who did not receive such care.[29]

Despite these compelling statistics, Riley soon found himself engaged in "extremely tough conversations" with some of his Republican colleagues. The Reagan administration did not want the resolution to pass, and had lined up a handful of Republican governors to fight it from within the organization. Governor Riley responded by appealing directly to moderate Republican governor Lamar Alexander, who was NGA chairman at the time, and whose wife, Honey Alexander, had served on the task force. Fortunately for Riley, Alexander was a "progressive thinker" with a "background of coming from the South and understanding the issue" and was thus "predisposed to be for it."[30] Alexander helped Riley rally support, and the governors ultimately endorsed the proposal unanimously.

MR. RILEY GOES TO WASHINGTON

Following the NGA meeting, Riley took the task force's proposal to Capitol Hill, working to line up support from Republicans and Democrats alike. He was particularly interested in securing an endorsement from his own state's senator, Republican Strom Thurmond. As Riley advisor Sarah Shuptrine later recalled, "We needed Senator Thurmond desperately. Somebody had to show leadership on the Republican side that was very high up. We were working with our Republican senators in the South and of course Senator Thurmond was key. At that time, he had a lot of power in Congress." During their meeting with Thurmond, Riley and Shuptrine emphasized the cost savings that would come from increased access to preventive care, to which the senator replied: "Well, you know, that just makes good sense to me." Thurmond then arranged for Riley to meet with Senate majority leader Robert Dole (R-Kansas), who was similarly supportive. "After that, it was just not going to be the thing to oppose anymore," said Shuptrine.[31]

At the press conference introducing the bill (the Medicaid Maternal and Infant Amendments of 1986) the conservative Thurmond joined liberal senator Edward Kennedy (D-Massachusetts) and several other Democrats at the podium. When Senator Kennedy got up to speak, he joked, "It's not normal for me and Strom to be on the same podium supporting the same legislation. I'm a little worried one of us has not read this bill."[32]

As Congress debated the bill throughout the spring and summer of 1986, one member after another spoke of the pivotal role the governors had played in bringing the measure under consideration. When Senator Kennedy introduced the legislation, he noted that "The Southern Governors Association has recommended the change in the law I am introducing today. The National Governors Association unanimously endorsed it. It is time for Congress to do its part."[33] Senator Lloyd Bentsen (D-Texas) commended Governor Riley and his task force for "developing a set of policy goals and for the educational campaign which they undertook in an effort to improve public understanding of the need for these changes."[34]

In addition to the NGA, a number of special interest groups, including the Children's Defense Fund and the American Hospital Association, testified in support of the proposed legislation.[35] One group that did not support the bill, however, was AFDC advocates, who felt threatened by the prospect of severing the link between the two programs. As Riley advisor Sarah Shuptrine recalls, AFDC advocates were "scared to death to lose the connection with Medicaid . . . for fear they would lose any support for increasing the AFDC payment level."[36] But AFDC advocates ultimately had to acknowledge that "increases in the AFDC eligibility levels weren't on anybody's radar screen. So all they were doing was holding the Medicaid program down."[37]

Congress enacted the task force's proposal as part of the Omnibus Reconciliation Act of 1986. The legislation gave states the option of extending coverage to pregnant women and children up to age five in families below the federal poverty level, even if they did not qualify for AFDC. And although it had not been a top priority for the governors, the legislation also gave states the option of paying the premiums and copayments of Medicare beneficiaries with incomes below the federal poverty level (Qualified Medicare Beneficiaries, or QMBs), thereby weakening the link between Medicaid and another cash welfare program: Supplemental Security Income (SSI) for the poor aged, blind, and disabled.

The decoupling of Medicaid eligibility from cash assistance was a major juncture in Medicaid's history—reducing the stigma associated with the program, and setting it on a distinct political trajectory from other welfare programs. One state official referred to OBRA 1986 as a "defining moment" and "the chink in the armor that broke that historical connection between welfare and Medicaid that had forced families to be on welfare to get access to preventive and primary care through Medicaid."[38]

The states' response to OBRA 1986 was remarkably swift. Within one year, half the states had expanded Medicaid eligibility to include poor children and pregnant women up to 100 percent of the federal poverty level; within two years, the number had risen to 44.[39] States that exhibited both a relatively great need—namely, those with the highest rates of low-birth-weight infants and infant mortality—and a relatively strong fiscal position were among the earliest responders.[40] States were generally slower to take advantage of the option to expand benefits for poor Medicare beneficiaries, however, seeing the need for, and cost-effectiveness of, expanded coverage as greater among children and pregnant women than among the elderly and disabled.[41] Nonetheless, the *New York Times* reported that when it came to health policy, the states seemed to have "seized the initiative from the Federal Government."[42]

Despite having weakened the link between Medicaid and AFDC, Governor Riley still was not satisfied. At the annual NGA meeting in August 1986, he asked his colleagues to join him in supporting another resolution urging the federal government to give the states several additional options to extend Medicaid coverage to pregnant women, infants, and children with incomes above the federal poverty level. By framing his proposal in a way that was universally appealing—describing it as not only "humane" and "pro-family" but also "cost-effective" and fiscally conservative"—he was able to win their support.[43]

The following year, Congress passed the Omnibus Budget Reconciliation Act of 1987, which, thanks to Henry Waxman, included a measure giving states the option to cover infants and pregnant women in families with incomes up to 185 percent of the poverty level. By 1989, fifteen states were electing to cover infants and pregnant women up to the new maximum.[44] The legislation also accelerated coverage for children who were mandated coverage under the Deficit Reduction Act of 1984, and extended the age limit from five to eight (Oberg and Polich 1988). Shortly thereafter, Congress passed the Family Support Act of 1988, which required states to extend a year of transitional coverage to families leaving the AFDC rolls due to earnings from work, and to cover all two-parent families with incomes below the AFDC standard in which the primary earner was unemployed (AFDC-UP).

Despite the rapid pace at which Congress was revising the Medicaid law, and the resulting encroachment on state budgets, few governors complained. As one state official explained:

> I think it was probably kind of a mixed feeling. On the one hand people recognized the value of the health coverage that Medicaid offered. And, as you know, the option to add coverage was politically attractive . . . But, there was a side to it that was a federal mandate. That there was an increasing draw against the state revenues was a bit of a problem . . . I must say . . . the fact that there were federal matching funds was probably the key . . . Were it not for that, it would have been a different discussion.[45]

Certainly, the barrage of changes in eligibility rules posed logistical challenges. One state official grumbled that the states got new federal rules "dropped on us in the middle of budget periods without any time to plan or budget for them."[46] But as Riley aide Sarah Shuptrine put it, it was "real hard" for governors to argue against extending health coverage for low-income pregnant women and infants;[47] indeed, the chief lobbyist for the National Governors Association remarked that no governor was willing to publicly oppose Medicaid mandates for these highly sympathetic groups (Posner 1998, 83).

Some governors even preferred mandates to options, seeing the federal requirements as a solution to the problems of uneven coverage and interstate competition. Governor Lawton Chiles of Florida explained that he "helped put some of the mandates on" because "some states weren't doing anything" when the expansions were optional.[48] Other governors, particularly those facing conservative legislatures, advocated mandates as a tool for overcoming political resistance within their own states.[49] Henry Waxman recalled that some "Southern governors were coming to us and urging that we start mandating some of these Medicaid proposals so that they could . . . get their states to go along with drawing down the federal dollars."[50]

However, after Congress shifted its focus from children and pregnant women to the elderly and disabled in 1988, the governors became increasingly vocal in opposing federal mandates. Ironically, the turning point was a piece of legislation primarily concerned with expanding not Medicaid, but Medicare—namely, the Medicare Catastrophic Coverage Act of 1988.

THE MEDICARE CATASTROPHIC COVERAGE ACT OF 1988

In the mid-1980s, there was a growing consensus that the Reagan administration's efforts to control national health-care expenditures had gone too far in eroding not only Medicaid coverage for the poor, but also Medicare coverage for senior citizens. Measures to scale back Medicare costs by increasing patient cost sharing and reducing payments to providers meant that the program's beneficiaries were paying an increasingly large share of medical costs. Between 1980 and 1985, Medicare beneficiaries' out-of-pocket hospital expenses rose 49 percent, while their physician and outpatient expenses rose 31 percent.[51] President Reagan's advisors came to see reducing out-of-pocket costs—particularly very large or catastrophic costs—as a way for Republicans to improve their waning popularity among senior citizens (Himmelfarb 1995). Republicans' need to reach out to this politically important group became even more imperative after the 1986 elections, when Democrats regained control of the Senate while retaining control of the House.

In 1986, President Reagan asked the secretary of health and human services, Otis Bowen, to come up with a plan to "address the problems of affordable insurance for those whose life savings would otherwise be threatened when catastrophic illness strikes."[52] Secretary Bowen responded with a proposal that Medicare cover all hospital and doctor expenses after a patient had paid $2,000 out of his or her own pocket. However, Reagan's economic advisors protested that the plan was too expensive, particularly in light of the rapidly rising national deficit, and too intrusive in private markets. Ultimately, the Reagan administration settled on a compromise that balanced political and economic considerations. The president gave Congress the green light to move forward, but with a major caveat: the new benefits would have to be budget neutral, meaning the financing had to come from beneficiary premiums rather than taxes.

The Democratic leadership in Congress—not to be outdone by the GOP when it came to social policy—was quick to augment the proposal. As one Democratic staffer explained, "once the President let that train leave the station, it was just a matter of how many boxcars we could hang on it."[53] Representative Waxman worked with Senator Bentsen and others to add several boxcars to the administration's proposal. The first was drug coverage, which was a major priority for the American Association of Retired Persons (AARP). Unable to resist the opportunity to use the Medicare bill as a vehicle to promote his Medicaid agenda, Waxman tacked on a second boxcar mandating that the states cover infants and pregnant women below the federal poverty level. A final provision required the Medicaid program to cover Medicare premiums and deductibles for "dual eligibles"—low-income seniors who qualified for both programs. Waxman later explained that Democrats "saw that a lot of the low-income seniors weren't going to get enough help in the Medicare Catastrophic bill. And so we wanted to then expand assistance in Medicaid to pay for the Medicare premiums and cost-sharing for people below poverty."[54] This was not a new idea: OBRA 1986 had given the states the option to help dual eligibles with cost sharing, and several states were already voluntarily doing so, having found it cost-effective to subsidize preventive care so as to reduce the incidence of high-cost illnesses (Rosenbaum 1993).

One benefit that was notably absent from the Medicare catastrophic bill was long-term care—the single largest category of catastrophic costs for the elderly and disabled. Many congressional Democrats favored the addition of a long-term care provision to the Medicare bill, but saw this goal as unattainable in light of the ballooning national deficit and resistance from the Reagan administration (Himmelfarb 1995). Thus, long-term care was to remain a shared federal-state responsibility under the Medicaid program.

From a financial standpoint, the bill was a mixed bag for the states. Although the cost-sharing provision for dual eligibles would mean increased costs for states that were not already voluntarily covering Medicare coinsurance, a Medicare drug benefit would reduce their financial burden since nearly all state Medicaid programs voluntarily covered prescription drugs for the poor elderly. Thus, the governors remained largely silent as Congress debated the bill throughout the spring of 1988.

The House passed the Medicare Catastrophic Coverage Act of 1988 by a margin of more than two to one; the Senate passed it by a margin of nearly eight to one. The AARP hailed the bill as "a watershed," and "a victory for the elderly."[55] Upon signing the bill in a Rose Garden ceremony in July 1988, President Reagan proclaimed that the legislation would "help remove a terrible threat from the lives of elderly and disabled Americans . . . replacing worry and fear with peace of mind."[56]

However, not everyone was pleased with the legislation. Several advocacy organizations—most notably, the National Committee to Preserve Social Security and Medicare—unleashed a barrage of criticism against the new law, and particularly its financing mechanism. The organization sent letters to millions of senior citizens denouncing the program, exclaiming: "A special tax on senior citizens! Have you ever heard of anything so outrageous in your life?"[57] Throngs of seniors responded to the letters by calling their representatives to complain. Many also expressed disappointment that the program would not cover long-term care.

Despite efforts by the program's supporters to characterize the attacks as "a very vocal minority sounding off,"[58] Congress caved under pressure— quickly considering a flurry of proposals and amendments, and engaging in chaotic debate before ultimately repealing catastrophic coverage in November 1989 (Moon 1990). The repeal of this legislation—the most significant social policy to come out of Reagan's eight years in office—marked one of the most dramatic legislative reversals in U.S. history.

However, to the governors' dismay, Congress retained the provisions of the law pertaining to Medicaid. Seniors had only complained about the measures financed by the surtax—not the parts for which the states were financially responsible—and congressional Democrats saw little reason to throw out the baby with the bathwater. But once Congress removed the drug benefit, the law was no longer a mixed bag for the states—it was a financial burden. Had Congress initially proposed the cost-sharing provision alone, the governors undoubtedly would have opposed it. Yet Congress removed the drug benefit so hastily that the governors did not have a chance to mobilize to protect it. (Years later, when Congress again enacted Medicare drug coverage in 2006, federal lawmakers solved the financing problem by forcing states to help pay for the benefits through a "clawback" mechanism—prompting several states to file an unsuccessful lawsuit arguing that it was unconstitutional to require them to help pay for a federal program.)

SUSPENSION RESOLUTION

The states' lack of enthusiasm for the mandated increase in spending on elderly and disabled dual eligibles immediately became evident as they dragged their feet in implementing the new policy. The law required the states to begin paying the out-of-pocket Medicare costs of poor seniors and disabled persons on January 1, 1989; by March, sixteen states still were noncompliant.[59] Henry Waxman called the delays unacceptable, and tensions escalated as the federal government threatened to cut off Medicaid funding completely if the states did not comply with federal law.

The governors grudgingly implemented MCCA 1988, but warned Congress not to enact any additional mandates. Testifying before Congress in June 1989, NGA executive director Raymond Scheppach explained that while the governors were "very proud" of the progress they had made in helping vulnerable populations in recent years, they were opposed to any further mandated eligibility requirements for specific populations on the grounds that "individual States are in the best position to decide how Medicaid funds should be spent."[60] As Henry Waxman later acknowledged in an interview, "the states were feeling that there was a lot being required of them in terms of putting up money for their share of the Medicaid [match]."[61]

The governors' change of heart reflected several considerations. First, unlike the earlier mandates, which had focused on children and pregnant women, MCCA 1988 targeted the elderly and disabled. Most governors considered caring for these populations a federal duty—in keeping with the federal government's assumption of financial responsibility for Social Security and Medicare—and resented being asked to help pay for Medicare's deficiencies. Some also worried that diverting resources to the elderly and disabled would squeeze out benefits for pregnant women and infants, which they considered a higher priority.[62] The elderly and disabled were an expensive and rapidly growing demographic, and investing in their care was widely seen as less cost-effective, compared to investments in preventive care for infants and pregnant women.

Second, by 1989, the national economy had begun to deteriorate, and a growing number of states were struggling with serious budget shortfalls. No category of spending caused more financial distress than Medicaid, which grew by 11.4 percent in 1989 and 18.4 percent in 1990 due to a combination of factors including the economic downturn, federal mandates, and medical cost inflation.[63] Combined with sluggish revenue growth, Medicaid's rapid expansion was making it increasingly difficult to balance the budget, as is required by law in nearly all states.

Third, as a result of its explosive growth, Medicaid was crowding out other state priorities. By 1990, Medicaid had surpassed higher education as the second-largest state spending category after K–12 education.[64] According to research by Kane, Orszag, and Apostolov (2005), the states that experienced the most rapid growth of Medicaid expenditures between 1988 and 1990 also experienced the largest reductions in higher-education spending. Additionally, many governors, including Governor Lawton Chiles (D-Florida), began to complain that Medicaid was crowding out other priorities as well.

> We are not able to do what we should be doing for education, what we should be doing for the environment, what we should be doing for transportation, what we should be doing in public safety in my state because all of our money is being taken now for Medicaid . . .[65]

Mandatory Medicaid spending was also increasingly crowding out optional Medicaid spending, limiting state leaders' discretion within the sphere of health policy (Grogan 1999).

At the 1989 annual meeting of the National Governors Association, Governor Richard Celeste (D-Ohio) introduced a measure titled "Suspension Resolution on Health Care," which called on Congress and the White House to "put a hold on any new Medicaid mandates for a period of two years." One governor after another spoke up in support of the resolution; many underscored the fact that their opposition to Medicaid mandates was pragmatic rather than philosophical. Governor Michael Dukakis (D-Massachusetts)—a staunch advocate of expanded access to health care—expressed his thoughts.

> I think we're all supportive of recent congressional expansions to the Medicaid program, which increased care to low income families. Most of us have asked Congress at one time or another at least to give us the option of expanding that coverage. But . . . there is a strong and growing consensus on the part of all of the governors that the time has now come to take a very fresh, comprehensive look at how we pay for health care in this country and to whom we provide it.

Others were more pointed in their criticism of the federal government's growing reliance on Medicaid mandates as a tool for accomplishing policy goals on the cheap. Governor James Blanchard (D-Michigan) was among those who complained.

> What we have happening right now because of the financial mess with the federal government and the federal budget, what we have is the President and the Congressmen dumping new functions upon the states without giving us the revenue. . . . Let's not kid ourselves. This is . . . a way to bleed revenue from the states for functions that the Congress, if they had any guts, would finance directly . . . It's bad enough they've been charging expenditures on the American people in the national debt; they're now doing it with the state credit card as well.

The motion to suspend health-care mandates for two years passed unanimously, and the governors vowed to "aggressively lobby for the moratorium" on Capitol Hill.[66]

"THAT SONUVABITCH WAXMAN"

Despite the governors' vigorous lobbying campaign, federal policy makers initially paid little heed to the moratorium. Henry Waxman, for one, was eager to continue expanding access to more poor Americans, and wanted to capitalize on the momentum the governors had, ironically, helped to create. Waxman was acutely aware that, despite his and others' efforts over the previous several years, millions of poor Americans still lacked health insurance. According to a staffer on Waxman's subcommittee, "Henry was a bulldog on this. He was in there for the long haul. He struck me as someone who would be happy spending his whole life protecting the health of moms and kids."[67] Representative George Miller (D-California) joked that when he first joined the House Budget Committee, he thought Waxman's first name was "sonuvabitch" because everyone kept saying, "Do you know what that sonuvabitch Waxman wants now?"[68]

Moreover, a wide variety of interest groups had rallied around the governors' initiatives over the previous several years, and continued to lobby for Medicaid expansion even after the NGA issued its request for a moratorium. In particular, a number of health-care industry and child-advocacy organizations had banded together to form the Children's Medicaid Coalition. The coalition included, among others, the Children's Defense Fund, the American Academy of Pediatrics, the American Medical Association, the American Hospital Association, and the Blue Cross and Blue Shield Association.

The health-care industry had many reasons to support Medicaid expansion. For one thing, insurers were concerned that the cost of treating the uninsured was putting upward pressure on insurance premiums, resulting in an "unfair tax on our policyholders." Providers and insurers were also worried that Congress might resurrect the idea of national health insurance, and viewed Medicaid expansion as the lesser of evils. As one health industry leader put it, "If we don't find a way to provide coverage for the nation's 31 million uninsured, the Federal Government may move to adopt some foolish, ill-advised, ill-conceived national health insurance strategy."[69]

The coalition urged Congress and the administration of newly elected president, George H. W. Bush, to continue expanding Medicaid despite the governors' objections. With a combination of respect and dismay, one White House official referred to the alliance of child advocacy and health-care industry groups as "an unbeatable political combination."[70] In June 1989, the Bush administration proposed mandating a modest extension of coverage for infants up to the age of one and pregnant women with incomes up to 130 percent of the federal poverty line. The proposal would also cover immunizations for children under age 6 who were receiving food stamps.

Henry Waxman, declaring the White House proposal inadequate, modified it to require the states to provide full coverage to pregnant women and children under age 6 up to 133 percent of the poverty line, and to pay for Early and Periodic Screening, Diagnosis and Treatment (EPSDT) services for children under 21 if a qualified provider deemed those services necessary. He tucked the measure into the Omnibus Reconciliation Act of 1989 (OBRA 1989), which President Bush signed into law in December.

Waxman's success was again due to his creative use of the reconciliation process. As Don Moran of the Office of Management and Budget put it, the administration had entered into "an interesting sort of Faustian bargain" with Waxman, whereby Medicaid expansion was "the price of getting a budget resolution through the House of Representatives."[71] OBRA 1989 also reflected a highly successful strategy which some observers began to call the "Waxman two-step" (Smith and Moore 2008, 178). Waxman would first offer the states an attractive option and then, a year or two later, mandate it for all states. By securing broad acceptance of optional expansion, and then waiting for a majority of states to take up that option before making it mandatory, he was able to minimize political resistance. As Waxman stated, "incrementalism may not get much press, but it does work" (Waxman 1989, 1217).

The governors begged with growing urgency for relief from the Waxman two-step. At the 1990 winter meeting of the National Governors Association, Governor George Sinner (D-North Dakota) implored House Speaker Tom Foley (D-Washington).

> Tom, we can't handle any more [mandates]. Can't you help us stop them? We have to prioritize our spending in the states. Some of us have horribly hurt economies. Prioritizing is extremely difficult. You just have to let us decide what our priorities are . . . We're grateful for the options . . . But can't Congress please let us run the states?[72]

Speaker Foley reassured Governor Sinner that "increasingly in the House and the Senate, there's a recognition, largely because of communications with the governors and the legislatures, that congressional mandates are an extremely serious problem."[73]

The Bush administration and Senate leaders—eager to slow the growth of federal Medicaid spending—happily agreed to respect the governors' wishes for a moratorium. But Representative Waxman pressed ahead with a proposal to require states to cover all poor children under the age of 18. During congressional hearings that fall, Alicia Pelrine, director of the NGA's human resources group, testified against the bill, underscoring the states' budgetary constraints.

> We feel the same swings and shifts in the economy that you do, and we don't know where we will find the money that the Federal Government has been unable to find . . . If Congress is firmly committed to moving forward with Medicaid expansions this year, we ask that they be options or that they be financed by the federal government . . . We share your goals, but at the same time must protect our states from collapsing.[74]

Even the governors who initially had pushed the hardest for eligibility expansions made a case against the measure, as Governor Clinton (D-Arkansas) ᐧ explained in congressional testimony.

> No governor would argue the merits of the policy to protect pregnant women and children. I was a southern Governor who voted for the 1985 resolution. My wife was on our Infant Mortality Task Force. We wanted the opportunity in the poor Southern States to cover more pregnant women and children . . . [But mandates have] stretched the States beyond their fiscal and administrative capacity.[75]

Despite the governors' objections, Waxman's amendments passed as part of the Omnibus Reconciliation Act of 1990. The legislation required the states to cover, by 2002, children through age 18 in families with incomes below the federal poverty level. It also required the states to pay Medicare cost sharing for dual eligibles with incomes between 100 and 120 percent of the federal poverty level. These beneficiaries were given the name Special Low-income Medicare Beneficiaries (SLMBs) to differentiate them from Qualified Medicare Beneficiaries (QMBs) below the poverty line, who had been made eligible by OBRA 1986.

When the governors gathered for their winter meeting in February 1991, they again passed a formal resolution calling for a two-year moratorium on new mandates. They invited House majority leader Dick Gephardt (D-Missouri) to the meeting and pleaded with him to be an "ally" to the states, which were "strapped" and needed to "get our budgets back in shape."[76] The governors also met with White House officials and other members of Congress, and found that their request for a moratorium was "favorably received" throughout Washington.[77]

Later that year, Congress passed the Budget Enforcement Act of 1990, which revised the budget process with the goal of reining in the federal deficit. The law established a pay-as-you-go process for entitlement programs, requiring that any increases in spending be offset by revenue increases or spending cuts so as to be deficit neutral. Some observers have suggested that this measure was deliberately designed as a restraint on Henry Waxman, although others have denied this claim.[78] Regardless of the law's intended purpose, it put an abrupt end to Waxman's Medicaid expansions.

CONCLUSION

The Medicaid program underwent a dramatic transformation in the 1980s. In each year from 1984 through 1990, Congress amended Title XIX to extend eligibility to additional pregnant women, infants, children, parents, elderly, or disabled persons. These laws, many of which were largely phased in during the 1990s, contributed to a dramatic increase in enrollment (fig. 4). The options and mandates passed during this period extended coverage to over half a million pregnant women, more than 4 million children, and more than 4 million elderly or disabled individuals (Rosenbaum 1993). Whereas the program had covered only 17 percent of births in 1985, by 1991 that share had nearly tripled to 45 percent (Coughlin, Ku, and Holahan 1994). Increases in Medicaid eligibility, in turn, were associated with reduced incidence of low-birth-weight births and a decrease in infant mortality (Currie and Gruber 1996), and improved health outcomes for children (Lykens and Jargowsky 2002).

Severing the link between Medicaid and AFDC helped policy makers expand health care without being weighed down by the connection to an increasingly unpopular cash-assistance program (Kronebusch 2001). In 1980, 80 percent of Medicaid recipients qualified by virtue of being on welfare; by 1992, this number had fallen to 60 percent; indeed, Medicaid's growth was particularly notable in contrast to AFDC's lack thereof. Between 1988 and 1992, the average annual growth rate of Medicaid enrollment among children and pregnant women was more than 150 percent, compared to only 3 percent for AFDC. Despite this rapid expansion, the program covered less

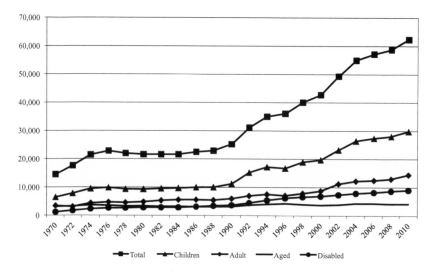

Fig. 4. Medicaid beneficiaries by eligibility group, 1970–2010. (Data from U.S. Department of Health and Human Services.)

than half of the nation's poor in 1991; those excluded were primarily adults without young children and members of two-parent families (Coughlin, Ku, and Holahan 1994).

Medicaid's expansion in the 1980s is largely attributable to the initiative of the governors—particularly Richard Riley and his Southern colleagues. Out of a combination of altruism and financial self-interest, the governors raised public awareness of the infant-mortality problem and pushed Congress to improve health-care access for poor children and pregnant women. In so doing, they secured billions of additional dollars in federal financial assistance at a time when federal grants were otherwise hard to come by. The program's expansion was also due in large part to Representative Henry Waxman's innovative use of the reconciliation process to jam legislation through Congress despite Republican opposition. Yet, as Waxman himself admits, he could not have accomplished all he did without the initiative of the governors, who ultimately would have to carry out the legislated changes.

Despite the governors' initial enthusiasm for Medicaid expansion, they soon found that the financial implications were onerous. Medicaid had a viselike grip on state budgets, and the vise was getting tighter each year. As the 1990–91 recession set in, the governors began to desperately seek ways to relieve the financial pressure. They soon discovered they could use creative accounting mechanisms to shift the program's ballooning costs back to the federal government—ushering in one of the most contentious periods in Medicaid's history.

CHAPTER 5
Creative Financing Mechanisms in the Bush Era

"Any governor who tells you he runs his state without trying to finagle money from the federal government is either a liar or a fool."[1]

AS FEDERAL MANDATES PROLIFERATED and the national economy deteriorated in the late 1980s and early 1990s, the states found it increasingly difficult to fund their share of the ballooning Medicaid program. Adding to the states' woes during this period were a host of other factors including medical cost inflation, the AIDS crisis, growing demand for nursing-home care, lawsuits initiated by providers seeking adequate reimbursement rates,[2] and Congress's passage in 1986 of the Emergency Medical Treatment and Active Labor Act (EMTALA), which requires hospitals to provide medical care to anyone needing emergency treatment, regardless of ability to pay or legal status.

Matching grants inevitably provide states with an incentive to engage in "supplantation," or the relabeling of expenditures so that they become eligible for federal matching funds—and the temptation to do so is particularly strong during periods of resource scarcity (Merriman 2006). In response to mounting financial pressure in the 1980s, many states began shifting state and locally funded school-based health programs into Medicaid, replacing spending on block-grant-funded health programs such as the Maternal and Child Health program with Medicaid spending in order to take advantage of the latter's more generous federal grant formula, and moving patients out of state psychiatric hospitals—where nonelderly adults were generally ineligible for Medicaid—into the community in order to make them eligible (Coughlin et al. 1999). As one state Medicaid director explains, there is a "conflict of interest" embedded in the program's financing arrangement: "you're still going to have to provide services and if you don't find a way to make them Medicaid-eligible, doggone it, you're going to be using [only] state dollars."[3]

As the states' fiscal crisis deepened, state officials devised several creative new mechanisms for exploiting the program's open-ended matching formula. In particular, they began to develop accounting gimmicks that enabled them to secure additional federal matching dollars without actually putting up any additional state funds. Through the use of provider donations, taxes, intergovernmental transfers, and other mechanisms, a state could make it appear as though it was spending money on Medicaid, thereby qualifying for the federal match. Although these creative financing mechanisms were technically legal, they were inconsistent with the spirit of the Medicaid law, which required each state to pay a specific share of the program's costs.

The governors' efforts to leverage matching funds caused federal Medicaid spending to skyrocket—much to the alarm of federal policy makers. In the early 1990s, the federal government issued a series of regulations and legislation attempting to close the legal loopholes that made the creative financing mechanisms possible. The National Governors Association played a critical role in protecting the states' interests—negotiating with the White House and lobbying Congress to delay implementation of the new rules and to leave certain loopholes intact. As a result, even after the new rules were in place, states were able to continue using financing mechanisms—albeit to a lesser extent—thereby fueling Medicaid's continued growth.

FEDERAL TUG-OF-WAR PRODUCES LOOPHOLES

Federal Medicaid policy in the 1980s was characterized by a tug-of-war between the executive and legislative branches and the parties that controlled them: the Reagan administration sought to cut Medicaid spending, while congressional Democrats sought to expand the program's scope—as documented in chapters 3 and 4, respectively. A significant by-product of this battle was the creation of several legal loopholes that enabled state officials to shift the program's costs to the federal government to an unprecedented degree.

Prior to 1981, federal law required state Medicaid programs to reimburse providers according to Medicare's reimbursement principles, which were based on a retrospective cost system. However, rapid medical cost inflation led to growing concerns that reimbursing providers based on their reported costs was inherently inflationary. Thus, Congress passed a measure—as part of the Omnibus Budget Reconciliation Act of 1981, or OBRA 1981—that repealed this requirement, freeing states to establish their own "reasonable and adequate" Medicaid reimbursement methodologies. The idea was to encourage states to adopt prospective payment systems, in which rates are set in advance and may be lower than the actual cost of service delivery.

However, Representative Henry Waxman (D-California) and other liberal members of Congress feared that removing the standard for an adequate rate—and thus permitting states to slash Medicaid payments to providers— might harm hospitals that served a disproportionate share of low-income patients. These concerns were heightened by recent evidence suggesting that hospitals serving large numbers of Medicaid and uninsured patients had higher operating costs.[4] Moreover, these hospitals were less able to shift the costs of uncompensated, or charity, care to insured patients, relative to hospitals serving wealthier populations. Thus, Waxman inserted a provision in the OBRA 1981 legislation requiring states to "take into account the situation of hospitals which serve a disproportionate number of low-income patients with special needs" and authorizing them to pay such hospitals a "disproportionate share hospital" (DSH or dispro) adjustment above the normal rate, and to receive the federal Medicaid match for such payments.

Congress left implementation of the DSH program up to the Health Care Financing Administration (HCFA), a regulatory arm of the Department of Health and Human Services that had been created a few years earlier to coordinate the growing Medicaid and Medicare programs. However, the Reagan administration was determined to limit Medicaid spending, so instead of establishing guidelines for state DSH programs, HCFA in 1983 issued a new regulation that made it harder for states to make DSH payments by setting an upper payment limit (UPL) to prohibit state Medicaid programs from paying more, in the aggregate, than would have been paid under the Medicare program.

However, several states quickly found creative ways around the upper payment limit in order to secure additional federal funds to support state hospitals. For instance, a state could make high payments to state-owned or -operated hospitals, but low payments to private or local-government-owned hospitals, so that the aggregate amount paid did not exceed the aggregate upper payment limit. In response, in 1987 HCFA created a separate UPL for state-owned facilities to prevent the states from using aggregation to their advantage.

Meanwhile, frustrated by HCFA's refusal to promulgate DSH rules, Representative Waxman and his Democratic colleagues again directed the regulatory body to define and identify DSH hospitals as part of the Deficit Reduction Act of 1984 (DEFRA 1984), but HCFA continued to resist. The failure of the regulatory approach led congressional Democrats to switch to a legislative strategy. In 1985, they inserted language in the Consolidated Omnibus Budget Reconciliation Act of 1985 (COBRA 1985) that established national qualifying criteria for DSH hospitals. The following year, in a provision of the Omnibus Budget Reconciliation Act of 1986 (OBRA 1986), Waxman inserted language clarifying that HCFA had no authority to limit states' DSH payments, thereby permitting states to make payments to DSH hospitals above the UPL. Thus, DSH payments became the only Medicaid payments that were not subject to the upper payment limit. Finally, in an effort to promote state participation, Waxman inserted a provision into the Omnibus Budget Reconciliation Act of 1987 (OBRA 1987) that required the states to submit a Medicaid plan amendment describing the criteria used to designate hospitals as DSH and defining the DSH payment formula.

There was little resistance to Waxman's provisions in Congress. Lawmakers assumed that the risk of states making overly generous supplementary payments to DSH hospitals was low since the states would have to come up with their own funds in order to receive matching federal funds (Gilman 1998). However, federal lawmakers failed to anticipate the creative ways in which state officials might finance the state share.

As state officials began to comply with the new law and set up DSH programs, they increasingly realized that the program was a potential windfall. As one state Medicaid director explained in an interview, the new rules "got Medicaid folks thinking in a particular direction that they really hadn't been thinking about before. And that was looking how to finance DSH payments . . . Are there ways to do this . . . in a way that legally allows a state to come out financially advantaged?"[5] Luckily for the states, the Reagan administration had recently passed a new regulation that unintentionally created an opportunity for exploitation.

Although most of the Medicaid regulations the Reagan administration issued in the 1980s were intended to restrain the growth of spending, one regulation had the opposite effect. In 1985, HCFA began allowing states to collect donations to help defray the state's share of Medicaid costs. The goal was to encourage support from charitable organizations such as the United Way, but the Reagan administration correctly predicted that the regulation would have little impact on the level of donations from such organizations, and thus on federal matching payments.[6] However, the White House overlooked the fact that the regulation's wording was vague enough to also include donations from health-care providers.

In a classic case of unintended consequences, resourceful state officials figured out how to turn these obscure rules into a golden goose. A state could collect a donation from a hospital and then immediately return the money to that hospital as reimbursement for Medicaid services, thereby qualifying for a federal Medicaid match without actually spending any state money. And the exemption of DSH payments from the UPL meant that the amount a state could collect was virtually unlimited. In short, the provider donation rule presented opportunities for exploitation on the "revenue side," while the DSH program presented opportunities on the "expenditure side" (Coughlin, Ku, and Holahan 1994, 94).

WEST VIRGINIA'S PROVIDER DONATION PROGRAM

In 1986, West Virginia became the first state to take advantage of the provider donation loophole (Thompson and Fossett 2008). For years, West Virginia had been grappling with one of the worst economic and budget crises in state history. The state's mining- and manufacturing-based economy, already struggling to cope with increased competition from foreign producers, had been hit particularly hard by the national recession of 1981–1982. In early 1983, the state's unemployment rate soared to nearly 18 percent—the highest in the nation—and hovered in the teens for the next several years. To make matters worse, mounting concern about acid rain and low oil prices due to a worldwide surplus were contributing to a widespread shift from coal—one of West Virginia's main exports—to oil. State lawmakers cut taxes in an attempt to stimulate the economy, but the main effect was to make it more difficult to balance the budget.

Throughout the mid-1980s, West Virginia lawmakers took increasingly desperate measures to close the budget shortfall, including temporarily closing 16 state colleges, halting welfare checks, and delaying Medicaid payments to hospitals. By 1986, the backlog of overdue Medicaid payments had reached nearly $40 million.[7] Since the state was unable to come up with its share of the matching funds, this meant West Virginia was relinquishing millions of dollars in federal matching funds. And given that West Virginia's income ranked 49th in the nation, qualifying the state for a three-to-one matching rate, this meant forgoing a considerable amount of federal funding at a time when revenues were desperately needed.

It was against this backdrop that West Virginia's Republican governor, Arch Moore, hatched a plan to eliminate the state's backlog of Medicaid payments at the federal government's expense. In October 1986, Governor Moore—a clever leader with a reputation for playing his cards close to his chest—held a secret meeting with hospital officials, and told them they had to make donations to the state treasury so that the state could collect federal funding, or else they would not be paid (Crouser 2006). The state would then return the donations as payment for Medicaid services, accompanied by federal matching dollars. The governor promised the hospital officials: "If you make that contribution . . . I will return it to you the next day. Within a matter of days, I will come back with the balance that is owed in each of the accounts that we are carrying with you."[8]

Because the state would not be putting up any of its own funds to cover its share, hospitals would be reimbursed for only the federal government's 72 percent share. To help compensate hospitals for the loss of state funds, Governor Moore offered to reimburse them at a higher rate than usual. Typically West Virginia's Medicaid reimbursement rate covered only 80 percent of the actual cost of service delivery, but Moore offered to reimburse hospitals at a rate of 95 percent for the remainder of the year.[9]

Governor Moore assured the hospital officials that he had researched the legality of his plan, and ultimately succeeded in convincing them to go along with it. As one hospital official put it, "We were so strapped by the Medicaid program that we were willing to put up our own money to get federal funds."[10] Another official noted that although it was not the "best deal in the world," a smaller amount of cash was better than a larger amount on the accounts receivable ledger.[11]

Thus, in November 1986, 63 hospitals donated a total of roughly $10 million to the state, which used the money to obtain $26 million in federal matching funds and then transferred both the donations and the federal funds back to the hospitals the next day, as promised. Governor Moore warned hospital officials to keep this arrangement as quiet as possible because he wanted to "continue to do it as long as I can get away with it."[12] Although he believed the deal to be legal, the governor did not want to draw attention to the plan, nor did he want it to catch on with other states, fearing that federal officials would pass a rule countermanding it.

It was only a matter of time before the scheme came to light, however. When Governor Moore ran it for a second time with another 52 hospitals in December 1986, the U.S. Department of Health and Human Services slapped West Virginia with a retroactive disallowance of its Medicaid program, accusing the state of giving "kickbacks" to the hospitals that had made donations.[13] Governor Moore defended his actions as consistent with federal rules, and complained that HCFA's legal action was intended "for one purpose and one purpose alone: that is to discourage the states looking positively toward this program."[14]

The legal battle between the federal government and West Virginia dragged out over the next several years, winding its way through federal district court, the U.S. Department of Health and Human Services Departmental Grant Appeals Board, and finally to the U.S. Court of Appeals. The battle grew increasingly acrimonious, with federal officials accusing the state of "illicit or unsavory activity" and the state's legal counsel—the Washington-based law firm of Covington & Burling—accusing federal officials of a "reprehensible attempt to discredit state officials."[15] Ultimately, the court found that HCFA's 1985 regulation on donations did not preclude states from providing an "inducement" for hospital donations, nor did it require donations to be "unconditional."[16] The court allowed West Virginia to keep the $60 million in federal matching funds it had acquired using provider donations, but prohibited the state from using the financing mechanism again in the future.

TENNESSEE'S PROVIDER TAX PROGRAM

Tennessee discovered the provider donation loophole shortly after West Virginia. In January 1987, Ned McWherter's first official act as the state's new governor was to set up a task force to study ways to expand Medicaid coverage. McWherter was a progressive Democrat and a champion of universal health coverage. Known as a "man of the people," he went on to become one of the most popular and powerful governors in state history.[17] He had won the election on a campaign to increase access to health care—but he had also pledged no new taxes. The state had no income tax, and sales tax revenues had been sluggish since the back-to-back recessions of the early 1980s, so the governor was looking for a creative way to finance the expansion.

The solution to this dilemma came to him from Steve Reed, an alert offi-

cial in Tennessee's Medicaid Bureau, who had come across the HCFA donation rule while scouring obscure federal legal documents.[18] Reed took the
idea to Medicaid director Manny Martins—who had a reputation as a brilliant and tireless public servant—and Martins quickly fashioned a provider
donation program for Tennessee.[19] In October 1987, 27 hospitals donated $19
million to the state of Tennessee, which used these funds to make a $63 mil-
lion payment back to the hospitals. Of this total amount, $24 million went
to increased DSH subsidies, $31 million went to expanded coverage for chil-
dren and pregnant women below the federal poverty level, and the remainder went to an increase in the hospital coverage limit from 14 to 20 days.[20]

HCFA disallowed Tennessee's donation program in June 1988, arguing
that the funds had not been donated according to the accepted meaning of
the term, but rather had been induced by the state in an effort to substitute
the hospitals for itself as the federal government's partner in funding the
Medicaid program.[21] The state of Tennessee appealed the decision, denying
that the donations had occurred as part of a quid pro quo. In fact, the state
had been careful not to condition eligibility for subsidies on a hospital's participation in the donation program; only 27 hospitals had made donations,
but a total of 36 hospitals had received increased payments. However, Mc-
Wherter later acknowledged privately that the donated funds were "hocus
pocus money" and that "truthfully, it was just raping the federal budget."[22]

In June 1988, the HHS appeals board ruled in Tennessee's favor, finding
that there was "absolutely no evidence in the record that the State gave pref-
erential treatment of any kind to hospitals that provided fund transfers." The
board found that Tennessee's provider donation program had been "applied
consistently and uniformly throughout the State to all hospitals with Medicaid patients."[23] Moreover, the board noted that the money had not been
used only to increase DSH payments, but also to expand coverage—consistent
with congressional intent.

In the meantime, while waiting for the appeal board's verdict, Manny
Martins had figured out how to develop a similar program using taxes instead of donations: the state could collect provider-specific taxes or fees, and
then return the revenues to those same providers along with federal matching funds. As Martins saw it, the mechanism was "in keeping with the spirit
of the law," and also reflected "the hospitals' willingness to be assessed a provider fee to generate revenue so the Medicaid program wouldn't be reduced."
A Tennessee Hospital Association official concurred: "There's no liability to
the state because the hospitals are putting up the money [and] it's a good

deal for the hospitals because they don't have to take the cuts" that might otherwise be necessary to balance the state budget.[24]

All told, creative financing mechanisms increased Tennessee's federal medical assistance percentage (FMAP) from the statutory rate of 68 percent to an effective rate of 83 percent during Governor McWherter's first term (Ogbonna 2007). Between 1988 and 1993, the number of enrollees nearly doubled from 540,000 to almost one million, while the state's Medicaid budget nearly quadrupled—from $692 million to $2.7 billion (Mirvis et al. 1995, 1235). As a share of total state expenditures, Tennessee's Medicaid program increased from 17 percent to 27 percent.[25]

LOUISIANA'S "DISPRO" PROGRAM

In 1988, Louisiana developed a creative financing mechanism based entirely on the Disproportionate Share Hospital program, without relying on the taxes and donations that had landed other states in court. Health care for the poor is largely delivered by state hospitals in Louisiana. Thus, when Congress mandated the DSH program, state health director Christopher Pilley called the resulting inflow of federal funds "God-given to Louisiana." With the blessing of the state's governor, Buddy Roemer—a Democrat who later switched to the Republican Party—Pilley used the DSH program to "leverage every federal dollar we could get our hands on."[26]

Louisiana's DSH mechanism worked in the following way: In addition to making Medicaid payments to the state, the federal government would send DSH subsidies to Louisiana state hospitals serving a disproportionate share of Medicaid patients. The state would then relabel these funds as the state's Medicaid payment to the hospitals for delivering Medicaid services, thereby qualifying for federal matching funds. In effect, the DSH program was a "conduit to change federal dollars into state dollars."[27] In some cases, the state recycled the same federal funds through a state-hospital account more than once. As Pilley pointed out, "it was a formula that never closed" because Congress had set no limit on DSH subsidies.[28]

Over a five-year period, Louisiana's health budget increased by 400 percent—from $1.6 billion in 1988 to $4.48 billion in 1993—despite the national recession of 1990–1991.[29] The DSH program was the main driver of growth. Prior to 1988, the state did not have a DSH program; by 1995, disproportionate share hospital payments comprised more than 20 percent of the state's total Medicaid payments.[30] The state's matching rate of 70 percent during this period meant that the state was supposed to receive less than $3 in federal funds for every dollar of state spending, but by 1992 it was receiving $6.68 per state dollar; by 1993, that figure had jumped to $13.90.[31]

State officials scratched their heads in disbelief that the federal government continued to let them get away with this Medicaid maximization strategy. As one state lawmaker put it, "When we first heard about this we thought, 'This is crazy. How can they let us do this?' The second was, 'How long is this going to last?'"[32]

TEXAS'S INTERGOVERNMENTAL TRANSFERS

In 1989, Texas devised a fourth type of financing mechanism based on intergovernmental transfers. Texas had one of the least generous programs in the nation—offering minimal coverage and relying heavily on local-government hospitals to bear the burden of caring for the poor. In the late 1980s, the economic downturn and other factors described at the beginning of this chapter exacerbated this burden, causing dozens of public hospitals to close. State leaders came under growing pressure from advocacy groups and health-care providers to expand Medicaid coverage and increase provider payments.

At the time, the state was governed by Republican Bill Clements, a wealthy former oil executive. Clements was passionate about expanding access to health care; after leaving office, he donated $100 million to a hospital affiliated with the University of Texas. However, he was also determined to keep the state's taxes low. Similarly, Lieutenant Governor Bill Hobby, a separately elected Democrat responsible for overseeing the budget process, was a strong advocate for the poor who wanted to leave a legacy of improved access to health care, but also had a reputation as a conservative fiscal manager. Creative financing mechanisms provided the perfect opportunity for Clements and Hobby to expand coverage without raising taxes. Throughout the late 1980s and early 1990s, they oversaw a series of Medicaid maximization strategies. The first one, launched in 1987, was similar to Tennessee's provider tax program. Two years later, the state implemented an inventive new variation involving intergovernmental transfers (IGT).

Intergovernmental transfers from cities, counties, special-purpose districts, and other local-government units—including health-care providers—to a state's Medicaid program are legal under federal Medicaid law.[33]

The 1965 Medicaid statute merely requires "financial participation by the State equal to not less than 40 per centum of the non-Federal share of the expenditures under the plan"—thus, up to 60 percent of the nonfederal share can come from local sources.[34] The underlying principle is that since local-government units are generally creatures of—and derive their taxing authority from—the state, local and state spending are of the same character when it comes to federal matching programs like Medicaid.[35]

However, state officials soon learned that intergovernmental transfers could also be used in an unintended and, federal officials would argue, illegitimate way. By transferring local funds in and out of state coffers, a state could increase the federal-financing share beyond the statutory federal matching rate. One of the main advantages of the IGT mechanism, relative to provider taxes and donations, was the flexibility to target payments to public institutions; indeed, a state could totally exclude private hospitals under an IGT-financed program.

The idea to use intergovernmental transfers in this creative new way originated with Texas comptroller Bob Bullock. A Republican, Bullock was campaigning for lieutenant governor at the time and, like Clements and Hobby, was looking for ways to expand state services at minimal state expense. Since a large number of hospitals in Texas were financed by special-purpose local governments known as hospital districts, it was only natural that Bullock turned to IGTs as a vehicle for creative financing. At his urging, the state legislature passed a bill in 1989 requiring local hospital districts to transfer an assessment equal to 1 percent of their total local ad valorem taxes to the state's disproportionate share fund. The legislation also applied a similar assessment to several state-university teaching hospitals. The assessments were then paid back to the participating institutions, along with federal matching funds.

In 1990, Texas used more than $6 million in intergovernmental transfers, plus $7 million in state funds, to draw down $22 million in new federal funds, and distributed the total amount—$35 million—to 108 hospitals. Bullock championed this program throughout his campaign for lieutenant governor, and won the 1990 election handily. The program worked so well that the hospital districts readily agreed to expand it. In 1991, the legislature passed a bill increasing the assessment from 1 to 5 percent of local ad valorem tax revenues, and substantially raising the assessments on state hospitals as well. The expansion generated $52 million in new federal funds.[36]

Texas hospitals experienced a dramatic turnaround as a result of these creative financing mechanisms. Throughout the 1980s, Texas had led the nation in hospital closures.[37] But at the end of 1991, when *Modern Healthcare* released a list of the 20 most profitable public hospitals and hospital districts in the United States, six of the institutions listed were in Texas. According to the administrator of one hospital district, the "enhancement" of federal Medicaid payments had been "the major factor" contributing to the turnaround.[38]

CREATIVE FINANCING TRACED TO MATCHING GRANTS AND "MANDATE MADNESS"

Many of the earliest exploiters of Medicaid loopholes were relatively low-income Southern states. Shortly after West Virginia, Tennessee, Louisiana, and Texas adopted their innovative financing mechanisms, other states including Missouri, Kentucky, Georgia, South Carolina, and Alabama adopted similar programs. In part, this was because poorer states qualified for higher federal matching rates than did wealthier states, so the payoff was bigger. For example, high matching rates provided a strong incentive in Alabama, which qualified for a rate of 75 percent—among the highest in the nation. Alabama's state Medicaid director went around to health-care providers making presentations on how, with their participation, she could exploit Alabama's high matching rate. "One of our charts was a little bag of [hospital] money and then a big bag of [federal] money," she explained. "My job was to maximize as much federal resources as we could maximize."[39] Similarly, a study of Texas concluded that "perhaps the single most influential factor" in the state's adoption of tax and transfer mechanisms in the late 1980s and early 1990s was the steady rise in the state's federal matching rate—from 54 percent in 1986 to 64 percent in 1992—following a sharp decline in oil prices, which reduced the state's income relative to the national average.[40]

Moreover, during this period low-income Southern states were having an especially difficult time finding the resources to pay for the expanded coverage required by the steady stream of mandates emanating from Congress. Mandates were particularly problematic for low-income Southern states because they typically had to expand coverage from a much lower base, as one federal official explains.

Texas had an income eligibility level of 18 percent of federal poverty standards. Going from there to 100 is a lot bigger jump than it was in New York
when they were at 85 to begin with. And so the southern states in particular
got really hosed by all the Medicaid expansions of '88 to '90 and the creative
financing stuff was really the mechanism by which they came up with the
math. And if you look at the states that ultimately became the biggest DSH
players like Louisiana, and say, "Well, why Louisiana?" . . . the answer is because they had this huge fiscal problem that this was the only way to fix.[41]

Many state and NGA officials explicitly pointed to federal mandates as
the catalyst, and justification, for state financing mechanisms. In an interview, one state Medicaid director explained: "we 'stole' money hand over fist
from the federal government using the justification that it was a federal
law . . . We thought the feds should pay for it."[42] Similarly, NGA director of
human resources Alicia Pelrine noted that state budgets had been strained by
"five consecutive years of federally mandated Medicaid eligibility expansions," and that "in an effort to stay afloat," many states had turned to creative financing mechanisms "for help in feeding the voracious beast Medicaid had become" (Pelrine 1992, 23). This link between federal mandates and
state-maximization strategies—and the resulting programmatic expansion—is a striking example of what Brown and Sparer (2003) call "catalytic
federalism," and Nathan (2005) refers to as "federal pull / state push."
    The governors were not alone in believing that the states were somewhat
justified in taking advantage of legal loopholes. Some members of Congress,
among them Representative Donald Ritter (R-PA), acknowledged that federal mandates had precipitated the use of financing mechanisms.

How have we gotten into this horrendous situation? Because many in Congress have seen fit to push one Medicaid mandate after another to the point
of diminishing whatever flexibility the States had for dealing with this situation on their own . . . [T]he mandate madness . . . forces States to go around
the spirit of the law.[43]

Bruce Vladeck, a health-policy expert who would later serve as HCFA administrator during the Clinton years, called the abuse of legal loopholes a "fraud"
and a "scam," but argued that "given the indifference of the last 10 years of
the executive branch to the needs of the states and their Medicaid populations . . . I think it serves them right."[44] Others pointed out that the federal

government was ultimately to blame for allowing the loopholes to remain open. Don Moran, who had served in the Office of Management and Budget under President Reagan, remarked: "if my former colleagues were idiot enough to leave the stuff up on the table, [state officials] had a statutory and constitutional responsibility to try and get their hands on it."[45]

Yet despite repeated attempts by the Republican-controlled White House to take the money off the table by closing the legal and regulatory loopholes that made creative financing mechanisms possible, the governors successfully lobbied the Democrat-controlled Congress for protection. As early as 1987, Tennessee governor Ned McWherter began soliciting the help of Representative Jim Cooper (D-Tennessee), who sat on the health subcommittee of the House Commerce Committee.[46] Cooper, in turn, worked with subcommittee chairman Henry Waxman to secure passage of a moratorium prohibiting HCFA from passing any new regulations on provider donations and taxes for a year—which they quietly slipped into the Technical and Miscellaneous Revenue Act of 1988. When the moratorium expired in May 1989, Governor McWherter solicited the help of Senator Jim Sasser (D-Tennessee), chairman of the Senate Budget Committee. Together with Senate Finance Committee chairman Lloyd Bentsen (D-Texas), Sasser succeeded in convincing HCFA not to amend the regulation pending further congressional review—buying time until they and Henry Waxman could push through a renewal of the moratorium through the end of 1990 as part of the Omnibus Budget Reconciliation Act of 1989.[47]

The Health Care Financing Administration—by this time overseen by Republican President George H. W. Bush—was not amused by Congress's delay tactics. Concerns about the escalating federal share of Medicaid costs were heightened by the beginning of the 1990–1991 national recession and ballooning federal budget deficit, which was rapidly approaching $300 billion—the largest since World War II. As one HCFA official complained, the states' financing mechanisms "speedily got the protection of Henry Waxman because his theory was every dollar that goes to a Medicaid program, that's a good thing."[48]

However, as more states adopted creative financing mechanisms and the federal budget outlook darkened, it became increasingly clear to Waxman and others that the loopholes' days were numbered. Thus, in November 1990, during late-night budget negotiations, Waxman worked out a compromise with HCFA administrator Gail Wilensky: a final extension of the moratorium until January 1992, at which point HCFA could implement new regu-

lations. The consensus view of this compromise—part of the Omnibus
Budget Reconciliation Act of 1990—was that it would ultimately pave the
way for elimination of federal matching for donations, although the implications for taxes and transfers were less clear.

STATES HOP ABOARD THE MEDICAID GRAVY TRAIN

The one-year grace period was "a signal for those states not already on the
gravy train to hop aboard before it was too late."[49] As one state official explained, "The door of opportunity is not going to be open for very long, but
we wanted to get our foot in it. Our hope is that when they close the door,
they'll grandfather in those states that were already doing this."[50] HCFA began to receive a flood of new state Medicaid claims and, due to the moratorium, had no choice but to authorize the payments.

Because creative financing mechanisms allowed states to maintain or expand services without raising taxes despite the mounting budget crisis, they
appealed to governors, regardless of party or ideology. In Massachusetts, for
example, the administration of Democratic governor Michael Dukakis began setting up an enormous DSH mechanism at the end of 1990, right before
Republican William Weld took over in 1991. According to a state Medicaid
official who served under both governors, the maximization strategy was
"absolutely" independent of party politics.

> The project had already been initiated the summer before in the Medicaid
> bureau. But it wasn't ready for prime time before Dukakis walked out the
> door. So Weld got the credit for it when he came in the door . . . this DSH rev-
> enue would have happened regardless of who was Governor at the time.[51]

New Hampshire's Republican governor Judd Gregg—a self-described
"skin flint" who was preparing to run for Senate in 1992 on a campaign platform of fiscal conservatism—saw creative financing mechanisms as a way to
close the state's budget shortfall without raising taxes. According to one official, the Gregg administration first figured out how much federal revenue
they needed to plug the budget gap, and then set the hospital tax rate ac-
cordingly.[52] The result was an increase in New Hampshire's matching rate
from the statutory 50 percent to an effective rate of 159 percent (Gilman
1998, 161). Throughout 1991 and 1992, New Hampshire used creative financ-

ing mechanisms to collect more than $400 million in federal funds, of which only a small fraction went to expanding Medicaid coverage. As one Republican state legislator who helped devise the mechanism put it, "It was a scam, no question about it. We're funding our state judicial system, our highway program and everything else out of a Medicaid loophole."[53]

Creative financing mechanisms were equally appealing to Pennsylvania's Democratic governor, Bob Casey, a believer in activist government and universal health insurance. Under Governor Casey's leadership, the state collected $365 million from 165 hospitals, and used the funds to extract $380 million from the federal government.[54] The transaction was completed in a single day, and in many cases the donations did not even leave the hospitals' bank accounts. "It was just bookkeeping," explained the state's Medicaid director.[55] Since it had worked for hospitals, the state ran similar schemes for nursing homes, mental hospitals, and intermediate care facilities for the mentally retarded.

Due to their widespread appeal, creative financing mechanisms were soon in place in a majority of states. In 1990, only 6 states had provider tax and donation programs; by 1992, 39 states had such programs (Ku and Coughlin 1995). The annual growth rate of total Medicaid expenditures skyrocketed to 27 percent in 1991, and DSH payments—a major driver of overall growth—expanded at the astonishing rate of 390 percent.[56]

As the literature on policy diffusion suggests, cross-state networking among policy entrepreneurs, facilitated by professional associations representing state-government officials, often fosters the dissemination of new policy innovations (Walker 1969; Grupp and Richards 1975; Savage 1985; Gray 1994; Mintrom 1997; Mintrom and Vergari 1998; Balla 2001; Miller and Banaszak-Holl 2005). In fact, the National Governors Association—along with the National Association of Medicaid Directors—played a critical role in promoting the rapid diffusion of Medicaid maximization strategies in the late 1980s and early 1990s. By bringing together high-level state officials from around the country several times a year, these associations provided a national forum for sharing information. Knowledge was also disseminated by the law firm of Covington & Burling, which advised a growing number of states, as well as the NGA, on the legal and technical aspects of Medicaid maximization during this period. By virtue of being uniquely involved in issues related to provider taxes and donations, intergovernmental transfers, and disproportionate share hospital payments, the law firm developed detailed expertise in structuring creative financing mechanisms.[57]

Missouri provides a striking example of the importance of policy networks. The state's Republican governor, John Ashcroft, was very active in the National Governors Association—serving as vice chairman in 1990-91, and chairman in 1991-92—and encouraged members of his administration to network with their counterparts in other states as well. According to Donna Checkett, then director of the Missouri Division of Medical Services, NGA and NAMD meetings served as a clearinghouse for information on creative financing mechanisms. "We would attend these meetings with the sole purpose of learning about what other states were doing. If we learned that HCFA had allowed something for another state that meant we could adopt it, too. States that stayed home simply didn't have access to this information."[58]

In 1989, the NGA and Covington & Burling helped Missouri figure out how to use provider donations and DSH payments to structure a creative financing mechanism modeled on Tennessee's (Friar 1999). At first, Missouri implemented a relatively modest $10 million program, but as the economy deteriorated and the federal government continued to issue new mandates, the state collaborated with the Missouri Hospital Association on a major expansion designed to avoid slashing Medicaid payments to hospitals. In 1991, the state used $65 million in provider donations to secure nearly $200 million in additional federal funds.[59]

BUSH ADMINISTRATION PROPOSES NEW RULES

By the spring of 1991, the federal share of Medicaid spending was growing too fast for the Bush administration to ignore any longer. When aides informed budget director Richard Darman that quarterly reports from the states indicated that the budget he had sent to Congress only two months earlier had underestimated federal Medicaid spending by billions of dollars, he went "ballistic" and demanded to know "how this could possibly happen."[60] Darman formed a SWAT team of budget experts, which concluded that the main reason for the unexpected increase in federal spending was that states were using "schemes" to exploit the program's open-ended matching grants.[61] Meanwhile, Richard Kusserow, inspector general of the Department of Health and Human Services, issued a series of reports referring to the creative financing mechanisms as "open season on the U.S. Treasury," and warning that "the proliferation of these programs threatens to bankrupt the Medicaid program."[62] In congressional testimony, HCFA administrator Gail Wilensky concurred that requests for new federal funding were "coming in so fast we are having trouble figuring out what they are representing and how much money is involved. What has happened in the last two or three months is really beyond belief in terms of requests coming in from the Governors."[63] She explained that in theory:

> In a matching program those responsible for expenditure decisions and the direct fiscal management of the program must have a reasonable stake in program costs. The shared responsibility works to shape decisionmaking to contain costs [and acts] as a restraint on the otherwise open-ended Medicaid program.

In practice, however, Wilensky argued that the states' use of creative financing mechanisms was "undermining the basic premise that funding be shared through a Federal match of State monies."[64]

By this time President Bush had already begun to float a proposal—similar to Reagan's in 1981—to slow the growth of Medicaid spending by converting the program into a block grant. In so doing, Bush hoped to root out the problem at its source by eliminating the open-ended matching grants that made creative financing mechanisms possible. But, as in 1981, the governors immediately rejected the proposal as an attempt to shift Medicaid costs to the states. When President Bush resurrected another of Reagan's proposals—a cap on the growth of federal matching payments—in 1992, the governors vehemently protested again, and the proposal quickly died in Congress.

Stymied by the Democrat-controlled Congress, the Bush administration realized the best hope for Medicaid cost containment was to crack down on creative financing mechanisms using a regulatory approach. In August 1991, HHS secretary Louis Sullivan and HCFA administrator Gail Wilensky signed a draft regulation stipulating that donations from medical providers would no longer qualify for federal matching payments. Provider taxes would no longer qualify for matching unless those taxes applied to all hospitals, nursing homes, facilities for the mentally retarded, and outpatient clinics, and the revenue collected did not automatically flow back to the taxed institution. Additionally, the proposed regulation imposed constraints on the use of intergovernmental transfers as a source of the state share of Medicaid spending.

The draft regulation provoked bipartisan outrage at the annual meeting of the National Governors Association. Governor Jim Florio (D-New Jersey) protested that the White House was "changing the rules in the middle of the game," and that the proposed changes would "cause great hardships to our people."[65] Governor Norman Bangerter (R-Utah) urged his colleagues to take a united, bipartisan stand against the White House.

> I say that if we really want to get serious about some of these federal-state issues, we better start sitting down and getting a little bit tough and say, no, you are not going to do it to us one at a time. We are going to stand together. And if you want Medicaid program to be funded on that level on that basis, you better pick up the tab because we can't play in your game anymore.[66]

The Bush administration found the governors' reaction predictable; as one senior official put it: "They don't like losing money . . . We knew that from the beginning."[67] Nonetheless, President Bush sent several senior officials to the governors' meeting in an attempt to drum up support for the regulations. Thomas Scully, associate director of the Office of Management and Budget, reportedly "walked the halls of the convention center and tried to placate angry governors by offering to cut deals with individual states" (Pelrine 1992, 24). But the governors refused and, at the close of their meeting, passed a resolution calling on Congress to protect the states' use of creative financing mechanisms.

When the Bush administration formally issued the new regulations in September 1991, governors sprang into action. Governor John McKernan, chairman of the NGA's human resources committee, sent his colleagues a letter imploring them to write or call their congressional delegations and respective party leaders in Congress "to inform them of how severely impacted both your state's budget and Medicaid program will be if the interim final regulation goes into effect," while NGA chairman John Ashcroft sent the governors a fax warning that "unless the interim final rule for Medicaid donations and tax programs is changed, every state will be adversely impacted," and urging them to "encourage strong legislative action."[68] Governors began flooding Congress with letters and phone calls warning that the new rules, which were scheduled to go into effect in January 1992, would decimate state budgets.

Under pressure from the governors, the chairmen of the congressional committees and subcommittees with jurisdiction over Medicaid and the budget sent HCFA a letter requesting the withdrawal of the regulations, arguing that they violated congressional intent. When it became clear that the Bush administration was not going to retract the rules, Representative Waxman introduced a bill calling for another one-year extension of the moratorium on HCFA regulations. However, the White House signaled that President Bush would veto such a measure if Congress passed it, and the Senate Finance Committee rejected it as too lenient. As a committee staffer explained, the House, with its comparatively urban focus, tended to support more expansive Medicaid policies than did the Senate as "a way to get money into the big cities."[69] Instead, the Senate Finance Committee recommended a three-month "dual moratorium" which would freeze not only HCFA regulations, but also any changes to state programs while the White House and state leaders negotiated a permanent solution. Committee leaders made it clear that they would only consider legislation based on a negotiated deal between the Bush administration and the states. As Raymond Scheppach, executive director of the National Governors Association, explained in an interview, "most folks on Capitol Hill didn't know much about Medicaid, so they figured if both sides could agree on a compromise, Congress would go along with it."[70]

The governors were divided. States that had not yet adopted creative financing mechanisms complained that the dual moratorium would prevent them from doing so. Those that had developed the most aggressive financing mechanisms were also disappointed, since Waxman's moratorium would have allowed them to continue for at least another year. However, many governors who had been struggling to manage the budget process in a difficult and highly uncertain environment were relieved that federal Medicaid policy would be clarified within a few months. Besides, many governors—particularly Republicans—liked the idea of negotiating with the White House instead of dealing with the Democrat-controlled Congress, which they resented for having imposed the series of mandates that had contributed to the states' budget problems. As executive-branch officials, some governors were generally distrustful of the legislative process, and predisposed to working with the federal executive branch.[71]

"EXECUTIVE FEDERALISM"

In mid-October, the Bush administration, represented by Gail Wilensky of HCFA and Thomas Scully of OMB, invited the National Governors Association to negotiate a compromise, on the premise that a deal reached with the governors "would carry the necessary political weight to prevail in legislation."[72] Other stakeholders excluded from the negotiations—such as the National Conference of State Legislatures, National Association of Counties, and groups representing Medicaid providers and beneficiaries—nervously awaited the outcome with the understanding that any agreement reached by the administration and the governors would surely be enacted by Congress. The governors' ability to directly negotiate the terms of federal policy with the White House, largely sidelining Congress and state legislatures, was a striking example of the rise of "executive federalism" in U.S. health policy (Gais and Fossett 2005).

The administration's desire to negotiate exclusively with the NGA underscored the governors' unique position of strength, particularly as the 1992 elections approached. By the fall of 1991, George H. W. Bush's reelection campaign was well underway, and his administration was feeling the pressure to remain on friendly terms with the governors—as one senior advisor explained.

> There was this strange kind of relationship with the governors . . . Bush [was] counting on the governors to develop the support [he] needed in those states. So those were always very interesting times in terms of negotiating . . . it was an enormously difficult issue for us in terms of keeping the governors happy . . . it was very tough for Bush who very much wanted to keep those guys in line.[73]

The governors told the White House that the continued flow of federal Medicaid payments was "a matter of political survival" as they prepared for their own reelection bids.[74]

The governors' negotiating team—comprised of NGA executive director Raymond Scheppach, NGA director of human resources Alicia Pelrine, NGA chairman John Ashcroft, and vice chairman Roy Romer, with the law firm Covington & Burling serving as informal counsel—faced the unenviable task of representing the divergent needs of 50 unique states that had developed a wide array of creative financing programs based on taxes, donations, or intergovernmental transfers. The team also sought to represent the interests of states that did not yet have creative financing programs, or had only developed small programs and wanted to be allowed to adopt or expand them before the window of opportunity closed.

Concerns that the NGA would not represent their states' unique interests led many governors to consider taking the Bush administration to court to prevent implementation of the regulations. Indeed, after HCFA leaked its interim rule in August, Covington & Burling had begun "collecting" states as clients, and when HCFA formally announced its rule in September, the firm began preparing a lawsuit on behalf of nearly 20 states.[75] Although many observers predicted that such a challenge would succeed in court, most states ultimately decided not to pursue litigation, feeling that the risks outweighed the potential benefits. Some state officials feared that if they sued the administration, they might get cut out of any deal that evolved from the NGA's negotiations with the White House. Others worried that a protracted legal battle would create too much uncertainty, interfering with the budget process and disrupting health-care service delivery.[76]

Concerns about how their states might fare under a negotiated settlement also led many governors to solicit special side deals during the negotiation process. Some states called in requests to the NGA's negotiating team. According to executive director Raymond Scheppach, "states would call in saying 'I need this,' and if it didn't cost a heck of a lot of money, we could sell it to the Administration."[77] Others, particularly Republicans, went straight to the administration. In early November, six Republican governors held a teleconference with Thomas Scully and pleaded for relief, complaining that they would have to call their legislatures back into session to deal with new limits on provider taxes and donations. The Bush administration agreed to push back phase-out deadlines for provider donation and tax programs to protect Alabama, West Virginia, and several other states. The administration also allowed a number of states, including Ohio and Connecticut, to create last-minute tax or donation programs, which would be grandfathered in. Observers depicted the administration's negotiating stance as "cutting deals state-by-state," and described HCFA Administrator Gail Wilensky as having her "checkbook" out.[78]

Other governors lobbied Congress—and particularly the Senate Finance Committee—for amendments that would benefit their states even before the NGA and Bush administration had reached a deal. In testimony before the Senate Finance Committee, Democratic governor Ann Richards of Texas warned that a negotiated agreement that did not protect the states' prerogative to fund Medicaid's nonfederal share with intergovernmental transfers would "cut the heart out of state budgets," and "break the hearts of real, live human beings who need the care that would have been provided under the existing rules."[79] She had a receptive audience in Senate Finance Committee chairman Lloyd Bentsen—a fellow Democrat and Texan. Republican governors were also quite influential with the fiscally conservative committee, as a committee staffer explained in an interview.

> Well, the scams of course had them outraged in the committee in terms of what the states were doing in terms of gaming us. But you also had a growing number of Republican governors . . . very, very outspoken Republican governors who—you know, had some sway. [They] essentially wanted absolute flexibility and no restrictions.[80]

Many governors got their states' senators to help them lobby the Finance Committee for side deals. As Senator Warren Rudman (R-New Hampshire) explained, "My attitude was that if that's the way the game is played, we'll play it too. If we were going to have this loophole, I wasn't going to see New Hampshire stand idly by." An aide recalls that Senator Rudman "argued it with the Finance Committee staff" on the logic that "any time we could do something for the state we were happy. This happened to be big."[81] Senator Rudman got the committee to agree to protect his state's tax program through 1993, allowing the state to collect an additional $367 million in federal funds over two years, of which only $44 million went to hospitals; the other $323 million went to plugging a hole in the state budget.[82]

MEDICAID VOLUNTARY CONTRIBUTION AND PROVIDER-SPECIFIC TAX AMENDMENTS OF 1991

After a closed-door negotiation process described by participants as "torpid," "rancorous," and characterized by "rampant distrust" and accusations of "bad faith," the Bush administration and the NGA announced a tentative agreement in November 1991 (Pelrine 1992, 25). In a letter to the governors, the NGA negotiating team noted that the Senate Finance Committee continued to have a "strong preference" for an agreement between the governors and the administration, and that the legislative clock was winding down, concluding: "This is our last, best opportunity to reach a settlement before Congress adjourns."[83] Within two days, the NGA had garnered the support of a supermajority of governors. As Raymond Scheppach observed, the governors' ability to "get around the uniformity problem" by negotiat-

ing individual side deals with Congress and the White House had been critical to reaching agreement.[84]

Congress quickly turned the compromise into legislation in the final 48
hours of the 1991 congressional session. The Senate approved the NGA-
administration agreement—with numerous amendments reflecting the side
deals that had been worked out in advance—on November 26, and the
House-Senate Conference Committee approved the plan the next day. The
provisions of the legislation—known as the Medicaid Voluntary Contribution and Provider-Specific Tax Amendments of 1991—are outlined below.

Provider donations: The legislation ended federal matching for provider
donations, effective January 1, 1992. However, it included a grandfather provision allowing states with preexisting donation programs to
continue those programs for six months to a year and a half longer,
depending on the state's fiscal year and the frequency of its budget
cycle.

Provider-specific taxes: The legislation required taxes to meet several new
criteria in order to qualify for federal matching: they must be broad-
based and applied uniformly to all providers in a class, they must not
have a "hold harmless" provision; that is, states could not provide
"credits, exclusions, or deductions that have as their purpose or effect
the return to providers of all or a portion of the tax paid," and they
could not comprise more than 25 percent of the state share. However,
a grandfather provision gave states with preexisting tax programs
time to comply with the new limits.

Intergovernmental transfers: The legislation included no limits on intergovernmental transfers, and prohibited HCFA from imposing limits,
specifying that "the Secretary may not restrict States' use of funds
where such funds are derived from State or local taxes (or funds appropriated to State university teaching hospitals) transferred from or
certified by units of government within a State as the non-Federal
share of expenditures under this title, regardless of whether the unit
of government is also a health care provider."[85]

Disproportionate share hospital payments: The legislation repealed the
prohibition against setting an upper payment limit on disproportionate share hospital payments. Starting in fiscal year 1993, DSH payments would be limited to 12 percent of total Medicaid spending.
However, "high DSH states"—those already above 12 percent—would

continue to receive their 1992 allotment, while "low DSH states" were allowed to phase in increases gradually.

The outcome was a mixed bag for the governors. On the one hand, many states had secured very generous transition provisions, and Texas and other states with intergovernmental transfer programs had clearly won an important victory. On the other hand, many observers felt the governors' desire to avoid short-run budget uncertainty had caused them to "cave in," especially given that the interim final regulations might have been successfully challenged in court.[86] Henry Waxman lambasted the Bush administration for putting the governors in an "untenable position." While acknowledging that they had "acted understandably" to avoid budget uncertainty, and that the negotiated agreement would serve them well financially in the "very short run," Waxman lamented that it would "do a great deal of disservice" to millions of poor, vulnerable Americans in the long run.[87]

Even after Congress passed the 1991 amendments, negotiations between the governors and the White House continued. As Alicia Pelrine of the NGA explained, the Office of Management and Budget had "seized control of the regulation writing process and wanted to interpret the law as literally and strictly as possible" (Pelrine 1992). For example, Arizona had negotiated an exemption from the 25 percent tax ceiling, yet in the spring of 1992 Governor Fife Symington found himself—accompanied by several members of his state's congressional delegation—at the White House, defending the legitimacy of his state's provider tax. In the end, he only got about half the $84 million in federal funds he sought.[88]

Many states also went to the White House seeking reversals of HCFA disallowances of tax and donation programs that had been deemed inconsistent with the new rules. As the 1992 presidential election approached, the White House was increasingly amenable to handing out special favors. In October 1992, Maryland's Democratic governor, William Schaefer, succeeded in convincing President Bush to release $75 million in payments that had been disallowed by HCFA; shortly thereafter, Schaefer endorsed Bush's reelection campaign. According to a Bush administration official, the election was the driving factor behind these deals—"these were political, not budgetary decisions."[89]

The side deals continued after Bush lost the election, and former governor Bill Clinton entered the White House. In February 1993, New Jersey's Democratic governor, Jim Florio—a prominent Clinton supporter who was preparing for his own reelection bid—made a personal pitch to the president and HHS secretary Donna Shalala. HCFA subsequently released $412 million in disputed Medicaid payments to the state. A HCFA official said the decision to release the funds had been made "at the highest level" of the administration.[90]

STATES EXPLOIT REMAINING LOOPHOLES

The 1991 amendments did not put an end to the states' use of creative financing mechanisms. Finding it difficult to establish provider tax and donation programs that met the new criteria, many states turned to intergovernmental transfer programs, which remained unregulated, in combination with DSH payments, which had been only loosely limited by the 1991 amendments. Almost overnight, dozens of states began transferring funds from state university hospitals and other public institutions to the state's general fund. One study of creative financing mechanisms in 39 states found that IGT revenue grew from $183 million in 1991 to $2.6 billion in 1994—an increase of roughly 1,300 percent (Ku and Coughlin 1995).

The intergovernmental transfer programs adopted by two states in particular soon began making headline news. In February 1993, North Carolina used $100 million in intergovernmental transfers from four state-run mental hospitals to qualify for nearly $200 million in federal matching funds. The federal funds were then deposited in the state's general fund, where they were used for schools, libraries, and other non-health programs.[91] In defense of the scheme, one state legislator explained that "if we don't get [the money], some other state will."[92] Shortly thereafter, Michigan secured $276 million in federal funds through an intergovernmental transfer to the state-owned University of Michigan hospital, which transferred the money back to the state the very same day. The state's Medicaid director explained the rationale in an interview.

> No one would ever claim that this was good public policy. But it was a legal thing to do, and from a state perspective we were really compelled to do these things. If you didn't you could be accused of . . . misfeasance for not having taken advantage of getting all the federal money the state was entitled to . . . as state officials representing the taxpayers of the state of Michigan we really had an obligation to do these things.[93]

Federal officials were aware of the growing abuse of intergovernmental transfers, but did not attempt to regulate them. Congress had restricted HCFA's authority to do so in the 1991 amendments, reaffirming the legality of transfers under the original 1965 Medicaid law. Moreover, the Clinton administration recognized that state and local governments had developed unique arrangements for sharing Medicaid costs, and that certain states—such as Texas—where health-care services for the poor were largely delivered by local hospital districts would be greatly harmed by such regulations.[94] As HCFA administrator Bruce Vladeck put it, "If we're serious about federalism, it's none of our goddamn business how the state raises money."[95]

Congress did rein in the creative use of DSH payments, however, as it was becoming increasingly apparent that some states were not using the DSH program for its intended purpose of providing financial assistance to safety-net providers. One study of DSH programs in 39 states in 1993 found that states were retaining one-third of DSH funds for other purposes (Ku and Coughlin 1995). Another study found that although DSH subsidies are associated with improved health outcomes for the poor, their impact is limited by the ability of state officials to divert the funds (Baicker and Staiger 2005). In August 1993, Congress included provisions in the Omnibus Budget Reconciliation Act of 1993 imposing new limits on the types of facilities that could receive DSH payments, and capping the amount of DSH payments any given facility could receive. However, a few days after signing the budget bill into law, President Clinton, under intense pressure from the governors, relaxed the ceiling on DSH payments at a cost of several billion dollars.

Creative use of the DSH program continued, and by 1996, DSH payments accounted for 1 out of every 11 dollars spent on Medicaid (Coughlin and Zuckerman 2002). In 1997, Congress again sought to impose tighter limits on the program. The Balanced Budget Act of 1997 (BBA 1997) established state-specific DSH allotments that were lower than had been permitted under previous law. However, under pressure from state officials, Congress gave special treatment to several states including Louisiana, New Jersey, and California. Federal policy makers had also grown increasingly concerned that the states were using DSH funds for purposes other than health care. Thus, BBA 1997 also placed an explicit ban on the use of federal matching payments for "roads, bridges, stadiums, or any other item or service not covered under a State [Medicaid] plan."[96]

Many states made up for the lost federal revenue by exploiting a loophole in the upper payment limit (UPL), which had been the basis for the states' very first creative financing mechanism—as noted at the beginning of this chapter. In the mid-1980s, many states had made large payments to state-owned or -operated hospitals, but small payments to private hospitals, so that the total amount did not exceed the aggregate upper payment limit. In 1987, the Health Care Financing Administration had responded by issuing a regulation establishing a separate UPL for state hospitals. However, HCFA had neglected to establish an upper payment limit for local hospitals. Thus, in the late 1990s, a growing number of states began paying local-government facilities at much higher rates than private facilities. The local-government facilities then returned the excessive payments to the state treasury through an intergovernmental transfer. By 2000, this practice was costing the federal government $3.7 billion per year.[97]

In January 2001, HCFA—which by this time had been renamed the Centers for Medicare and Medicaid Services—issued a new regulation establishing upper payment limits for county and city facilities. However, a number of states successfully lobbied for special loopholes. Eighteen states were permitted to phase out their UPL mechanisms over a transition period of up to eight years. Meanwhile, Congress, under pressure from state officials, offset revenue losses due to the closing of the UPL loophole by postponing the DSH cuts scheduled for 2001 and 2002 under the Balanced Budget Act of 1997.

CONCLUSION

Medicaid's open-ended matching grants are an "invitation to fiscal entrepreneurship by the states," particularly during times of fiscal stress (Thompson and Fossett 2008, 161). In the late 1980s and early 1990s, the mounting pressures of federal mandates and a national recession prompted state officials to develop a wide array of creative financing mechanisms involving provider donations, provider-specific taxes, intergovernmental transfers, disproportionate-share hospital payments, and upper payment limits. Although federal policy makers have narrowed many of these loopholes, their use persists to this day—albeit on a smaller scale than in the early 1990s (Coughlin, Zuckerman, and McFeeters 2007). Indeed, in 2004, the Office of Management and Budget reported that:

Medicaid's open-ended financing structure encourages efforts to draw down Federal matching funds in any way possible, some of which are not appropriate. These financing practices undermine the Federal-State partnership and jeopardize the financial stability of the Medicaid program.[98]

Rather than closing the loopholes, federal lawmakers have repeatedly bowed to political pressure from the powerful intergovernmental lobby.

The escalation of creative financing mechanisms in the late 1980s and early 1990s had two important implications for the subsequent direction of Medicaid policy. First, federal efforts to narrow legal loopholes meant that states that had come to rely heavily on creative financing mechanisms had to either scale back coverage, or find a new source of funding. Many states chose the latter approach, and applied for "research and demonstration waivers" as a means of securing additional federal funds—as is discussed in chapter 6. Second, as a congressional staffer explained in an interview, creative financing mechanisms "made the overall financing of the program less stable" and thus "set up the program to be scrutinized for reform."[99] In particular, the rapid escalation of federal Medicaid costs in the early 1990s increased interest among federal policy makers in converting Medicaid from an open-ended matching grant to a block grant—the subject of chapter 7.

CHAPTER 6

Waivers in the Clinton Era

THE EARLY 1990S were trying times for state Medicaid programs. The combination of federal mandates, a national recession, and the tightening of the legal loopholes that had permitted states to develop creative financing mechanisms—as discussed in chapter 5—meant that the states simultaneously had to cope with the explosive growth of expenditures, and the loss of billions of dollars of federal funds.

It might seem that such financial pressures would lead the states to cut optional eligibility groups and services, and indeed, some did. But a surprising number of states responded by voluntarily expanding coverage—in some cases, to hundreds of thousands of people—in an effort to secure additional federal matching funds to meet the growing need for health care. The main vehicle used to expand coverage during this period was research and demonstration waivers, which permit states to circumvent federal Medicaid rules in order to experiment with alternative approaches to health coverage. These waivers enabled state-level policy entrepreneurs to exploit Medicaid's open-ended financing mechanism in creative new ways, bringing in hundreds of millions of new federal matching dollars.

RESEARCH AND DEMONSTRATION WAIVERS

Research and demonstration waivers predate the creation of the Medicaid program by several years. In 1962, President John F. Kennedy urged Congress to allow the states more freedom to tailor their welfare programs such as Aid to Families with Dependent Children in response to an alarmingly high national poverty rate. In an impassioned speech, he argued that the difficulty of the problems the nation faced required imaginative solutions, and that the federal government should "encourage experimental, pilot, or demonstration projects that would promote the objectives of the assistance titles [of the Social Security Act] and help make our welfare programs more flexible and adaptable to local needs."[1]

That year, Congress added to the Social Security Act a new provision—section 1115—which allowed the secretary of the U.S. Department of Health and Human Services to waive requirements for a state's compliance with federal statutory and regulatory provisions governing state-administered welfare programs to allow experimentation. Specifically, the provision stated that

> in the case of any experimental, pilot, or demonstration project which, in the judgment of the Secretary, is likely to assist in promoting the objectives [of a welfare program] the Secretary may waive compliance with any of the requirements [of that program] to the extent and for the period he finds necessary to enable such State or States to carry out such project.

Moreover, the provision specified that state spending to implement a demonstration project that would not otherwise qualify for federal matching payments would qualify for such payments "to the extent and for the period prescribed by the Secretary."[2] A few years later, when Congress created Medicaid, it amended section 1115 to specify its applicability to that program.

Federal lawmakers apparently intended for section 1115 to be beneficent, but narrow (Williams 1994). In his speech to Congress, President Kennedy noted that demonstration projects might "not come cheaply" and warned the states against using waivers to make "ruthless and arbitrary cutbacks."[3] Similarly, during congressional hearings, no lawmaker or witness suggested that section 1115 might be used to reduce eligibility or services. However, Senate reports suggested that projects should focus on limited geographical areas and limited time frames, and that the secretary should avoid duplication of a project across multiple states.

Research and demonstration waivers allowed states to secure federal financial assistance for coverage expansions that would otherwise not qualify for matching payments. For instance, states could use waivers to extend coverage to an otherwise ineligible population, such as adults without small children, or to offer a narrow set of benefits to a target population, such as family-planning services for women with incomes too high to qualify for the full package of covered services. A state can also get permission to cap enrollment of the population covered under the waiver to avoid the financial risk that accompanies an open-ended entitlement. In addition, waivers permit states to enroll Medicaid beneficiaries in managed-care delivery systems without regard to certain contracting requirements under federal law.

In Medicaid's early years, demonstration projects tended to be limited in scope—focusing on, for instance, the introduction of school-based early periodic screening, diagnosis, and treatment (EPSDT) services, or home-based long-term care for subgroups of the Medicaid population (Vladeck 1995; Schneider 1997). In fact, prior to 1982, not a single state implemented a comprehensive statewide research and demonstration waiver. However, over time, mounting financial pressures created incentives for states to devise new and far-ranging experiments.

ARIZONA HEALTH CARE COST CONTAINMENT SYSTEM[4]

In 1982, Arizona revolutionized the use of the research and demonstration waiver. At the time, Arizona was the only state that had not yet adopted a Medicaid program. As one federal official explained in an interview, the politically conservative state "just did not want to have any part of Medicaid . . . for various reasons, including not wanting to have to contribute to the costs of care for their Native American population."[5] Instead, Arizona had come to rely on county governments to deliver health care for the poor. But as demand for long-term care increased, medical cost inflation soared, and state revenues dwindled, Arizona's counties began to run into serious financial difficulties. Between 1975 and 1980, county spending on health care more than doubled from $59 million to $123 million, and soon ate up as much as half of some counties' budgets.[6] The budget crisis only intensified after 1980, when a taxpayer revolt led the state to adopt a constitutional amendment limiting property-tax increases.

County officials lobbied the state to adopt a Medicaid program throughout the 1970s, criticizing state lawmakers for forgoing hundreds of millions of dollars in federal aid and pointing out that Arizona residents were paying federal taxes to support other states' Medicaid programs without benefitting from the program themselves. In 1974, lawmakers succumbed to pressure and passed legislation authorizing a Medicaid program, but Republican lawmakers repeatedly refused to appropriate any state funds. However, by the early 1980s, it had become clear that the situation was untenable. In January

1981, the state's Democratic governor, Bruce Babbitt, warned the legislature that without an infusion of federal and state funds, the counties would be bankrupt within two years. Under pressure from the governor and county officials, Republicans were finally "dragged, clawing and howling" into allocating state funds for the program.[7]

Arizona's Republican-controlled legislature did not want to adopt a traditional Medicaid program for fear that it would turn into a "bottomless pit" of state spending.[8] Thus, in May 1982, the state applied for a waiver to receive federal matching funds for a program of its own creation, designed to deliver fiscal relief to counties while minimizing financial risk to the state (Brecher 1984). The Reagan administration shared the state's interest in experimenting with new ways to contain Medicaid costs, and thus was willing to negotiate a special arrangement. The state's waiver request was approved in July 1982 and implemented in October of that year.

The plan, known as the Arizona Health Care Cost Containment System (AHCCCS, pronounced "access") differed from the typical Medicaid program in several respects. The state used a competitive bidding process to select private managed-care providers, and paid them based on a capitation system. The state also limited certain services, such as nursing-home care and family-planning services, and required beneficiaries to make copayments. Despite its high start-up costs, the program began to deliver cost savings as it matured, enabling the state to gradually extend coverage to include additional groups and services over time (McCall et al. 1994).

Arizona's use of the research and demonstration waiver was a dramatic departure from what President Kennedy and Congress had envisioned in 1962. For one thing, the program was not temporary; the federal government has repeatedly renewed Arizona's waiver to keep the program running for the past three decades. Moreover, the scale of the demonstration was enormous; AHCCCS covered 1.35 million people as of 2011.[9] As one federal official notes, "The Arizona Medicaid program was not a pilot or demonstration project in the original use of the term [but] it's very elastic language and they are running with it as far as they can to advance their policy agenda."[10]

BUDGET NEUTRALITY

The Arizona experiment led the Reagan administration to overhaul the waiver process, as the administration realized that large-scale, permanent, and costly programs such as Arizona's would require more oversight than the federal Health Care Financing Administration (HCFA) had traditionally provided. In fact, HCFA had never established any formal guidelines for reviewing waiver applications, or estimating and tracking their costs (Andersen 1994). HCFA subsequently began to require more supporting information and documentation from the states.

Moreover, fearing that the states might use waivers to experiment in ways that would deplete the federal treasury, the Office of Management and Budget (OMB) in 1983 introduced a principle known as "budget neutrality," which specified that a waiver must not lead to greater federal Medicaid spending than would have occurred in the absence of the waiver. To enforce the budget neutrality provision, OMB required any state that wanted a research and demonstration waiver to agree to a cap on federal Medicaid payments. Following the adoption of these reforms, waiver activity declined precipitously (Dobson, Moran, and Young 1992). Many state officials simply did not want to accept the increased financial risk that would accompany a cap on federal matching funds. Those states that did apply for waivers were often denied, particularly if the application included a significant expansion of coverage. Indeed, for more than a decade following Arizona's experiment, not a single statewide waiver was approved (fig. 5).

The additional red tape was a major source of irritation for the governors, and increasingly so in the late 1980s and early 1990s as federal mandates and a deteriorating economy increased the states' demand for flexibility and federal funding. With a mounting sense of urgency, governors of both parties pressed federal leaders for "an expedited process for granting waivers in the medical field so that the states may immediately begin to address the problems using innovative ways to improve health care delivery for our citizens."[11] Arkansas's Democratic governor, Bill Clinton, was a particularly vocal critic of the virtually insurmountable hurdles to acquiring a waiver, complaining that after "two years of back and forth" the Reagan administration had rejected his waiver request as too expensive.[12] Upon winning the 1992 presidential election, Clinton's frustration with the waiver process was still fresh in his mind. As a Clinton administration official later explained in an interview, "When he became President years later he remembered that. And one of his objectives that was articulated right off the bat . . . was to get those [OMB and HCFA] people out of the way."[13]

On February 1, 1993—less than two weeks after taking office—the new Democratic president met with the governors at the White House for three

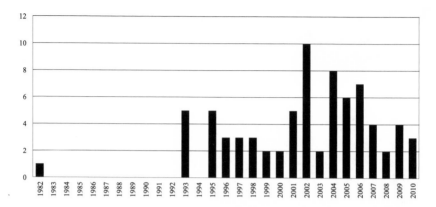

Fig. 5. Number of comprehensive statewide Medicaid demonstration waivers approved by year, 1982–2010. There were no comprehensive statewide demonstration waivers prior to 1982. (Data from U.S. Department of Health and Human Services.)

and a half hours—an extraordinarily long time by the standards of previous presidents. Calling federal Medicaid rules "Byzantine and counterproductive," Clinton noted that "for years and years and years, governors have been screaming for relief from a cumbersome process by which the federal government has micromanaged the health care system affecting poor Americans."[14] He expressed hope that state experimentation could lead to both expanded coverage and cost savings, noting that "states very often believe that they can provide more services at lower costs if we didn't impose our rules and regulations on them."[15]

Following his meeting with the governors, President Clinton announced several revisions to the waiver process, including limits on HCFA's ability to request additional information from the states, as well as automatic approval of certain types of waiver requests such as those copying another state's successful program. He also ordered HCFA to consult with the National Governors Association and develop additional recommendations to streamline the waiver process. Governors of both parties expressed elation as they left the White House, noting that the president's experience as a governor "on the front line" had increased his "sensitivity" to the states' interests.[16]

Support for liberalization of the waiver process was also growing among congressional leaders of both parties. Many Democrats in Congress hoped that relaxing the waiver policy would help states expand health coverage for the poor. Senate majority leader George Mitchell (D-Maine) explained that based on "a significant number of meetings with individual Governors and groups of Governors," he had come to conclude that "there ought to be a liberal waiver policy" to help the states "meet the health care needs of their citizens."[17] Meanwhile, many Republican members hoped that state experimentation might yield cost savings, helping to reduce the ballooning federal deficit. However, others expressed skepticism about the potential for an expedited waiver process to lower the program's cost. Outgoing HCFA administrator Gail Wilensky predicted that "What the president will find out is that a lot of what the states want to do costs money."[18]

Indeed, during the NGA-HCFA consultations that took place in the spring and summer of 1993, the governors' top goal was liberalization of the budget neutrality provision. Following President Clinton's orders, HCFA complied with this and other demands. Thus, in addition to agreeing to provide early consultation and additional technical assistance, and to commit the internal resources necessary for a "sound and expeditious review" (within 90 days if possible), the administration announced that it would abandon the traditional, stringent approach to budget neutrality. Specifically, it would "assess cost neutrality over the life of a demonstration project, not on a year-by-year basis, since many demonstrations involve making 'upfront' investments in order to achieve out-year savings." Moreover, recognizing the "difficulty of making appropriate baseline projections of Medicaid expenditures," the administration declared itself "open to development of a new methodology in that regard."[19]

At the annual meeting of the National Governors Association in August 1993, NGA chairman Carroll Campbell (R-South Carolina) proclaimed that after "nearly six months' negotiations between the states and the administration" and "some very tough talks," the governors had "not gotten everything that we need to make the waiver process user friendly, but we have gotten a lot."[20] The governors' ability to negotiate significant federal policy changes with the White House was—like the negotiations over creative financing mechanisms a few years earlier—another striking example of the growing prominence of "executive federalism" in U.S. health policy (Gais and Fossett 2005).

THE OREGON HEALTH PLAN

Oregon was the first state to apply for a waiver from the Clinton administration. Throughout the late 1980s and early 1990s, Oregon had repeatedly tried to secure a waiver from President George H. W. Bush's administration in order to experiment with a new approach to health coverage for low-income residents. At that time, Oregon's Medicaid plan capped eligibility at 58 percent of the federal poverty level, leaving hundreds of thousands of low-income Oregonians uninsured. Even so, the state still struggled to pay the program's growing and volatile cost—particularly as the economy deteriorated. A series of budget crises forced the state to dump tens of thousands of enrollees from the program, which in turn led increasing numbers of the uninsured to turn up in emergency rooms, requiring acute care for conditions that could have been avoided with less expensive preventive care.

In 1989, Oregon state senate president—and, later, governor—John Kitzhaber, a Democrat and former emergency-room doctor who had witnessed these problems firsthand, developed a proposal to cover more people by covering fewer services than were required under federal Medicaid law. As Kitzhaber explained, "everyone deserves to be in the health-care lifeboat," but "if we can agree that society cannot afford to buy everything for everyone who might conceivably benefit from it, then we have to develop a process to determine what level of care everyone should have access to."[21] Under the proposal, the state would draw up a prioritized list of services, with low-cost, preventive, or "essential" services—such as mammograms and immunizations, near the top, and costlier or "less important" services—such as organ transplants and treatment for certain terminal cancers considered unresponsive to medical care, near the bottom. When preparing each year's budget, state lawmakers would decide how much money to allocate for Medicaid, and then draw a line on the prioritized list below which the state would not pay for services—thereby both trimming and stabilizing annual Medicaid appropriations. Kitzhaber hoped to use the resulting savings to expand coverage to all state residents below the federal poverty level—an additional 120,000 people.[22]

Although the plan enjoyed strong support from the Oregon Medical Association, organized labor, organized business, the general public, and state lawmakers—having passed almost unanimously in both houses of the state legislature—the Bush administration had rejected Oregon's waiver application in 1992. One problem was that Oregon's plan was expensive, at least in the short run, due to the proposed coverage expansion. Oregon officials estimated that covering an additional 120,000 people would cost the state an extra $95 million, and the federal government an extra $110 million in matching payments over the program's first five years—a sizeable cost increase compared to the $350 million total annual cost of the state's existing Medicaid program. Moreover, the Bush administration had been skeptical about the projected long-term cost savings, and thus the budget neutrality, of the demonstration project, and concerned that approving the program would lead other states to request similar waivers, draining the federal treasury. As one administration official explained: "The general view is it's interesting. We'd like to do it. But there's a fundamental problem. The state contribution comes up short by probably a couple of hundred million dollars."[23] Oregon's proposal was also politically controversial—triggering a national debate over the rationing of medical care, and leading advocates for the disabled to argue that it discriminated against them—a political hot potato that the Bush administration hoped to avoid touching in an election year.

Oregon's luck changed in 1993, when Democrat Bill Clinton took office after twelve years of Republicans in the White House. Recognizing a window of opportunity, Democratic governor Barbara Roberts resurrected Oregon's waiver application, and pushed the Clinton administration to approve it under the newly liberalized waiver process. In particular, Oregon officials took advantage of the Clinton administration's agreement to evaluate cost neutrality over five years, arguing that lower spending growth in later years would compensate for higher spending in earlier years. Moreover, Oregon officials insisted on using not only the state savings, but also the federal savings to finance expanded coverage. As one HCFA official put it, "we were enormously pressed" by Oregon, which wanted to "use the savings from the waivers to add patients to the waivers," adding that Oregon officials were "torturing us endlessly" to cover more people.[24]

The Clinton administration approved Oregon's waiver request on March 20, 1993. Under the five-year experiment, all poor Oregonians would qualify for Medicaid—thereby increasing the state's Medicaid rolls by 50 percent, from 240,000 to 360,000. Oregon quickly passed a ten-cent-per-pack tax on cigarettes to fund the state share of the cost; implementation began on February 1, 1994.

Fears about the rationing of health care turned out to be misplaced (Bodenheimer 1997). Contrary to expectations, the benefit package covered by the Oregon Health Plan was more generous and comprehensive than the package covered under the state's previous Medicaid plan, and even superior to private insurance in Oregon in many respects (Oberlander, Marmor, and Jacobs 2001, 1585). Rationing did not occur for several reasons. First, health-care providers found ways to evade the rules, such as diagnosing patients suffering from illnesses not covered under the prioritized list with comorbidities covered under the prioritized list. Second, the federal government limited the state's flexibility in scaling back services in response to fiscal pressures. For example, in 1996, the Clinton administration denied the state permission to cut several services from the covered list, warning that "further reductions in services would result in a benefit package that would not be sufficiently comprehensive to meet the basic needs of the Medicaid population" (Leichter 1999, 154). Third, the political controversy around rationing forced state officials to make concessions and move services up the list "by hand" to appease constituents (Oberlander, Marmor, and Jacobs 2001, 1586).

Largely due to the lack of rationing, the Oregon Health Plan failed to deliver the enormous cost savings that state officials had hoped for. Estimates suggest that rationing only saved the state 2 percent of total expenditures in the first five years, relative to what the state would have spent under the pre-existing system, although moving patients into managed-care plans delivered additional cost savings (Jacobs, Marmor, and Oberlander 1999). Due to the negligible cost savings and political controversy surrounding Oregon's demonstration project, no other state has emulated its rationing model.

One promise the Oregon Health Plan did deliver on, however, was eligibility expansion. The demonstration project brought more than 100,000 newly eligible individuals into the Medicaid program, helping to lower the state's uninsured rate from 18 percent in 1990 to 11 percent in 1997, at a time when the national uninsured rate rose from 14 to 16 percent (Oberlander, Marmor, and Jacobs 2001, 1586).

For these reasons, the Oregon Health Plan proved to be costly. The cost of the state's Medicaid program nearly doubled from $1.3 billion to $2.4 billion between 1993 and 1999.[25] When the 2001 recession hit, the state was forced to scale back and ultimately close enrollment until 2008, when it introduced a lottery system in which more than 80,000 people competed for 3,000 slots in the plan (Oberlander 2007). Despite these challenges, the program continues to be significantly larger than before the reform, enrolling over 650,000 people, and covering a more comprehensive set of services.[26]

In short, a program that supporters had heralded as a cost-saving experiment and a beacon of American health policy for other states to emulate—

and that opponents had lambasted as a reprehensible attempt to cut costs by rationing care—turned out to be a fairly straightforward expansion of coverage financed through increased state funding and federal matching dollars. Once again, Medicaid's federal-state financing structure proved to be an engine of incremental expansion.

EXPANSIONARY INCENTIVES

Oregon was only the beginning; following the Clinton administration's revision of the waiver process, the applications began pouring in. As one HCFA official put it, "all the states had gotten the message: Okay, this is an administration that is willing to work with you. And it turned out that there was pent-up demand to do various things."[27] In addition to Oregon, four other states—Hawaii, Kentucky, Rhode Island, and Tennessee—applied for and received Medicaid waivers in 1993. Since then, states have submitted several statewide research and demonstration waiver applications each year, and the majority of these applications have been approved (fig. 5).

The states had powerful financial incentives to seek additional flexibility in administering their Medicaid programs to cope with the national recession, federal mandates, and other financial pressures of the early 1990s. As one state Medicaid director put it, "when it comes to waivers, it's a budget thing, it's how to save money . . . the tighter the finances, the more people are open to some innovation."[28] Three specific financial motives for seeking waivers were particularly common in the 1990s (Holahan et al. 1995). First, many states hoped to deliver services more efficiently—typically by replacing the traditional fee-for-service system with fixed capitation payments to managed-care plans—and use the potential savings to expand coverage to new populations normally ineligible for Medicaid matching dollars. Second, some states wanted to fold state-financed health-insurance programs into Medicaid in order to receive federal matching funds, but these programs provided coverage that conflicted with federal Medicaid rules. Third, as Congress began cracking down on creative financing schemes in the early 1990s, many states feared losing their disproportionate-share hospital payments, and hoped to use waivers to divert these federal funds from subsidizing hospitals to financing expansion of coverage.

Interestingly, the one thing the states did not seem interested in using waivers for was to scale back enrollment; in fact, most early waiver applications greatly expanded Medicaid eligibility.[29] A 1995 federal government report underscored the surprising fact that "while federal and state budgetary constraints highlight the urgency of containing costs, a number of states are pressuring to expand the program and enroll hundreds of thousands of new beneficiaries."[30] In part, the states' interest in waivers reflected a desire to reduce the rising uninsured rate. Facing balanced budget rules and strong voter opposition to higher taxes, state officials also saw waivers as a way to get additional federal money flowing into the state. Indeed, empirical evidence indicates that states with higher matching rates were more likely to apply for waivers in the 1990s—controlling for income, economic conditions, and other state characteristics—suggesting that the allure of additional federal funds was a significant consideration (Satterthwaite 2002).

The incentives to shift health-care costs to the federal government were so powerful that even progressive states with a demonstrated willingness to expand coverage at state taxpayers' expense—such as Minnesota and Hawaii—lined up for waivers. Throughout the early 1990s, Minnesota lawmakers struggled to expand coverage with the ultimate goal of providing universal health insurance. Although there was widespread support for broadening access to health care, lawmakers had strained to find a way to pay for it. The Clinton administration's liberalization of the waiver process enabled Minnesota to fold existing state-financed health-care programs into Medicaid and use the savings to expand coverage to a number of groups, including all adults up to 125 percent of the federal poverty line. As Minnesota's Medicaid director put it, just because the state is socially liberal "doesn't mean that it's not also about money."[31] Hawaii used a waiver for a similar purpose, folding an existing state program into Medicaid and expanding coverage to all adults up to 100 percent of the FPL. Both states have since repeatedly amended these demonstration projects to further expand coverage.

State-level policy entrepreneurs' creative use of the waiver process—and the Clinton administration's openness to such creativity—reflected a clear departure from the congressional intent behind section 1115. HCFA administrator Bruce Vladeck acknowledged that several of the administration's policies, including "encouraging big statewide programs" and "letting states use other states' waivers for applications as templates" were "directly contrary to the spirit of the statute."[32] Another HCFA official admitted that the administration was granting waivers that were "not really demonstrations" in the sense of learning something new, but rather were designed to "dramatically change policy."[33]

Despite the mounting cost to the federal government, a liberal interpretation of section 1115 was consistent with the president's campaign pledges to promote state experimentation and expand access to health care. It also reflected a strategic calculation based on the administration's keen understanding of how Medicaid's federal-state financing structure shaped state leaders' incentives—as Bruce Vladeck explains.

> At some point relatively early we figured out that all the states were going to take all the Medicaid bene[ficiarie]s they could and dump them into managed care and that it was better if they would use the savings gained thereby to expand coverage rather than just pocketing them—because they clearly had the legal opportunity just to pocket the savings.[34]

Nonetheless, the Clinton administration's reinterpretation of budget neutrality led a number of states to manipulate the waiver process for financial gain. Although demonstration projects were still supposed to be budget neutral, the new rules made it possible for states to create the illusion of budget neutrality by manipulating the projected cost of running the demonstration project, the baseline spending projections to which the project's cost would be compared, or both. As one HCFA official put it, the liberalization of budget neutrality led states to begin "inflating the cost of their current experience and deflating the costs of their expected experience."[35]

First, some states underestimated the cost of their proposed demonstration project by exaggerating the savings that could be achieved from experimental approaches to health-care delivery. For example, several states argued that managed care would save hundreds of millions of dollars despite the fact that, at the time, empirical evidence of cost savings from Medicaid managed care was inconclusive.[36] In a few cases—such as Kentucky and Florida—the Clinton administration approved such a waiver application only to have a conservative state legislature refuse to implement the project on the grounds that the promised cost savings were unlikely to materialize. Some states also underestimated the number of people likely to enroll in the demonstration project and then negotiated a budget neutrality cap calculated on a per-capita basis—thereby shifting the financial risk of higher-than-expected enrollment to the federal government.[37]

Second, a number of states overestimated the budget baseline to which the demonstration project's cost was compared, using two main approaches to inflating the baseline: the hypothetical expansion argument and the historical cost inflation argument.[38] Several states—including Hawaii, Rhode Island, and Kentucky—argued that their baselines should include the cost of extending Medicaid coverage to optional groups that hypothetically could have been—but were not actually—covered by the state's Medicaid program. The basic argument was that in the absence of the waiver, the state could have expanded coverage in a more traditional way and received additional federal financial assistance—and thus that expanding coverage under the waiver would not cost the federal government any more money, relative to this hypothetical counterfactual. Moreover, several states—including Tennessee and Florida—projected baseline spending growth in excess of national Medicaid growth projections on the grounds that their states' past spending growth exceeded the national average—despite the fact that recent increases in cost growth were largely driven by two trends that were not expected to continue: mandates and creative financing mechanisms.

These alleged abuses came under fire from political conservatives. The right-leaning *Washington Times* lambasted the Clinton administration for allowing the states to manipulate the waiver process, calling waivers a "cash cow" for the states, and noting that "Governors in the states know a good thing when they see it. And, right now, they see a very good thing—a way to get a lot of money to pay for helping more people in their states."[39] Although the White House publicly refuted such criticisms, federal officials privately acknowledged that the states' manipulation of cost estimates was threatening to undermine the administration's waiver policy.[40]

Concerned about the potential cost to the federal government, Congress asked the Government Accounting Office to investigate. In April 1995, Comptroller General Charles Bowsher testified before Congress that "the administration's method for determining budget neutrality may allow States access to more Federal funding than they would have received without the waiver." An accompanying GAO report noted that "by using unique methods in each state, the administration has created the potential for budget-neutrality decisions to be based on the technique most favorable to a particular state." Singling out the hypothetical eligibility argument in particular, the report argued that what states are doing should be the basis for determining budget neutrality—not what states might do.[41] The comptroller general also questioned the administration's practice of allowing states to apply the federal share of savings from managed care to finance coverage of additional populations instead of using the savings to reduce federal spending. The report concluded that allowing states to expand coverage to hundreds of thousands of additional individuals without congressional consultation was "inappropriate" and "could lead to a heavier financial burden on the Federal Government."[42]

Despite the comptroller general's warnings, Congress continued to provide little oversight of the waiver process. As one congressional staffer explained in an interview, "it is very hard for Congress to rein it in" in part because of pressure from the governors. "If the waiver is something a Governor wants, the Governor can protect his waiver through his state's delegation in the House and the Senate."[43]

TENNCARE

Waivers proved to be a particularly big cash cow for Tennessee. The state had come to rely heavily on creative financing mechanisms based on provider taxes and disproportionate-share hospital (DSH) payments in the late 1980s and early 1990s—as documented in chapter 5. Thus, when Congress passed the 1991 amendments narrowing the loopholes that made provider-tax schemes possible—requiring Tennessee to end this practice as of July 1992—the state was hit particularly hard. Tennessee stood to lose $1 billion, or roughly one-third of its $3 billion Medicaid budget.[44] The state's Medicaid budget, in turn, comprised more than one-quarter of total state spending (fig. 6). Governor Ned McWherter warned that as a result of the impending loss of federal Medicaid funds, "the entire state government in Tennessee remains in jeopardy."[45]

At first, the state made up for the lost DSH revenue by replacing the illegal tax scheme with a legal tax. After a bitter battle, Tennessee hospitals agreed to a 6.75 percent "privilege tax" to raise roughly $500 million in revenues, and $800 million in federal matching funds. In an eleventh-hour compromise, the hospital industry reluctantly agreed to the tax on several conditions: that the state not cut Medicaid coverage, that the tax be temporary, and that the state begin working on "true Medicaid reform."[46] The state legislature agreed to impose the tax for only 18 months, and Governor Ned McWherter set up a task force to study long-term solutions.

However, this temporary fix soon ran into a number of political and fiscal hurdles. First, the health-care industry's tenuous support for the tax immediately began to unravel. In early 1993, the Tennessee Hospital Association voted to seek its repeal, five hospitals filed a lawsuit challenging the

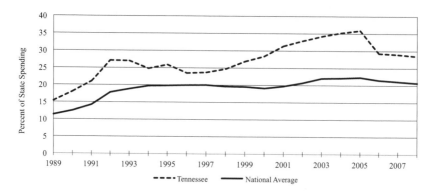

Fig. 6. Medicaid spending as a share of total state spending: Tennessee vs. national average, 1989–2010. (Data from National Association of State Budget Officers.)

tax's legality, and many others simply refused to pay the tax. Second, the tax brought in considerably less revenue than expected as a result of both hospital noncompliance and a sluggish economy. Third, the Medicaid program's costs continued to escalate, and by the spring of 1993 Governor McWherter acknowledged that even with the hospital tax, funding would be $764 million short of the amount needed to continue the program at its current level.[47]

In March 1993, Governor McWherter's task force identified three long-term options to solve the state's Medicaid crisis: raise taxes, slash coverage, or fundamentally reform the program. The health-care industry vehemently opposed the first two options. The Democratic governor wanted to expand—not cut—coverage, and although he was willing to raise taxes, many legislators, particularly Republicans, opposed a permanent tax increase, comparing raising taxes for Medicaid to "feeding a monster."[48] Fundamental reform seemed to be the only option.

The following month, the governor unveiled a proposal to treat the state's poor the same as its public-sector employees, who had been enrolled in a managed-care plan since 1988. Whereas Tennessee's Medicaid budget had been growing at a rate of 15 percent per year, the cost of care for the state's employees had declined by 1.2 percent in 1992.[49] The governor's budget team estimated that the cost savings from moving all of its nearly one million Medicaid beneficiaries into managed care would be so large that the state could extend coverage to at least two-thirds of the state's 750,000 uninsured residents. To further cut costs, enrollees with higher incomes would be asked to pay copayments and deductibles on a sliding scale.

The state's health-care industry vehemently protested the governor's proposal. Tennessee's provider reimbursement rates were already below the national average, and providers feared that managed care would push them even lower. Medical associations threatened boycotts and lawsuits, and launched public relations campaigns to discredit the program. But Governor McWherter—who, as an enormously popular leader ineligible for reelection under Tennessee's term-limit laws, had little to lose—pressed ahead, saying of the health-care industry: "I don't care if they call me a few names."[50] To circumvent the health-care lobbyists, he planned to implement the program with an executive order while the legislature was out of session that winter. But first, he needed a waiver from the Clinton administration.

The McWherter administration submitted its "TennCare" waiver application to the Health Care Financing Administration for review in June 1993. In addition to Governor McWherter—whom HCFA Administrator Bruce Vladeck described as "smart as hell, with a twinkle in his eye"[51]—the proposal's authors included Tennessee's "brilliant" state finance director, David Manning, and "very skilled" Medicaid director, Manny Martins (Hurley 2006, w223).

In its waiver request, the McWherter administration proclaimed that TennCare would provide comprehensive health coverage for every Tennessean, while eliminating the need for the state hospital tax. The letter acknowledged that "The obvious question is how can Tennessee finance universal coverage without the hospital taxes, if we can't adequately finance Medicaid with those taxes?" The answer, at least as far as the Clinton administration was concerned, was by shifting costs to the federal government.

The TennCare waiver request boldly proposed to cut state Medicaid contributions, but to continue receiving federal matching funds at the same level. Specifically, state officials proposed to repeal the hospital tax—thereby cutting the state's contribution roughly in half in the first year, from $920 million to $480 million—and to convert Tennessee's current level of federal funding into a block grant that would grow by 8.3 percent per year. Nonetheless, state officials claimed that the plan was not only budget neutral, but would actually save the federal government $1.5 billion over five years.[52]

The Clinton administration was skeptical, however, arguing that these changes would "simply increase the Federal share of a less expensive Medicaid program," and in fact would raise the state's effective federal match from 67 to 85 percent. The administration accused Tennessee officials of making "overly optimistic assumptions about managed care savings," and using an "aggressive approach for defining the baseline" for federal funds the state would be able to draw down in the absence of the waiver in order to justify the initial allocation and 8.3 percent annual increase in federal funding. Tennessee's Medicaid costs had been escalating faster than those of almost every other state due to its aggressive use of creative financing mechanisms. The Clinton administration pointed out that "with such a high base rate of inflation, it is not hard to show out-year savings from cost controls," but that "growth in Tennessee's Medicaid program is likely to slow down anyway" due to recent federal efforts to crack down on financing schemes.[53]

After the Clinton administration rejected Tennessee's block grant proposal, Manning and Martins went back to the drawing board. Determined to keep federal funds flowing into the state, they desperately began to search for any spending that federal officials might be persuaded to recognize as state Medicaid expenditures eligible for matching. They came up with several creative "contributions," including a proposal to underpay hospital costs by a designated amount that would be labeled "certified public expenditures" eligible for federal matching. They also proposed to treat patient revenues as state expenditures. Instead of going directly to managed-care plans, TennCare enrollees' premium payments would be captured by the state, and then dispensed to the managed-care plans in order to qualify for the federal match.[54] To keep the cost of reform low, state officials also proposed to pay managed-care organizations capitation payments that were significantly lower than the state's already low payment levels under Medicaid, despite warnings from the Tennessee Medicaid Association that these rates were "actuarially unsound," and would "not provide for adequate, high quality patient care."[55]

The negotiation process over the terms of the TennCare waiver dragged on for six months, despite the Clinton administration's pledge to approve waivers within 90 days. One HCFA official explained, "there was a lot of nervousness about TennCare" because it involved creating an entirely new health system and was thus "far more complicated than even Oregon."[56] The Clinton administration was particularly concerned that the state would be unable to meet the proposed January 1, 1994, target date for implementation. One federal official elaborated:

there was a great desire to have this thing active on certain dates. But the technical people who were looking at this basically all came to the same conclusion. They can't do it. They don't know what they're doing. They don't have all the elements lined up. They don't even have a list of names of people—of the beneficiaries who they must contact. They didn't have a good process for enrolling people.[57]

Moreover, there were only two managed-care organizations in the entire state at the time. The McWherter administration's plan was to create ten more "out of the ether" before the end of the year.[58] One observer likened the situation to "building the plane while flying it."[59]

However, the McWherter administration insisted that the implementation date was nonnegotiable. One state official explained, they "had to do it quickly. If it didn't happen quickly it would have never happened at all."[60] The governor was under enormous pressure from health-care providers to let the privilege tax expire as scheduled on December 31, but without additional federal funds coming into the state starting January 1, he would be forced to either extend the tax or slash coverage. Moreover, the state legislature would be back in session by January 15, giving health-care lobbyists an opportunity to kill the controversial managed-care reforms.

Finally, through a combination of "smoke and mirrors," "under-the-table deals" and "sheer intimidation," the McWherter administration convinced the Clinton administration to grant its waiver request in November 1993.[61] Despite concerns about the federal price tag—as well as the "dangerous" precedent it set for other states to emulate—the administration had several compelling reasons to support the demonstration project.[62] First, the president had recently begun touting a nationwide health care reform proposal—the Health Security Plan—that shared many features in common with TennCare, and thus felt pressure not to turn down a state initiative similar to what he was trying to do nationally. Second, administration officials worried that disapproval of the waiver would "trigger a State financing crisis," and that the State was "laying the groundwork to blame such a crisis on the Federal government."[63] Third, President Clinton and Governor McWherter were close friends; indeed, when the governor encountered initial resistance to his financing plan from HCFA officials, he insisted on negotiating directly with the president.

On January 1, 1994, only six weeks after the administration had approved

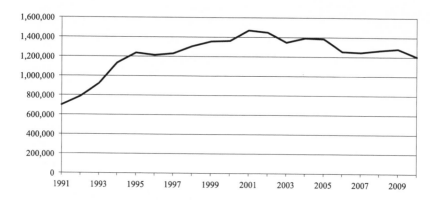

Fig. 7. Tennessee's Medicaid/TennCare enrollment, 1991–2010. (Data from U.S. Department of Health and Human Services.)

the waiver, TennCare went into effect. Within a year, the program had 1.2 million enrollees, and by 2001 that number had expanded to nearly 1.5 million—more than one-quarter of the state's total population (fig. 7).

There were many positive signs in the program's early years, including steep declines in inappropriate hospitalization and emergency-room utilization. Moreover, one study concluded that "there is little question that those who previously were uninsured have benefited from TennCare in terms of access, cost, quality, and satisfaction" (Conover and Davies 2000, 9). However, there were also many problems. The state was forced to temporarily close enrollment on several occasions because it simply could not afford to cover everyone who qualified. Moreover, due to Tennessee's low capitation rates, the state's managed-care organizations struggled to survive financially, and some folded. Under pressure from the powerful health-care lobby, the state gradually relaxed the cost discipline of managed care and reassumed greater financial risk. Thus, despite its successes in expanding coverage and improving health outcomes, TennCare earned a reputation as a "low-budget semi-disaster cobbled together on the fly."[64]

TennCare's financial problems only intensified following the 2001 national recession. Tennessee's inability to raise capitation rates to a sustainable level reflected, in part, the fact that it was one of only seven states without an income tax. Republican governor Don Sundquist—despite having won the 1994 election on an antitax platform—repeatedly urged the state legislature to adopt an income tax, citing TennCare as the primary reason, but lawmakers refused. As one observer noted, "The antitax people argued that we didn't need a tax, we needed to get rid of TennCare" (Hurley 2006, w219). The governor sought to scale back coverage but was stymied by the courts. In 2004, Sundquist's successor, Phil Bredesen—a Democrat—announced that he would completely dismantle TennCare, and return to the original Medicaid model. However, political resistance and fiscal realities led him to instead submit an amendment to the waiver in order to scale back the program, cutting several hundred thousand people from the Medicaid rolls, and trimming covered services for the remaining enrollees.[65]

Although these cuts are the largest in Medicaid's history, they must be considered in the context of the TennCare program's broad scope. TennCare continues to cover 1.2 million people—more than 20 percent of the state's population—placing it among the top ten states in terms of share of the population covered by Medicaid (fig. 7).[66] Also, Medicaid continues to comprise nearly 30 percent of the state's budget—considerably higher than the national average (fig. 6). This is particularly noteworthy when one considers Tennessee's relatively conservative political culture—as the state's former Medicaid director explained in an interview.

> TennCare [is] remarkable for having ever started or having ever been sustained, because there are many forces in Tennessee that would love to get rid of TennCare . . . the reason TennCare has survived is that the state doesn't know how to live without it. None of the critics on the Right, at least, have figured out how to replace the funding stream that TennCare secures. Without TennCare, if the state would go back to the regular financial arrangements . . . that money which once was DSH money would be lost . . .[67]

Despite succumbing to substantial cuts, TennCare's resilience serves as a compelling example of the powerful financial incentives that propel Medicaid's growth and undermine efforts at retrenchment.

GOVERNORS RESIST NATIONAL HEALTH REFORM

As the TennCare experience illustrates, Medicaid's built-in potential for incremental expansion—thanks to its open-ended financing arrangement and broad state discretion over eligibility and coverage policies—was further augmented by the liberalization of the federal waiver process. Medicaid's inherent propensity for growth stands in stark contrast to the persistently steep obstacles to fundamental health care reform in the United States, as exemplified by the Clinton Administration's failure to enact a federal reform package that was similar to TennCare in many ways.

Amidst the flurry of waiver activity in 1993 and 1994, the Clinton administration was working on its own plan to make health care accessible and affordable to all Americans, with the dual goals of reining in cost growth and solving the problem of the uninsured. In the summer of 1993, the president's Task Force on National Health Care Reform—chaired by his wife, Hillary Rodham Clinton—recommended a Health Security Plan which would—among other things—dismantle Medicaid, and integrate low-income Americans into the same system of mandatory coverage in private managed-care plans that would cover higher-income people. The states would be required to help the federal government subsidize the costs of covering low-income people.

As the Clinton administration began to pitch its proposal, White House officials grew concerned that the states' increased use of Medicaid waivers might pose "significant risks" to nationwide reform. For one thing, "proliferation of state program variations reflecting different principles" could further accentuate variation and fragmentation among the states, making it "difficult to preserve the infrastructure necessary for national health reform." A second concern was that opponents could use waivers to "slow down nationwide reform" by arguing that "we need to see the results of these demonstrations before we proceed with national reform."[68] Third, the Clintons had framed their reform plan as an urgently needed solution to a national health-care crisis, but allowing Tennessee and other states to forge ahead with large-scale reforms of their own might "let the air out" of the national solution (Hurley 2006, w219). Fourth, the White House worried that "States will consider waivers as an alternative to reform . . . if it is to their financial advantage," sapping a potential source of political support for the initiative.[69] Reports surfaced that the administration was so concerned that they were considering shutting down the Medicaid waiver process, although officials denied these rumors.[70]

Since the health care reform plan would require a potentially controversial overhaul of the federal-state partnership, the president was desperate to secure the governors' support in order to increase his leverage on Capitol Hill. To this end, he added four governors to the health reform task force, noting that "their input, their advice, their perspective is essential to our success."[71] In speeches, he repeatedly reassured the governors that his plan would be fair to the states, telling them "I remember what it was like being in your shoes."[72]

It might seem that the governors would be open to a reform plan that dismantled Medicaid. As one governor put it, "If you ask every governor, 'What's your biggest cost problem,' they'd pick the word Medicaid."[73] Indeed, in January 1994 the governors issued a policy resolution calling upon the president and Congress to pass health care legislation that year to alleviate "immediate budgetary pressures caused by the Medicaid program."[74]

However, the governors ultimately refused to support the Health Security Plan. Although Medicaid was breaking the states' backs, the governors feared that the Health Security Plan might prove to be even costlier. While most governors expressed optimism that President Clinton would not forget his roots and dump costs on the states, their recent experience with federal mandates led many to express distrust of the Democrat-controlled Congress; Governor John Engler (R-Michigan) was among them.

> I'm concerned that there's going to be a big attempt to shift costs back to the states and it may not be the fault of the Administration. The problem we've got are members of Congress who . . . consistently try to solve their problems by pushing the burdens and the responsibilities back to the states . . . It's not so much where the Administration starts out, it's where Congress takes things that's so frightening. If we're not careful, we could have a very, very expensive plan . . .[75]

Such concerns were not unique to Republican governors; many Democratic governors acknowledged that they were similarly "gun-shy" about what might happen "when Congress gets the plan."[76]

Moreover, as the White House feared, many governors expected to achieve greater savings under state demonstration projects than under federal health care reform; indeed, governors who were already using waivers to implement large-scale Medicaid demonstration projects were among the most outspoken critics of nationwide reform. For instance, Barbara Roberts, governor of Oregon—eager to protect federal funding for the Oregon Health Plan—objected that federal health care reform might prevent the states from serving as "laboratories" and exploring "different ways to do things."[77]

Furthermore, given the failure of most previous attempts at comprehensive reform, many governors predicted—correctly—that the Clinton plan would never make it through Congress, and saw continuation of the incremental, state-based approach to reform that was already underway as a more viable option. Even the most optimistic governors predicted a long, drawn-out process and—given the pressure that Medicaid was placing on their budgets—did not have the luxury of waiting for a federal reform that might be several years in the making. As NGA executive director Raymond Scheppach put it, "they're not waiting around doing nothing, and my advice to them is not to wait."[78]

Of course, in addition to financial considerations, some governors opposed the Clinton plan for political reasons. As the 1994 election approached, the GOP put intense pressure on Republican governors to toe the party line on health care reform, which had become the single most important issue in the election. A growing chorus of Republican governors began attacking the Clinton plan, calling it "a disaster," and "not in the best interest of the country."[79] Acknowledging that he needed the governors' support to win approval in Congress, President Clinton repeatedly warned them not to "let health care reform fall victim to partisan bickering."[80]

However, Republican governors also refused to endorse the GOP's alternative to the Clinton plan, which—among other things—sought to constrain the growth of health-care costs by imposing a cap on federal Medicaid contributions. In the summer of 1994, the NGA sent Senate minority leader Bob Dole a letter explaining that governors of both parties had "a very strong position against caps on Medicaid" because "a cap on the Federal share of Medicaid spending would assure that states bear a disproportionate share of a program that was intended as a state and Federal partnership. This action imposes a significant unfunded mandate on states and could result in state budget crises."[81]

By refusing to endorse either party's reform proposal, the governors effectively supported continuation of the status quo. Despite Medicaid's skyrocketing costs, it afforded the states considerable flexibility and federal funding—particularly under the liberalized waiver policy. When faced with the prospect of a potentially costlier and more cumbersome reform option, the governors chose to protect rather than dismantle Medicaid. The governors preferred the devil they knew, just as they had during the new federalism negotiations with the Reagan administration in the early 1980s (discussed in chapter 3).

Ultimately, the Clinton health care reform plan failed as conservatives and special-interest groups successfully shifted the focus of debate from the expansion of health coverage to the expansion of federal government power and spending (Skocpol 1997). The reform's failure contributed to an emerging consensus that, given the steep obstacles to federal reform, "turning the states into bustling laboratories" through the use of Medicaid waivers was a "quicker, quieter way to overhaul America's health care system."[82] Thus, Medicaid in the early 1990s yet again exhibited a self-reinforcing quality, whereby incremental change and continued reliance on established institutions—not wholesale reform—proved to be the path of least resistance.

CONCLUSION

The states continued to use waivers to expand access to health care throughout the 1990s. Due to waning enthusiasm for managed care (Fossett and Thompson 1999), and political backlash against the "rationing" of health care (Jacobs, Marmor, and Oberlander 1999), these waivers tended to be less ambitious than the early projects implemented in Tennessee and Oregon, typically extending coverage to tens—rather than hundreds—of thousands of low-income individuals. Waivers approved in the late 1990s included extensions of comprehensive coverage to low-income adults without young children, and the creation of family-planning programs for low-income uninsured women of childbearing age.

The states' use of waivers to expand coverage continued in the 2000s, as Clinton's successor in the White House, Republican George W. Bush—a former governor and advocate of states' rights—chose not to return to the restrictive waiver process that had prevailed under Republican presidents in the 1980s (fig. 5). Nor did the Bush administration terminate the ambitious demonstrations launched in the Clinton years as they came up for renewal—although the administration did occasionally threaten to do so, as is discussed in chapter 8. In fact, the new president authorized the creation of several new variations on the section 1115 waiver, including Pharmacy Plus, which allows states to secure additional federal matching funds to help cover the cost of prescription-only programs for seniors who otherwise would not qualify for Medicaid. Although the Bush administration also invited states to submit waivers that would cut costs by trimming covered services, and several states took advantage of this opportunity, such cases were the exception rather than the rule. In part, this was because the Bush administration continued to apply Clinton's loose definition of budget neutrality, allowing states to manipulate the cost projections underlying expansive waiver applications in order to secure extra federal matching funds.[83]

In sum, research and demonstration waivers have, by bestowing greater flexibility and funding on the states, contributed significantly to Medicaid's incremental expansion. As one study of recent Medicaid demonstration projects concludes, "waivers have not been a major force for subterranean program erosion" as one might expect, given the pressure Medicaid imposes on federal and state budgets. On the contrary, research and demonstration waivers have strengthened "political forces that, seemingly against the odds, sustain Medicaid" (Thompson and Burke 2007, 999–1000).

CHAPTER 7

Block Grants and the 1994 Republican Revolution

IN 1995, congressional Republicans drafted legislation that would have converted Medicaid's financing arrangement from an open-ended matching grant to a block grant. By offering the states substantial flexibility over the design of eligibility and benefit policies and delivery systems, congressional leaders hoped to entice state leaders into accepting explicit limits on federal funding. By breaking the link between state effort and federal funding—an inherent feature of open-ended matching grants—they hoped to rein in the states' expansionary incentives and bring federal Medicaid outlays under control.

That conservative national leaders wanted to block-grant Medicaid was nothing new; Presidents Ronald Reagan and George H. W. Bush had advocated similar reforms in the 1980s and early 1990s. What was new was that an unprecedented number of governors expressed support for the idea of trading greater discretion for less money. This turnaround was due to a unique set of political and economic factors that characterized the mid-1990s, including a large number of Republican governors, heightened party polarization, a recent spate of federal mandates, and a strong national economy.

Although gubernatorial support for a Medicaid block grant in the mid-1990s was stronger than ever before, it was by no means universal or unqualified. Democratic governors resisted the idea, fearing that without the federal government's open-ended financial commitment, the states would have insufficient resources to maintain current eligibility and benefit policies. Many Republican governors who publicly supported the proposal privately expressed similar reservations. Even the handful of conservative Republican governors who wholeheartedly embraced the principle of a block grant found themselves engaged in a bitter formula fight over the distribution of funds. Ultimately, these internal divisions among the governors doomed the proposal's prospects in Washington. Despite unprecedented support for a Medicaid block grant at both federal and state levels of government, the program's institutional design once again shielded it from retrenchment.

REPUBLICAN REVOLUTION

Following the 1994 midterm elections, the GOP gained control of the House of Representatives, the Senate, and a majority of governorships for the first time in Medicaid's history (figs. 8, 9, and 10). This so-called Republican revolution was widely viewed as a referendum on President Clinton's shaky first two years in office, and particularly his failed attempt to enact comprehensive health care reform. It also reflected widespread support for the Contract with America—a Republican manifesto championed by new House Speaker Newt Gingrich (R-Georgia) that promised, among other things, floor votes on a balanced budget requirement, tax cuts, spending cuts, and welfare reform. The sudden surge of Republican power across the nation provided the GOP with a rare window of opportunity to carry out this ambitious agenda. As Senate majority leader Robert Dole (R-Kansas) acknowledged, "if we blow it, we may be denied the opportunity for another 10, 15, 20 years."[1]

Despite Medicaid's rapid growth, the Contract with America did not include Medicaid reform due to uncertainty over the fate of the Clinton health care reform initiative as well as a desire to avoid politically sensitive and divisive policy areas such as health care for children and other vulnerable populations (Weaver 1996).[2] But as the new Republican Congress began working out the details of an ambitious plan to eliminate the federal budget deficit while also cutting taxes, it became increasingly clear that all entitlement programs, including Medicaid, would be on the chopping block.

Moreover, following the election, a small but vocal group of Republican governors—emboldened by their party's surge to power—began extolling the virtues of converting Medicaid (as well as Aid to Families with Dependent Children) into a block grant to allow both levels of government to scale back spending. This group was led by Michigan governor John Engler—a "portly man with an air of great certainty" who was "treated as a demigod in certain quarters on Capitol Hill"—and rounded out by Wisconsin governor Tommy Thompson, and Massachusetts governor William Weld (Drew 1997, 83). The three "captains of conservatism" were known for their crisp ideol-

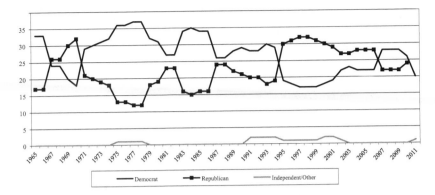

Fig. 8. Number of governors by party affiliation, 1965–2012. (Data from U.S. Census Bureau.)

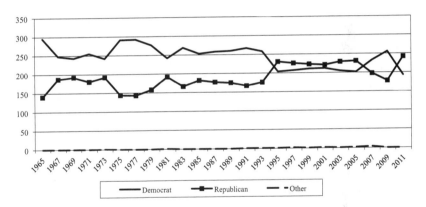

Fig. 9. Party composition of the U.S. House of Representatives, 1965–2012. (Data from U.S. Census Bureau.)

ogy and bold risk-taking style (Katz 2008, 83). They were particularly visible and influential due to their seniority as well as their key leadership positions within the National Governors Association and Republican Governors Association.

Congressional leaders were delighted by the conservative governors' support for a Medicaid block grant, since state leaders had repeatedly stymied similar reform efforts in the past; indeed, history suggested that without the buy-in of the governors—the ones who would ultimately have to

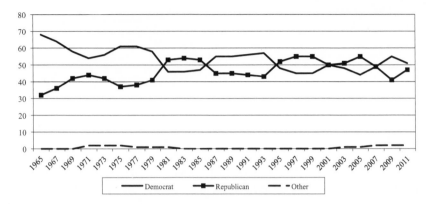

Fig. 10. Party composition of the U.S. Senate, 1965–2012. (Data from U.S. Census Bureau.)

implement the reforms—swing voters in Congress (not to mention President Bill Clinton) would refuse to go along. In addition, since the governors were closer to the electorate, congressional Republicans saw them as "hugely helpful" in communicating to the public that Medicaid reform was "the right thing to do" (Drew 1997, 84). Finally, only a handful of members of Congress knew much about Medicaid, making state leaders—with their practical experience running the program—a critical source of expertise on the technical details of structuring a block grant.[3]

Most Republican governors were willing to join Engler, Thompson, and Weld in publicly supporting a Medicaid block grant—despite having joined their Democratic colleagues in rejecting similar proposals in the past—due to an extraordinary confluence of economic and political factors during the mid-1990s. The first was the changing political landscape, which was characterized by not only lopsided Republican control of federal and state governments, but also increased party polarization. As one gubernatorial aide explained in an interview, Republican governors saw Medicaid reform as "part of a national movement [and] wanted to be helpful and supportive . . . there was a whole political ideological side here that was extremely compelling to the Republican Governors."[4]

Second, the Contract with America altered the Republican governors' strategic calculus. If federal spending cuts were inevitable, they might as well seek to extract as much programmatic discretion as possible in exchange. One state official elaborated:

> If you're going to balance the budget, it means everyone's going to take a cut: every single interest group, every state. And the worst case scenario is if you were to just take a fifteen to twenty percent cut across the board, but keep in place every single string [or] mandate that went with all the programs. (Weaver 1996, 58)

Since the new congressional leadership was aiming to balance the budget not immediately, but over a seven-year period, the governors hoped to negotiate few strings and a lot of money in the short run, even if it meant less money in the long run.[5] As NGA executive director Raymond Scheppach explained in an interview, some Republican governors supported the block grant because, as politicians, they had a "short-term focus" and saw the long-term reduction in federal funding as "a problem for next governor to deal with."[6]

Third, the recent spate of federal Medicaid mandates contributed to gubernatorial interest in a block grant. Most Republican governors disliked being forced to use an increasingly large share of state resources to pay for health care for the poor instead of corrections, transportation, and other priorities. They criticized Medicaid as a "covert attack on the States' fiscal health," and warned that if no action was taken the program would "consume literally every dollar that is appropriated in state budgets" within a few decades.[7] They hoped that a block grant without strings would give the states more flexibility to scale back their own Medicaid spending, freeing up funds for other programs, even if it also meant making do with less federal money.

Finally, the importance of the economy cannot be underestimated. Unlike 1981 and 1991, when Republican presidents had proposed Medicaid block grants during national recessions and governors of both parties had vehemently resisted, the mid-1990s saw the longest peacetime expansion in U.S. history. Thanks to increased productivity, employment, and income, state budgets were in good shape—diminishing the salience of the states' need for federal funding. In fact, the states were so flush with resources that they collectively cut taxes in 1995 by more than they had in nearly two decades.[8] With state coffers full, many Republican governors began to tell Congress: "We don't need more money. We need the flexibility to manage programs."[9]

However, in many cases, Republican governors' public enthusiasm for Medicaid reform belied private reservations. According to NGA executive director Raymond Scheppach, moderate Republican governors were "weak-kneed" at the thought of losing billions of dollars in federal funds, and "although they might not say so publicly, it was clear most of them weren't going to push the proposal forward."[10] A few moderates even voiced their concerns out loud, despite intense pressure to toe the party line. For example, Minnesota governor Arne Carlson warned that since most states were looking at double-digit growth rates in their Medicaid budgets, capping the federal government's contribution would be "financially damaging" for the states.[11]

Moreover, 12 of the 30 Republican governors had entered office in January 1995 as part of the Republican revolution and simply had not had sufficient time to carefully consider the ramifications of block grants; these governors tended to defer to their more senior colleagues. As a result, Engler, Thompson, and Weld dominated the public conversation and gave the appearance of unity among not only Republican governors, but the National Governors Association as a whole. As a January 1995 internal NGA memo noted, "public discussions and comments over the past few months appear to assume that there is broad agreement among the Governors on the need for block grants" but in fact "the Governors have not fully discussed the implications."[12]

FEAR OF A TROJAN HORSE

Most Democratic governors, like their Republican counterparts, saw the flexibility of a Medicaid block grant as "extraordinarily appealing."[13] Nonetheless, the Democratic governors ultimately opposed a Medicaid block grant for several reasons. First, they expressed distrust of the conservative new congressional leadership, and fear that the block grant was merely a veiled attempt to shift costs to the states. Indiana governor Evan Bayh compared block grants to a Trojan Horse, noting: "It looks pretty good right now, but what's waiting inside that could be potentially harmful?"[14] Florida governor Lawton Chiles accused House Speaker Newt Gingrich of finding "a few G.O.P. governors—Judas goats—to go along with the idea," referring to an animal used to lead others to slaughter.[15]

Second, left-leaning governors rejected the block grant proposal because it would eliminate Medicaid's entitlement status. Entitlement status is complex in federal-state programs; in addition to the individual entitlement—whereby individuals who meet eligibility criteria have a right to benefits specified in law—there is also an implicit state entitlement that protects state governments against unexpected reductions in federal funding (Weaver

1996). According to NGA chairman Howard Dean (D-Vermont), Democratic governors felt that "the individual entitlement must stay because it protects children and because it provides a safety net for the State taxpayers and State budgets."[16] This desire to retain Medicaid's entitlement status was consistent with the NGA's traditional stance against block-granting Medicaid due to "both differences in the treatment of individual entitlements under the federal budget process and the fact that individual entitlements are often particularly sensitive to cyclical changes in the economy."[17] In addition to exposing the states to increased economic risk, converting Medicaid into a block grant would move the program to the discretionary side of the federal budget, subjecting it to annual review in the appropriations process. As executive director Scheppach explained in an interview, "once they break the entitlement, there's nothing to preclude Congress from saying I'll give you $150 billion one year and $100 billion the next."[18]

Third, many Democratic governors expressed concern that if the federal government no longer required the states to put up their own matching funds in order to receive Medicaid grants, state-level political pressures would compel them to shift state funding to other areas, harming vulnerable populations. Such concerns were particularly acute in the South, where many governors, such as Florida governor Lawton Chiles, faced conservative legislatures reluctant to allocate funds for Medicaid.

> You just give me a block grant, hell, I can spend the money anywhere. There are a lot of places that my legislature would like to spend that money that would not be taking care of children. I have just gone through a budget situation in which I saw everybody wants to build prisons in my State. That is the popular thing.[19]

Such concerns highlight the extent to which Medicaid's institutional structure insulates the program from retrenchment in the face of competing budget pressures, despite the constituency's lack of political power.

Due to the governors' partisan divide, the NGA fell short of the three-fourths vote needed to take an official position. Instead, the NGA released a vague policy resolution that acknowledged the "enormous opportunity to restructure the federal-state relationship," and urged Congress to "both examine the allocation of responsibilities among the levels of government and to maximize state flexibility in areas of shared responsibility." In a bow to Republican governors, the statement expressed a willingness to consider

"reasonable restrictions" on future Medicaid growth in exchange for "significant statutory flexibility in program delivery." However, the resolution
also reflected Democrats' fears, warning federal lawmakers that "the federal
budget must be balanced by true savings, not by shifting costs to the states."[20]

The governors' inability to speak with one voice meant that the NGA was
largely sidelined throughout 1995. Governors Engler, Thompson, and Weld
stepped into the vacuum and conferred with congressional leaders as they
worked out the details of their first federal budget resolution. House Speaker
Newt Gingrich acknowledged that the input of these three governors made
the congressional leadership "much bolder than we would have been without them" (Drew 1997, 84). The budget resolution that ultimately emerged
from Congress would transform Medicaid from an entitlement program
funded with open-ended matching grants to a block grant ("Medigrant")
capped at an average annual growth rate of 4 percent—a sharp reduction
from the current rate of 10 percent. All told, it would slash $182 billion in
federal Medicaid funding over seven years.

Democratic governors immediately rejected the budget resolution. In
addition to their concerns about the loss of Medicaid's open-ended funding
and entitlement status, they resented having been excluded from consultations during the drafting process. According to Raymond Scheppach, "Gingrich asked the Republican governors 'how many Democratic governors can
you get on board?' and the answer was none. Since they hadn't been included in the negotiations, they weren't willing to go along."[21]

The Clinton administration, congressional Democrats, and a handful of
moderate congressional Republicans also opposed the proposed changes,
which President Clinton declared "far, far more than the health care system
can handle." The White House estimated that, by 2002, the Republicans'
plan would cut 4.4 million children and 350,000 nursing home residents
from the Medicaid rolls.[22] However, Democrats were in a state of demoral-
ized shock following the 1994 elections, and did not put up much resistance
as the Republican leadership pressed ahead.

FORMULA FIGHT

The budget resolution established total federal spending targets but did not
specify how each state's Medicaid block grant would be calculated. Throughout the summer of 1995, as federal lawmakers debated how to reallocate

funds among the states, they sought input from the governors. Replacing the open-ended federal commitment with a lump-sum payment designed to meet a federal deficit-reduction target created a zero-sum game that pitted the states against one another as they struggled over a fixed pot of money. Although Republican governors had expressed support for a Medicaid block grant in principle, agreeing on a specific formula was another matter altogether. According to Raymond Scheppach, moderate Republican governors grew increasingly "edgy" and "wishy-washy" about the reform as Congress started getting into the details.[23]

Whereas disagreements over the general principle of a block grant were primarily partisan in nature, the formula fight largely broke down along geographical lines. The governors of midwestern and northeastern states—which tend to have generous Medicaid programs—urged Congress to base the block grant formula on a state's current level of spending. However, Southern states argued that this would unfairly lock in large interstate variations in federal aid. For example, federal Medicaid spending was $2,400 per capita in New York compared to $700 in Florida at the time.[24] Southern governors argued that block grants should not reward states that had been granting "excessive benefits," while northeastern and midwestern governors argued that Congress should not privilege states that had been "miserly" and "unwilling to commit resources."[25]

An additional source of regional tension was that in the South and Southwest "Sun Belt" region, the poor elderly and disabled population was growing much more rapidly than in the Northeast or Midwest. Florida governor Lawton Chiles, whose Medicaid budget was growing at a clip of 13 percent per year—more than three times the rate that would apply under the cap—complained "It's no wonder the Governors of Wisconsin, Michigan and Massachusetts are on this bandwagon," because their states would suffer little financial harm.[26] The leaders of these fast-growth states lobbied Congress to base the block grant formula on state demographic characteristics rather than current spending.

Governors with large disproportionate share hospital (DSH) programs and section 1115 demonstration projects—who "had a good thing going, and wanted to keep the funds flowing"—sought to protect these special payments under the new formula (Smith and Moore 2008, 238). Governor George W. Bush (R-Texas) argued that his state's DSH funds—which accounted for 18 percent of the state's total Medicaid spending—should be included in Texas's formula. Similarly, Governor John Kitzhaber (D-Oregon) worried that if a state's block grant was based on its spending in fiscal year 1994, as congressional leaders were considering, it would wipe out the enormous influx of federal funds that had occurred when his state's demonstration project was implemented in 1995. At Kitzhaber's urging, the state's congressional delegation asked the president to veto any bill that threatened the Oregon Health Plan.

Finally, many governors argued that the formula should take into account unique aspects of their states' Medicaid populations. Governor George Pataki (R-New York) wanted the formula to address the fact that New York's Medicaid population suffered disproportionately from HIV, mental illness, and substance abuse. Governor Pete Wilson (R-California) made the case that the formula should account for his state's large population of poor illegal immigrants and the resulting strain on California's emergency rooms.

By the time of the annual meeting of the National Governors Association in August 1995, the formula fight had reached a fever pitch. At the meetings, congressional leaders repeatedly urged the governors—"the guys who have to implement the reforms"—to overcome their differences and agree on a formula so that Congress could move forward with a proposal.[27] Senator Robert Dole (R-Kansas) told state leaders, "We can't do it without you . . . if there's a big split with[in] the Governors, it makes it more and more difficult."[28] The governors themselves worried that their difficulty in reaching a consensus was counterproductive to their collective interests in securing maximum flexibility and funding. Incoming NGA chairman Tommy Thompson warned his colleagues: "If we don't do something, it's going to be to our detriment. Congress will do something, and we're not going to like it."[29]

Nonetheless, the governors left their annual meeting unable to reach an agreement. Executive director Raymond Scheppach observed that the organization was simply too pluralistic to agree on a formula that would cut as much as 20 percent from the single largest source of federal aid to the states (Smith 2002, 49). In a classic case of path dependence, attempts to move away from the status quo allocation of resources were encountering seemingly insurmountable obstacles.

"LET'S MAKE A DEAL"

The congressional debate over the allocation of Medicaid block grant funds in the fall of 1995 was a striking example of the power of state financial interests in national lawmaking. In the House, the Commerce Committee voted mostly along party lines—with only one Democrat joining the Republican majority—to replace Medicaid's open-ended entitlement with a block grant. Bowing to pressure from the governors of Sun Belt states, the committee endorsed a funding formula based on a state's number of poor residents, caseload severity, and medical cost inflation rather than current spending levels. As a result, the formula generated higher caps for fast-growth states that had historically spent less on Medicaid and lower caps for slower-growth, higher-spending states. Northeastern and midwestern governors rejected the proposed formula as "unfair, harmful and completely unacceptable,"[30] while Democratic governors and representatives alike objected that the bill ended vulnerable Americans' entitlement to medical assistance.

Democratic, northeastern, and midwestern governors fared somewhat better under the relatively liberal Senate Finance Committee bill. Voting along party lines, the committee chose a formula more favorable to slower-growth, higher-spending states. Two powerful committee members from New York succeeded in amending the formula so as to lower the state share of Medicaid costs for high-income states from 50 to 40 percent. To free up the funds needed to finance this provision, the bill excluded a portion of DSH payments from the formula, disproportionately harming Southern states such as Texas and Louisiana. To win the support of moderate committee member John Chafee (R-Rhode Island), the committee agreed to retain the individual entitlement for particularly vulnerable groups including poor pregnant women, children under the age of 13, and the disabled (Smith 2002). The bill also retained spousal asset protections so that spouses of nursing-home residents would not have to relinquish all family funds and assets before Medicaid would start paying nursing home costs.

As the Finance Committee's bill headed to the Senate floor for debate, Republican and Southern governors sprang into action. Twenty-four Republican governors wrote a letter to Senate Majority Leader Robert Dole complaining that the bill contained "overly prescriptive and onerous provisions that will militate against the states' ability to implement reforms."[31] Sun Belt state leaders objected that the bill provided insufficient funding relative to the House version. Governor George W. Bush and Senator Kay Bailey Hutchinson (R-Texas) were particularly vocal in their criticism. Governor Bush protested that it was unfair to allocate only 6 percent of federal Medicaid funds to Texas, since the state was home to nearly 10 percent of the nation's Medicaid enrollees. A Senate Finance Committee staffer recalls a series of "very unpleasant in-your-face screaming match sessions" with Hutchinson,[32] who insisted that Texas receive "not one dollar less" under the Senate bill than under the House bill.[33]

Since the Senate vote was much closer than the House vote, Senators who withheld support had considerable bargaining leverage, resulting in what one GOP aide described as "Let's make a deal, with Bob Dole as your host."[34] One of Dole's staffers explained that the majority leader—who was running for president at the time—was "terrified about . . . breaking with the governors because they were so critical" to building his election campaign.[35] After Dole helped Bush and Hutchinson secure an additional $5 billion for Texas, the leaders of several other Southern states including Arizona, Georgia, and Kentucky made similar demands, whittling away at the Republicans' deficit-reduction target.

Ultimately, under pressure from the governors, the Conference Committee reconciled differences between the House and Senate versions of the bill by allowing states to choose between the House and Senate formulas based on which would provide them with more funding. The compromise mandated coverage for poor pregnant women, children under the age of 13, and the disabled, but allowed states to determine the benefit package as well as the definition of "disabled." Due to financial concessions to the states, the estimated federal savings fell from $182 billion to $163 billion (Smith 2002).

In November, President Clinton offered a last-minute compromise: a seven-year balanced budget plan which, as an alternative to the Medigrant proposal, would retain the individual entitlement but impose a per-capita cap on federal spending, trimming a relatively modest $54 billion. However, Republican governors denounced the proposal as "the worst of evils," warning that cutting federal funding while retaining the entitlement would "impoverish the states."[36] Having drawn a line in the sand against any bill that slashed federal funding of health care for vulnerable Americans, President Clinton vetoed Congress's budget reconciliation bill on December 6, 1995. In a symbolic touch, he used the same pen that President Lyndon Johnson had used to sign the Medicare and Medicaid legislation in 1965. As Republicans returned to the drawing board, the Democratic president warned that "If necessary, I'll veto these deep cuts in health care for children again and again and again."[37] Without a budget, the federal government was forced to shut down for the second time in two months.

GOVERNORS EMERGE AS A "THIRD HOUSE OF CONGRESS"

As the federal budget impasse dragged on through the winter, the nation's governors grew increasingly alarmed. In the absence of a compromise between the president and Congress, the states had no idea how much federal Medicaid money they would receive or how much flexibility they would have in spending that money, making it difficult to budget for the coming year. The governors also felt partly responsible since their inability to reach a consensus had contributed to the stalemate.

To help break the logjam, the NGA created a task force of six governors—three Republicans and three Democrats—with the goal of developing a bipartisan proposal that would serve as a "middle ground" between Congress and the White House.[38] The Republican governors were John Engler, Tommy Thompson, and Mike Leavitt (Utah); the Democrats were Lawton Chiles (Florida), Bob Miller (Nevada), and Roy Romer (Colorado). They met repeatedly between November 1995 and February 1996. According to Romer aide Alan Weil, the task force "met an incredible number of times for well into the hundreds of hours trying to craft a compromise . . . there was a genuine desire to do so despite the fact that there were some genuine differences between the Republican and Democratic Governors in their views."[39]

The primary challenge was to come up with a plan that balanced Republican governors' desire for the flexibility of a block grant against Democratic governors' preference to retain Medicaid's entitlement status and open-ended federal financial assistance. To minimize tension, the task force members decided not to use divisive buzz words; as Governor Thompson put it, "we don't say entitlement, and we don't say block grant. We say plan X and program Y."[40] The task force also agreed on four overarching principles that would guide their Medicaid reform plan, reflecting a combination of Republican priorities (flexibility and cost containment) and Democratic priorities (protecting vulnerable populations and protecting states against unanticipated costs).[41]

After a long and arduous negotiation process—during which nearly every member stormed out at least once—the task force finally reached a compromise designed to achieve these four overarching principles.[42] Bowing to Democrats' demands, the proposal would guarantee coverage for poor pregnant women, children under the age of 13, elderly meeting SSI income standards, and persons with disabilities who met standards to be defined by the state; other groups covered under current law would no longer be entitled to coverage. However, in a reflection of Republicans' priorities, states would have broad discretion over the amount, duration, and scope of covered services.

The task force's plan called for a federal grant formula that delicately balanced the governors' competing demands. Each state's allocation would be equal to the sum of four factors: a "base allocation" that reflected a state's prior spending level—states could choose between 1993, 1994, or 1995—a "growth factor" to account for estimated changes in the state's caseload, "special grants" for specific populations such as illegal immigrants and Native Americans, and an "insurance umbrella" to account for Medicaid population growth arising from unanticipated business cycle fluctuations, changing demographics, and natural disasters. With the exception of special grants, states would be required to share in the program's cost up to a maximum of 40 percent—as in the Senate bill. The plan would repeal federal restrictions on provider taxes and donations and would include a state's current DSH spending in the base allocation.[43]

When the task force presented its plan at the governors' 1996 winter meeting, NGA chairman Tommy Thompson urged his colleagues to support it unanimously. He warned that the president and Congress were unlikely to resolve their impasse unless the governors rallied around the task force's plan, and that the uncertainty of a prolonged stalemate would have "cataclysmic" implications for state budgets, and "make it very difficult for states to give people the services they expect."[44] Congressional Republicans in attendance encouraged the governors to reach a bipartisan agreement, signaling that they would support virtually any reconfiguration of Medicaid recommended by state leaders.[45] The Clinton administration was less encouraging, reportedly asking Democratic governors to withhold their support from any agreement that would fundamentally restructure Medicaid. Administration officials denied these reports, however, noting that "we do not and cannot control what Democratic governors want or don't want."[46]

Despite the administration's concerns, Democratic governors—eager to put an end to the budget impasse and realizing that a better deal was unlikely—joined their Republican counterparts in unanimously approving a resolution to support the task force's plan. After the vote, one governor after another marveled that the NGA had pushed politics aside and set an example of bipartisan cooperation for Congress to follow. Governor Thompson told his colleagues he had "never been prouder to be a member of this organization."[47] The news media exclaimed that the nation's governors had "stepped into the Washington fray in an unprecedented fashion" and emerged "almost like a third house of Congress."[48]

Despite their unanimous vote, however, governors of both parties continued to express serious concerns about the proposal. Shortly after the vote, Governor George Allen (R-Virginia) told his colleagues, at the risk of "ruining this lovefest," that he had voted for the NGA plan despite "grave reservations" that it might result in "the same old Medicaid program, but this time, with capped entitlements and unfunded mandates on the states."[49] On the other hand, some Democratic governors felt that the plan's coverage guarantees were insufficient. For instance, Governor Parris Glendening (D-Maryland) noted that he had reservations about the proposal because "as a progressive Democrat, I happen to believe that guarantees are important."[50]

In fact, the most critical factor that had enabled the governors to reach a unanimous, bipartisan agreement was that the plan was quite vague. As Romer aide Alan Weil put it, the document was "a fairly general statement" of only four pages; "how you would actually do it I think would be very, very difficult."[51] Governor Thompson acknowledged that it was a "very, very fragile package" and that if Congress tinkered with it too much, the governors' unanimous support would quickly fall apart.[52]

The NGA plan clearly reflected the states' financial interests, leading many congressional Democrats to assail it as a self-serving attempt to protect state budgets rather than the health of vulnerable populations. Representative Henry Waxman (D-California) acerbically noted that "the constituency for Medicaid is not the governors—the constituency for Medicaid is the elderly, the disabled and low-income mothers and children."[53] Child advocacy groups and civil-rights organizations echoed these criticisms. The president's health advisors also opposed to the NGA plan because it would eliminate guaranteed coverage for children above the age of 13; give total discretion to states to alter the amount, duration, and scope of services; and allow the states to cut $200 billion from the program over seven years.[54] However, realizing that the president was "very close to the governors" and might be influenced by their proposal, his health care team was "scared to death" that he might feel compelled to support it.[55]

It was not until President Clinton invited Governors Engler and Thompson to a meeting in the Cabinet Room in late February that his advisors learned of his position on the NGA plan. In a surreal touch, the president had met earlier with some officials from New Orleans who had presented him with some Mardi Gras beads, which he was still wearing during the meeting. HCFA Administrator Bruce Vladeck recalls: "We walked in that meeting and we didn't know for sure what the President was going to say. And, you know, after five minutes of teasing us which, you know, was part of his style, he came out very strong about why this was unacceptable."[56] In particular, the president objected that the NGA plan stopped short of fully preserving Medicaid's status as an entitlement program.

The president's firm rejection of the NGA plan reflected the changing political climate in Washington. The year before, the shell-shocked White House had offered only mild resistance as the new Republican leadership had worked with Republican governors to draft a balanced budget blueprint. But after the second government shutdown, voters had increasingly turned against Newt Gingrich and his Contract with America. According to Vladeck, "the contrast between February '95 and February '96 was so dramatic. February '95 . . . the Administration was just in total funk. And a year later the world was looking up again."[57]

As the president dug in his heels, Republican leaders in Congress did the same. Although they praised the NGA plan, announced their intention to convert it into legislation, and held a "Hearing on the Governors' Bipartisan Medicaid Proposal," they excluded Democratic governors and NGA officials from the drafting process, again consulting only with a handful of Republican governors. In May 1996, they introduced a bill that did not resemble the NGA plan so much as their original block-grant legislation which President Clinton had vetoed in December. Despite the governors' efforts, the Washington stalemate continued.

GOVERNORS' FRAGILE CONSENSUS CRUMBLES

As the Democratic governors pored over the GOP's bill, comparing its provisions to what they felt they had agreed to, they expressed outrage at the "tremendous differences" between the two.[58] The three Democratic members of the NGA task force sent a letter to congressional leaders complaining that the legislation was inconsistent with the NGA plan. In particular, they objected that the bill—hailed by congressional Republicans as reflecting the governors' bipartisan compromise—deviated from their proposed formula for distributing funds, which they referred to as "the main artery of the Governors' package."

> Governors spent hours crafting a compromise that has dollars following indi-
> viduals and that maintains the Federal government as our partner . . . [W]hile
> you have used many of the terms in our agreement . . . you have created a
> block grant for this program with essentially the same language and param-
> eters of the vetoed bill.[59]

In June, the Democratic task force members continued to criticize the legislation in testimony before the Senate Finance Committee.

> We want to say in the clearest terms possible: the bill before you does not re-
> flect the NGA agreement as it pertains to Medicaid. We know. We were the
> governors who negotiated that agreement . . . The most obvious failing in the
> bill is in the financing formula . . . The funding formula is critical because a
> guarantee to provide coverage without sufficient funding is a meaningless
> guarantee.

The Democratic governors pointed out several aspects of the bill which they
found particularly problematic. The "growth factor" was not based on estimated caseloads, was "severely constrained by floors and ceilings," and thus
was "entirely inconsistent with the NGA policy which is based upon the
principle that federal funds should follow the people served by the program." Moreover, the umbrella fund was "entirely different and inadequate"
compared to what the governors had proposed, in part because it only covered unanticipated caseloads for a period of one year. In addition,

> Some of the features of the bill so fundamentally change the nature of that
> guarantee that one cannot say that those guarantees remain—certainly not
> in a form anything like what the NGA proposal contemplated. Specifically,
> permitting unlimited copayments and deductibles, residency requirements,
> family financial responsibility, and other similar provisions completely
> undermine[s] the guarantee of health care services to our most needy citi-
> zens.

Democratic governors accused congressional leaders of "adopting the positions Republican Governors felt were most critical, while rejecting the most
important issues for the Democratic Governors," and then attempting to
"pin our bipartisan name" on a bill that reflected the preferences of a single
party.[60] Announcing that the governors' compromise had collapsed, Gover-

nor Romer proclaimed that Democratic governors would all ask the president to veto the bill if Congress passed it.

Republican governors on the task force bitterly accused their Democratic colleagues of posturing to give the president political cover to veto the legislation, and accused the White House of pressuring Democratic governors to renege; indeed, White House documents suggest that the Clinton administration had urged them to reject the Republican proposal. Notes from a phone call between White House chief of staff Leon Panetta and the three Democrats on the NGA task force indicate that even before the Republicans released their bill, Panetta was urging them to "very publicly walk away," and offered the services of a "Medicaid swat team" to "help you criticize their flawed, 'partisan' approach." During the call, Panetta inquired, "How are the other Democratic governors doing?" and urged Romer, Chiles, and Miller to make sure their colleagues did not cave under pressure and support "a Medicaid plan that would have to be vetoed."[61]

In the end, most Democratic governors were happy to cooperate with the White House. In fact, many were relieved when the bipartisan compromise began to collapse, having had misgivings about Medicaid reform from the start—as Romer aide Alan Weil explained.

> Democratic Governors got way out ahead of their party and their President and agreed to fundamentally redoing this program and then had to say, 'Oops. Gulp. We might actually get what we asked for or at least very close to it,' and had to make a lot out of the pieces that were missing.[62]

Some moderate Republican governors were also secretly relieved, having tentatively supported their party's proposal in public despite privately fearing the loss of open-ended financial support, as noted earlier.

After the governors' bipartisan consensus crumbled, the prospects for a Medicaid block grant looked increasingly dim in the summer of 1996, but the AFDC block grant proposal remained alive and well. Negotiating an AFDC block grant was a simpler undertaking for several reasons (Weaver 1996). First, AFDC was a smaller program—with a budget approximately one-sixth the size of Medicaid's—and growing much less rapidly. The lower stakes meant both that the governors were more open to the principle of a block grant and that the formula fight was less intense. Second, as a cash-assistance program that was widely seen as discouraging work and promoting dependence, AFDC enjoyed considerably less political popularity than Medicaid. Third, the governors received support from powerful allies—most notably hospitals and nursing homes—in lobbying against the Medicaid block grant but not the AFDC block grant. Fourth, since the Contract with America had included welfare reform but not health care reform, congressional Republicans were determined to block-grant AFDC but did not feel as committed to Medicaid reform. Finally, President Clinton, who had promised universal health coverage during his 1992 campaign, was steadfastly opposed to a Medicaid block grant, but saw an AFDC block grant as consistent with his pledge to "end welfare as we know it."

In a last-ditch effort to force the president to sign off on their Medigrant proposal, congressional Republicans—with the blessing of conservative Republican governors—packaged the Medicaid and AFDC block grants together in a single piece of legislation, gambling that the president would not go back on his welfare reform pledge right before the 1996 election. Democratic governors were outraged by this maneuver. In a letter to congressional leaders, they wrote: "We are within striking distance on welfare reform and we cannot agree to a partisan strategy that holds welfare hostage."[63]

In packaging the two reforms together, Republican leaders had initially viewed welfare reform as "a powerful little tugboat that would pull the leaky barge of Medicaid reform to the safe harbor of legislative passage and presidential endorsement." But as the president called the Republicans' bluff and continued to threaten a veto, it became increasingly clear that "the Medicaid barge would have pulled welfare reform down with it" (Weaver 1996, 82). The congressional leadership finally caved in and stripped the Medicaid provisions from the bill, paving the way for passage of a welfare reform bill. In August 1996, the president signed the Personal Responsibility and Work Opportunity Reconciliation Act (PRWORA), replacing the open-ended AFDC program with a more restrictive block grant known as Temporary Assistance for Needy Families.

The opposition of Democratic governors had been critical to the demise of the Republicans' Medigrant proposal. One Clinton administration official elaborated:

There is no question that we would not have succeeded in the block grant fight in '96 if a couple of the Democratic governors hadn't stepped up. Lawton Chiles for a couple of weeks held the Democratic governors at bay just by

saying we won't disagree with the president without looking at [the bill]. And
then, Governor Romer of Colorado got very involved and spent a lot of time
and ultimately was able to bring the rest of them along.[64]

The Democratic governors' backing gave the president the political cover he
needed to credibly threaten to veto the block grant legislation despite intense congressional pressure. Once again, the governors' efforts to protect
their states' financial interests also served to preserve the Medicaid program's
institutional structure.

ECHOES OF THE BLOCK GRANT DEBATE

Medicaid came closer to being fundamentally restructured and retrenched
in the mid-1990s than ever before due to a unique set of political and economic factors including a large number of Republican governors, heightened party polarization, a recent spate of federal mandates, and a strong national economy. Ultimately, however, the governors' enormous financial
stake in the status quo proved to be an insurmountable obstacle and, due to
state leaders' emergence as "leading players" in the national policy-making
process, the Medigrant proposal failed (Derthick 1996). Three subsequent
episodes in Medicaid's history—the creation of the Children's Health Insurance Program in 1997, the failure of President George W. Bush's block grant
proposal in 2001, and the temporary increases in federal matching rates enacted by Congress in 2003 and 2009—serve to underscore these lessons from
the Medigrant experience.

Children's Health Insurance Program

The block grant debate of 1995–96 resumed the following year when President Clinton proposed a major new expansion of health coverage for low-
income children. In striking contrast to the Medigrant debate a year earlier,
governors of both parties strongly supported the idea. Block grants were
widely seen as less threatening this time around since, unlike the earlier proposal, which had been a potential replacement for the Medicaid program
accompanied by a 20 percent cut in federal funding, the 1997 debate concerned a supplement to Medicaid: a new program that would ultimately be
called the Children's Health Insurance Program (CHIP). Since the debate

concerned allocation of new funds rather than redistribution of existing funds, there was no status quo bias, so the formula fight among the states was relatively mild compared to 1995–96.

The Clinton administration's proposal to extend health coverage for low-income children emerged largely from concern that, given the historical linkage between Medicaid eligibility and AFDC eligibility, PRWORA was causing many children to lose health coverage as their parents left the welfare rolls. Moreover, welfare reform had been unpopular with many Democrats, and Clinton was looking for ways to redeem himself with them (Smith 2011). And after the embarrassing failure of his comprehensive health care reform proposal in 1994, Clinton was seeking a more gradual, politically palatable way to expand coverage. Focusing on children—a highly sympathetic group—also happened to be an effective political strategy, as many congressional Republicans felt that the federal government had a "moral responsibility" to help protect kids.[65] Thus, in his State of the Union speech in February 1997, the president announced a proposal to extend health coverage to an additional five million children.

The Clinton administration initially proposed to pay for half the cost of the new coverage by establishing a per-capita cap on federal Medicaid contributions so as to free up additional federal funds. Predictably, the governors' response was swift and resolute. In a statement, the NGA warned that "Any unilateral Federal cap on the Medicaid program will shift costs to state and local governments that they simply cannot afford. The governors adamantly oppose a cap on Federal Medicaid spending in any form."[66] After the governors came out against it, the president quickly dropped the proposal, acknowledging the need for new federal appropriations.

The national debate over how to go about extending coverage to millions of uninsured children focused on two main alternatives: expansion of Medicaid coverage, or creation of a new stand-alone block-grant program, which would give the states a lump sum of money and broad discretion over its use. Not surprisingly, Congress was split mostly along party lines. Most congressional Democrats shared President Clinton's preference for Medicaid expansion, fearing that a block grant would not provide sufficient carrots and sticks for the states to spend money on covering uninsured children, while Republicans preferred the block grant approach for ideological and fiscal reasons.

By contrast, governors of both parties lobbied hard for block-grant funding for the new children's health initiative. They told Congress they did not want to be constrained by Medicaid rules and feared taking on another uncontrollable individual entitlement and the financial risks it entailed. Even governors such as Lawton Chiles (D-Florida), who had fought hard against block-granting Medicaid the year before, argued that the approach was favorable because under matching grants, few states would be able to afford the "entry fee"—that is, the state spending required to qualify for federal matching funds. Senator John D. Rockefeller (D-West Virginia), one of the co-sponsors of the Medicaid expansion proposal, reported that "an amazing number of governors" had been calling his office to protest.[67]

After the National Governors Association rejected the Medicaid expansion plan, Congress abandoned that approach and instead settled on a bipartisan compromise designed as a "midway" between a block grant and Medicaid expansion (Smith 2011, 25). The State Children's Health Insurance Program (SCHIP; later shortened to simply CHIP) included numerous provisions specifically designed to address the governors' concerns. The legislation entitles states—not individuals—to federal financial assistance, thereby minimizing states' risk. States receive annual allotments determined by a formula based on the number of low-income and low-income uninsured children, as well as a state medical-cost factor. Although the legislation retains the matching grant structure in order to induce states to spend some of their own funds, it offers enhanced matching rates ranging from 65 to 83 percent. However, to control the federal cost, the total amount of federal funding is capped, as under a block grant, at roughly $4 billion per year. The legislation also allows states to choose among three benefit options: enroll children in Medicaid, create a stand-alone SCHIP program, or devise a hybrid of the two approaches.[68]

Governors were generally quite pleased with this outcome. At the annual NGA meeting in July 1997, they issued a bipartisan statement hailing the new program.

> In charting a new course toward expanding coverage to more uninsured children, Congress and the President are giving states the ability to build on their successes in designing health insurance programs that meet the unique needs of their states. With state flexibility to design more meaningful and comprehensive benefits packages, coverage numbers will increase substantially.[69]

At the conclusion of the meetings, NGA chairman George Voinovich (R-Ohio) congratulated his colleagues on securing "more money for children . . . with as little strings as possible."[70]

Congress's strategy of enacting a "financially generous alternative" to the Medicaid entitlement was widely viewed as "brilliantly successful," as states "responded to the lure of good money with few strings attached by rapidly implementing SCHIP and extending assistance to several million additional uninsured low-income children" (Rosenbaum, Markus, and Sonosky 2004, 3). All 50 states eagerly chose to participate in the program, and after 10 years, 6 million children—roughly 80 percent of the eligible population—were enrolled.[71]

This chapter in Medicaid's history provides a powerful illustration of the program's self-reinforcing nature. Whereas federal lawmakers' attempts in 1995 and 1996 to convert Medicaid into a block grant failed due to gubernatorial resistance and formula fights, in 1997 the governors unanimously and wholeheartedly embraced the creation of a new block grant to finance expanded coverage for low-income children. This striking contrast suggests that the Medicaid program has persisted for decades as an individual entitlement funded with open-ended categorical matching grants—despite numerous federal attempts at reform—not because governors prefer that structure but rather as a result of a path-dependent process, whereby early decisions about the program's institutional design constrained subsequent opportunities for change.

Block Grant Redux

As this chapter has argued, the governors' unprecedented openness to trading more flexibility over Medicaid policy for less federal funding in the mid-1990s reflected not only the transformation of the political landscape following the Republican revolution, but also the strong national economy, which reduced the salience of the financial risk that such a reform would entail for the states. In fact, a few years later, when federal policy makers proposed a nearly identical Medicaid block grant in the wake of a national recession, the governors' reaction was strikingly different.

Following the 2001 recession, plunging tax revenues and swelling Medicaid rolls contributed to the largest state budget shortfalls in several decades. Compounding the states' problems was the fact that many had chosen to undertake major Medicaid expansions in the 1990s in response to strong revenue growth and the availability of creative financing mechanisms and research and demonstration waivers—as documented in chapters 5 and 6. Although many states responded to the downturn by trimming optional benefits or enrollees or cutting provider reimbursement rates, state leaders were reluctant to undertake major reductions in coverage. As one budget analyst noted, "Medicaid was a big moneymaker. Now, if they cut spending, it reduces the federal matching funds."[72] Moreover, federal standards limited the states' discretion to reduce coverage.

As the recession intensified, the governors grew increasingly desperate for both greater flexibility and—as is discussed in the next section—more money. In early 2003, a handful of Republican governors—among them the president's brother, Governor Jeb Bush (R-Florida)—sent a letter to the president requesting more flexibility to implement beneficiary cost-sharing and to undertake targeted coverage reductions without having to go through the lengthy research and demonstration waiver application process.

The Bush administration—sensing an opportunity for a quid pro quo— proposed to grant the requested flexibility in exchange for limits on federal Medicaid funding. States would receive block grants that would grow by a certain percentage each year. This proposal was similar in many respects to the Republicans' 1995 proposal, but differed in one important respect. Learning from the 1995 experience, the Bush administration made the block grant financially advantageous to the states in the short run, increasing federal funding by $12 billion dollars over the first several years, and cutting it by the same amount thereafter. The proposal essentially amounted to an offer of short-term financial assistance in exchange for elimination of the federal government's open-ended financial commitment.

The Bush administration aggressively courted the governors' endorsement of the block grant proposal. Strong gubernatorial support was essential for passage, especially since many members of Congress—sensitive to their states' dire financial predicament—initially expressed little enthusiasm for the plan. As one White House official noted: "It will be hard for Congress to pass any legislation unless it has strong bipartisan support from governors . . . If [governors] don't want to do it, it's not going to happen."[73]

Despite intense pressure from the White House, governors of both parties flatly rebuffed the proposal. Although they wanted the temporary infusion of federal funds as well as the increased flexibility to cut state spending, they feared that a block grant would not provide sufficient protection against financial risks arising from economic downturns like the one they were experiencing at the time, as well as demographic changes, outbreaks of disease, or medical cost inflation. Even the president's brother, Jeb Bush, was "right there with the other governors" in rejecting the Medicaid reform proposal for lacking "a safety net to address the possibility of a phenomenal or catastrophic event."[74]

Instead of endorsing the president's proposal, the governors established a bipartisan task force to negotiate a better deal with the White House. The task force proposed a modified version of the president's plan with higher federal funding caps and greater state flexibility. Most significantly, the governors proposed that the federal government absorb the $40 billion per year that states were paying toward health care for six million elderly and disabled people who were eligible for both Medicaid and Medicare. They argued that these dual eligibles—who accounted for nearly one-third of total Medicaid expenditures, largely due to the high cost of long-term care—should (like Medicare and Social Security) be the responsibility of the federal government, not the states. The White House balked at the "massive cost" of the governors' counteroffer, and the negotiations ended without a deal.[75]

"Compensatory Federalism"

Not only did the governors block the proposed elimination of open-ended matching grants in the wake of the recession, they also managed to secure additional matching funds. Starting in the fall of 2001, governors of both parties repeatedly lobbied Congress and the president for a temporary increase in Medicaid matching rates at a cost of $10 billion. NGA executive director Raymond Scheppach acknowledged that there was no precedent in recent history for state officials seeking such a large increase in federal aid.[76] Even conservative Republican governors like John Engler—who just a few years before had argued forcefully that the states could make do with less federal Medicaid money—told federal lawmakers that an increase in federal support for Medicaid was "critical."[77]

President George W. Bush was cool to the governors' requests. White House officials told state leaders that the federal government—which was struggling with its own budget deficit—had never provided the states with additional Medicaid funding during previous recessions. The Bush administration pointed out that "the federal government is shouldering half the cost in Medicaid spending now, and we're not favoring a change in that situation."[78]

The governors' frustrations reportedly boiled over into partisan bickering at the winter 2003 meeting of the NGA, as Democratic governors accused the White House of "callousness toward state needs," and Republican governors called their colleagues "big-government liberals." Media reports suggested that the governors "narrowly averted a partisan rupture" during a closed session described by one governor as a "come-to-Jesus meeting" in which NGA chairman Dirk Kempthorne (R-Idaho) urged state leaders to "put pragmatism ahead of partisanship," and focus on their shared goal of securing additional federal funding.[79] However, one insider suggested that the partisan posturing had been largely for show, noting that "behind closed doors" the governors—with their common need for federal aid—"exhibit a lot more similarity than folks are being led to believe."[80]

As President Bush continued to rebuff the NGA's funding requests, governors of both parties turned their attention to Congress, with Governor George Pataki (R-New York) taking the lead. Not only was New York struggling to pay for one of the most expensive Medicaid programs in the nation, it was also reeling from the terrorist attack on the World Trade Center, which cost the state billions of dollars in lost revenue. Pataki worked closely with Democratic senators Charles Schumer and Hillary Clinton to secure congressional support for a temporary increase in the Medicaid matching rate as a way to replace this lost revenue. Given federal lawmakers' resistance to a 9/11 bailout for the state, Schumer saw increased Medicaid funding as "another way to skin the same cat."[81]

Despite being controlled by Republicans, Congress—ever attuned to state needs—proved to be more receptive to the governors' pleas than the White House. In May 2003, Congress passed $20 billion in temporary federal fiscal relief for the states as part of the Jobs and Growth Tax Relief Reconciliation Act. Of that amount, $10 billion came through a temporary 2.95 percentage-point increase in each state's matching rate for 18 months; the other $10 billion consisted of temporary grants that could be used for Medicaid or other purposes.

This temporary increase in matching rates in response to a recession—or "compensatory federalism"—set a precedent for the next national downturn: the Great Recession of 2007–2009 (Thompson 2011). Following an intense bipartisan lobbying campaign by the governors, Congress allocated $140 billion for increased state aid, of which $87 billion consisted of a temporary increase in Medicaid matching rates, as part of the American Recovery and Reinvestment Act of 2009. The formula included three factors: a hold-harmless provision to prevent states' matching rates from declining automatically due to changes in state income, a 6.2 percent increase in all states' matching rates, and an additional increase of up to 11.5 percent for states with high unemployment rates. All told, the average state's match grew by more than 10 percent—significantly larger than the increase in 2003. The measure was originally scheduled to last nine quarters, from October 2008 through December 2010, but the recession dragged on longer than anticipated and—under pressure from governors of both parties—Congress agreed to extend it through June 2011 at an additional federal cost of $16 billion.[82]

In both 2003 and 2009, Congress required states to comply with maintenance of effort requirements: in order to receive the additional federal funds, states had to maintain Medicaid eligibility standards no more restrictive than those in place in September 2003 and July 2008, respectively. Without such mandates, states could have adjusted their Medicaid plans so as to use the new federal funds to supplant, rather than supplement, their own Medicaid spending, thereby freeing up state funds for use in other areas. Of course, the fact that such strings were necessary to prevent cost-shifting under Medicaid's federal-state financing arrangement further served to protect the program against retrenchment.

CONCLUSION

When it comes to Medicaid, state leaders want two things: more money and fewer mandates (Gormley 2006). Converting Medicaid from an entitlement program funded with categorical matching grants to a block grant would afford the states greater discretion over eligibility, benefits, provider reimbursement, and delivery systems, which is greatly appealing to most governors. However, a block grant would also shift enormous financial risks from the federal government to the states—risks that many state officials are not willing to assume. Moreover, converting Medicaid to a block grant poses a thorny transition problem: since states are pitted against one another in a distributive fight over a fixed pie, and are determined not to lose funding relative to the status quo, it is virtually impossible for them to agree on a block grant formula. When the block grant is accompanied by proposed funding cuts, the pie shrinks and the formula fight becomes even more intractable. Although Republicans had an historic opportunity to transform Medicaid's institutional structure in the mid-1990s—as a host of political and economic factors aligned in favor of reform—these obstacles proved to be insurmountable. Just as Senate majority leader Robert Dole had predicted, Republicans would not have another such opportunity for decades to come.

CHAPTER 8

Health Care Reform in the 2000s

IN 2006, Republican governor Mitt Romney signed legislation providing universal health coverage for Massachusetts residents. Four years later, Democratic president Barack Obama signed the Patient Protection and Affordable Care Act of 2010, expanding health coverage to 34 million uninsured Americans. The two reforms share many features in common, including an individual mandate, an employer mandate, health-insurance exchanges through which individuals may purchase private insurance, and expanded Medicaid coverage. These similarities are no accident—the Obama administration explicitly used the Romney plan as a template for federal reform—a fact that later haunted the Republican governor as he ran for president in 2012, and struggled to find a coherent way to tout his own reform program while attacking the Democratic president's plan.

In addition to their similar provisions, the two reforms share another, less obvious characteristic: in both cases, policy makers used Medicaid's federal-state financing arrangement as a mechanism for cutting and shifting costs. In Massachusetts, Governor Romney's desire to minimize the need for new taxes led him to develop a health care reform plan that relied on federal Medicaid funds for more than half of its financing. Similarly, by expanding Medicaid to include 17 million additional Americans, federal policy makers took advantage of state cost-sharing, as well as savings from the program's low provider reimbursement rates and administrative costs, to minimize the need for politically unpopular tax increases during the Great Recession. The nation's governors emerged as a formidable lobbying force, however, and succeeded in convincing Congress to provide supplemental funding for the newly eligible enrollees and the Supreme Court to make the expansion optional rather than mandatory.

The successful enactment of these two programs stands in stark contrast to the failure of dozens of previous efforts at comprehensive health care reform in the United States due to the antigovernment ethos that pervades U.S. political culture—and the accompanying resistance to tax increases needed to finance reform—as well as a decentralized political system full of checks and balances that makes it easy for opponents to block change (Sparer 2009). However, institutional fragmentation also creates rich opportunities for policy entrepreneurs to expand coverage incrementally through the back channels of the policy process (Hacker 2002). One particular form of institutional fragmentation—fiscal federalism—enabled policy entrepreneurs in Massachusetts to develop a reform model that avoided the pitfalls that typically sink efforts at comprehensive health reform. By exploiting Medicaid's federal-state cost-sharing arrangement, Massachusetts policy makers were able to bridge partisan and ideological divisions and minimize resistance among taxpayers and interest groups. The Massachusetts reform, in turn, provided a working model that federal policy makers were able to scale up to the national level. The Medicaid program has thus proven to be a convenient vehicle for "incremental universalism," or getting to universal coverage by filling the gaps in the existing system rather than starting from scratch (Gruber 2008).

HEALTH CARE REFORM IN MASSACHUSETTS

In April 2006, when Governor Mitt Romney signed legislation providing universal health coverage to Massachusetts residents, it was the culmination of three waves of health care reform spanning three decades (McDonough 2004; McDonough et al. 2006). Although the first two waves—spearheaded by Democratic governor Michael Dukakis in the 1980s and Republican governor William Weld in the 1990s—drew less fanfare than the third, they laid critical groundwork for the eventual passage of universal coverage.

Medicaid played an integral role in all three waves, as state leaders of both parties, facing stiff political opposition to tax hikes, found exploiting the program's open-ended federal matching grants to be the path of least resistance. In a striking case of path dependence, political actors' efforts to minimize the burden on state taxpayers and businesses—through use of creative financing mechanisms and waivers—early in the state's march toward comprehensive health care reform shaped political actors' opportunities and constraints later in the process. In fact, Romney has acknowledged that his plan would not have worked had he been unable to build on earlier governors' efforts to exploit Medicaid's financing arrangement (Romney 2010). Thus, Massachusetts's groundbreaking universal health care reform—and how Medicaid came to play such a critical role within it—can only be fully understood in historical context.

First Wave of Reform

Massachusetts's first wave of reform was initiated in the mid-1980s by Governor Michael Dukakis (McDonough et al. 1997). At the time, Dukakis was a popular leader—having been reelected by nearly 70 percent of voters—presiding over a financial-services and high-tech-fueled economic expansion known as the Massachusetts Miracle. A liberal Democrat and passionate advocate of national health insurance, Dukakis was preparing a bid for the White House, and looking for ways to increase his national profile.

In the summer of 1986, Governor Dukakis unveiled an ambitious plan to guarantee health coverage to every resident in the state. The centerpiece was a "play-or-pay" employer mandate which would have required employers to either participate in the employer-sponsored health insurance system or help subsidize government-provided coverage through payment of a $1,680 fine per uninsured employee per year. The plan also included several smaller provisions designed to fill holes in the safety net, including expanded Medicaid coverage of children and pregnant women; a program called Healthy Start to cover low-income pregnant women and new mothers who were not poor enough to qualify for Medicaid; a program called CommonHealth to cover disabled children and adults who did not qualify for Medicaid; and a Medical Security Plan to cover individuals collecting unemployment compensation. The goal was to provide near-universal coverage by 1992.

Dukakis's proposal—and, particularly, the employer mandate—faced stiff opposition from groups representing business and taxpayer interests. To minimize political resistance, Dukakis agreed to scale back private-sector contributions to a preexisting arrangement—the Uncompensated Care Pool—whereby hospitals could bill the state for the cost of providing care to low-income, uninsured patients. Since its inception in 1985, the pool had been funded through a surcharge included in all private payers' hospital bills, but Dukakis agreed to cap and gradually phase down the private-sector liability, with the rationale that the employer mandate would reduce the need for uncompensated care. In a fateful decision, he committed the state to make up for any shortfalls by contributing public funds to the pool.[1]

In April 1988, the Democrat-controlled state legislature narrowly passed chapter 23 of the Acts of 1988—An Act to Make Health Security Available to All Citizens of the Commonwealth and to Improve Hospital Financing—making Massachusetts the first state to enact a law that would guarantee health care for all. However, few observers predicted that the legislation would ever be fully implemented. As the leader of a taxpayer group explained, the law was "incredibly divisive," and its passage had required "a huge amount of arm twisting and a lot of bitterness."[2] Even members of the governor's staff who publicly promoted the reform privately predicted that "it was all going to fall apart as soon as Dukakis left the State House."[3] Indeed, following Republican William Weld's victory in the 1990 gubernatorial election on a platform of pro-business policies, tax cuts, and the repeal of universal health care, the state legislature—where the margin of support had been narrow to begin with—repeatedly postponed implementation of the central component of the reform: the employer mandate.

However, state lawmakers put most of chapter 23's other, less controversial provisions into place right away. Expansion of Medicaid coverage was relatively low cost for state taxpayers and businesses—making it relatively attractive to politicians—thanks to the availability of federal matching funds. Thus, state lawmakers immediately expanded coverage to infants and pregnant women up to 185 percent, young children up to 133 percent, and older children up to 114 percent of the federal poverty level. Other expansions of coverage (Healthy Start, CommonHealth, and the Medical Security Plan) were initially funded out of state coffers, but as the state's economic and budget situation deteriorated, state leaders found ways to fold these programs into Medicaid in order to qualify for federal matching funds—as discussed in the next section.

State lawmakers also immediately implemented the cap on private-sector contributions to the Uncompensated Care Pool in response to pressure from business groups. However, in the absence of an employer mandate, the anticipated decline in the number of uninsured—which was to have alleviated financial pressure on the pool—failed to materialize. To the contrary, the economic downturn caused a spike in the uninsured rate, elevating the state's liability to the pool and exacerbating the state's already-grim budget situation.

When William Weld entered the governor's office in 1991, the Uncompensated Care Pool was desperately underfunded, but the new governor was eager to keep his campaign pledge of no new taxes. Luckily for Weld, a number of other states had recently figured out how to use creative financing mechanisms to shift Medicaid costs to the federal government—as discussed in chapter 5. Governor Weld notified the U.S. Health Care Financing Administration that he believed Massachusetts was entitled to collect $500 million in retroactive disproportionate-share hospital (DSH) funds to support the pool dating back to 1988, and several hundred million more per year going forward. After a lengthy and contentious negotiation process, "the feds went down kicking and screaming," according to one state official.[4]

Although the creative financing mechanism provided an enormous infusion of federal funds to support health care for the poor in Massachusetts, helping the state avoid a fiscal crisis in the short term, its long-term significance remained unclear for more than a decade. Ultimately, this pot of federal funds would play a pivotal role in bringing about universal coverage in Massachusetts.

Second Wave of Reform

In the mid-1990s, Governor Weld came under increasingly intense pressure to address the problem of the uninsured. The Democrat-controlled state legislature hammered him for allowing the uninsured rate to rise from 8.5 percent to 11 percent following the 1990–1991 recession (fig. 11). Although they had repeatedly delayed implementation of the employer mandate, state lawmakers refused to repeal it altogether in the hopes that keeping it alive would pressure the governor to act. With the mandate hanging over his head, Governor Weld was eager to come up with a plan of his own. As one Weld administration official acknowledged, "We realize that Chapter 23 is coming. If we're not going to support that, we need to put an alternative on the plate."[5]

Thus, the Weld administration began to develop a new initiative advertised as "universal coverage without an employer mandate." Because the governor had vowed not to raise taxes, the initiative relied heavily on funding from the federal government. In short, Weld wanted to "reduce the number of Massachusetts residents who lack health coverage by hundreds of thousands without costing an extra penny in state funds."[6]

In the spring of 1994, the Weld administration applied for federal approval of a section 1115 demonstration project known as MassHealth. The

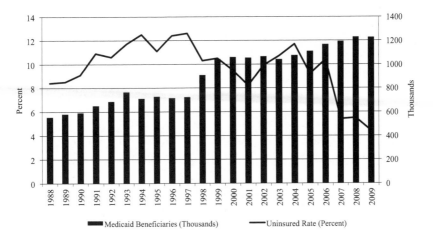

Fig. 11. Massachusetts's Medicaid beneficiaries and uninsured rate, 1988–2009. (Data from U.S. Census Bureau.)

proposal created several new Medicaid eligibility categories including the long-term unemployed. It also expanded income limits for existing eligibility categories: children, pregnant women, parents, and disabled individuals who had been covered up to 86–185 percent of poverty prior to the waiver were to be covered up to 150–200 percent of poverty. The Weld administration also requested federal approval to absorb several fully state-funded health programs into Medicaid—shifting half of the cost of these programs to the federal government, and thereby freeing up state funds to help pay for the expansion of coverage. In addition, the proposal featured tax credits to encourage employers to offer insurance and subsidies to encourage low-wage workers to enroll in employer-sponsored insurance plans.

As part of the waiver proposal, state officials also requested a special pot of federal money designated for the two largest and most powerful public safety-net providers in the state: Boston City Hospital (now Boston Medical Center), and Cambridge City Hospital (now Cambridge Health Alliance). These providers saw the transition to managed care as a potential threat to their financial stability, fearing that reimbursement rates would be lower than under the existing fee-for-service system and that patients would have greater flexibility to seek treatment elsewhere.[7] Bowing to pressure from these powerful health care providers, the Weld administration supported the creation of managed-care organizations (MCOs) by the two providers and asked the federal government to give them supplemental payments in excess of the Medicaid upper-payment limit. Moreover, the state proposed that the nonfederal share of the supplemental payments be funded through intergovernmental transfers from the cities of Boston and Cambridge, thereby drawing down additional federal matching funds without putting up any new state dollars.

In order to win federal approval of the MassHealth experiment, state officials had to demonstrate budget neutrality.[8] To this end, the Weld administration proposed to limit Medicaid cost growth to 4 percent per year through managed-care savings and other cost-containment measures. The administration claimed that its demonstration project would actually save the federal government more than half a billion dollars over five years—a projection that proved to be overly optimistic.[9] Most significantly, the Weld administration argued that the project would so greatly reduce the need for uncompensated care that the state should be allowed to funnel two-thirds of the funds in the Uncompensated Care Pool—which was primarily comprised of federal DSH funds—into MassHealth.

With the help of influential U.S. senator Edward Kennedy (D-Massachusetts), a liberal advocate of universal health care with close ties to the Clinton administration, Massachusetts won approval of its demonstration project from the U.S. Health Care Financing Administration in 1995—yielding an increase in federal funding of $331 million per year. This infusion of federal funding neutralized the political debate over the financing issue, allowing state leaders to focus the debate on the less controversial matter of children's health-care needs (Greenberg and Zuckerman 1997).

In addition to federal approval, the MassHealth experiment required authorization from the state's Democrat-controlled legislature, which favored an even more generous expansion of coverage than did Governor Weld. In July 1996, state lawmakers approved—over the governor's veto—the Act Providing for Improved Access to Health Care (chapter 203 of the Massachusetts Acts), which added to Weld's plan additional Medicaid coverage of low-income children, and a prescription drug program for low-income seniors. The legislation raised cigarette taxes by 25 cents per pack to help finance the additional expansions.

Implementation began on July 1, 1997. Within two years, Massachusetts's Medicaid program had grown by more than 40 percent—from approximately 700,000 to one million beneficiaries (fig. 11). Despite initial concerns that it might merely crowd out private insurance, the MassHealth experiment contributed to a significant reduction in the state's uninsured rate (Zuckerman et al. 2001).

Third Wave of Reform

The third wave of health reform in Massachusetts began in the wake of the 2001 national recession, shortly after Republican businessman Mitt Romney won the gubernatorial election on a platform of eliminating the state's budget shortfall without resorting to tax increases. Although his campaign platform had made no mention of health care reform, upon taking office Romney identified it as one of the major goals of his administration. In his autobiography, Romney explains that he did so despite initial concerns that "I'd have to break my promise not to raise taxes, because after all, getting everyone insured would cost hundreds of millions of dollars, if not billions" (Romney 2010, 170).

Fortunately, the ambitious goal of universal health insurance would be less costly for Massachusetts than for virtually any other state in the nation. For one thing, the state already had one of the lowest uninsured rates in the country, due in large part to the first two waves of reform. Less than 10 percent of the population—roughly 500,000 people—lacked insurance at the time, compared to an average of 15 percent nationwide.[10] Moreover, many of the state's uninsured residents were already receiving extensive care thanks to the Uncompensated Care Pool. The governor realized that since "someone was already paying for the cost of treating people who didn't have health insurance . . . the cost of insuring everyone in the state might not be as expensive as I had feared" (Romney 2010, 171).

Thus, the Romney administration began to explore the possibility of using the Uncompensated Care Pool as a ready-made source of funding for universal health coverage. Specifically, state officials hoped to redirect the pool's DSH monies from hospitals that served a disproportionate share of uninsured individuals to the individuals themselves to help them purchase private health insurance. However, as Romney acknowledged, "The plan would work only if we could get our hands on the money that was then being used to pay for the health care of the uninsured, most of which came from the federal government" (Romney 2010, 173).

Unfortunately for Romney, President George W. Bush's administration was in Medicaid retrenchment mode. The recession, tax cuts, and war in Iraq had caused the federal deficit to spiral out of control, and the Bush administration was looking for ways to scale back domestic spending. Having failed to implement a Medicaid block grant—as discussed in chapter 7—the administration turned its attention to cracking down on the states' use of section 1115 waivers and creative financing schemes.

Although a few years earlier the Bush administration had renewed the MassHealth waiver without modification through mid-2005, in 2004, budget pressures led the White House to begin threatening to cut off the extra federal money—a total of $585 million per year—to support the demonstration project thereafter. Federal officials argued that the state was receiving more than its fair share of federal Medicaid funds, objecting in particular to the $385 million in annual supplemental payments to Boston Medical Center and Cambridge Health Alliance. This money represented nearly one-tenth of the state's Medicaid budget, so its loss would have been devastating—particularly at a time when the state was facing a projected budget gap of $1 billion.[11] Without these federal funds, Massachusetts would not only be hard-pressed to solve the problem of the uninsured but also would have to scale back Medicaid coverage for hundreds of thousands of people.

The magnitude of this financial threat spurred state leaders into action. Romney's secretary of health and human services, Timothy Murphy, recalls that the potential loss of the MassHealth waiver set off "a lot of high level scrambling" among the governor's staff, state legislative leaders, and members of the state's congressional delegation in Washington. An initial wave of feelers sent out to the Bush administration returned only bad news. Said Murphy: "The feds simply wanted the money off the table. They were running deficits—they could use the money."[12]

The state's urgent need to keep its Medicaid waiver led to the formation of an unusual political alliance: in late 2004, Romney joined forces with Senator Edward Kennedy. The Democratic senator had worked with another Republican governor—William Weld—to secure federal approval for the waiver several years earlier, but Kennedy's collaboration with Governor Romney was even more remarkable because, as Romney put it, the two men "disagreed on almost every major issue of public policy," and had waged a "knock-down battle" for Kennedy's Senate seat in 1994 (Romney 2010, 173–74). This highly unlikely partnership between political rivals illustrates the states' powerful incentives to secure federal financial support to meet state health care needs. As Senator Kennedy explained, getting "the matching funds which Massachusetts is entitled to" was "obviously a matter of enormous importance to everyone in Massachusetts."[13] According to one of his staffers, "We needed to stay together and everybody needed to be on board, working collectively toward a common goal because all the money was at risk."[14]

United by their shared stake in preserving the inflow of federal Medicaid funds, Governor Romney and Senator Kennedy joined forces to "double team everyone in Washington who might be able to influence the waiver decision."[15] After lengthy negotiations with U.S. secretary of health and human services Tommy Thompson in January 2005, they won an agreement to keep the funds flowing to Massachusetts, provided that the state redirect the money from supporting politically powerful providers to subsidizing individuals' purchase of health insurance. If the plan worked, Romney and the Bush administration could both claim credit for reforming health care with market-based ideas and without raising taxes.[16] Thompson gave the Romney administration until January 2006 to present a plan to federal officials, and July 2006 to implement it.

The July 2006 implementation deadline was, as one of Romney's health advisors put it, "a real time bomb that importantly affected state deliberations" (Gruber 2006, 16). The Romney administration quickly put forward a "market-based" plan that included an individual mandate requiring all residents to have health coverage. The redirected federal funds from the waiver would subsidize the purchase of private insurance by low-income individuals. To make insurance more affordable, the governor also proposed to relax state regulations to allow insurance companies to offer less expensive policies with fewer benefits. Romney also wanted to redouble efforts to enroll already-eligible individuals in Medicaid. One-fifth of the state's 500,000 uninsured residents already qualified, and since half of the cost was paid by the federal government, it was a relatively cheap way for the state to expand coverage. Although enrolling 100,000 additional people in Medicaid would require Massachusetts to put up an additional $150 million of its own funds in order to receive the federal match, Romney hoped that the state could recoup most of that money through savings from "aggressively managed treatment."[17]

House Speaker Salvatore DiMasi, a liberal Democrat, shared Romney's desire to guarantee coverage to all Massachusetts residents, but thought it impossible to do so without raising taxes. DiMasi favored an employer mandate requiring businesses with more than 10 employees to pay a payroll tax if they failed to provide coverage to their workers, much like Dukakis's proposal two decades earlier. He also wanted to extend Medicaid eligibility to an additional 130,000 people, and proposed to finance the state's share of the cost with a 50-cent increase in the cigarette tax.

However, Governor Romney, Senate President Robert Travaglini—a moderate Democrat representing the Boston area—and interest groups representing businesses and taxpayers immediately rejected DiMasi's proposed tax increases. As the stalemate dragged on throughout the winter of 2006, the Bush administration gave the state an extension of a few months, but warned, "Anything that happens after the First of July means dollars lost to the state of Massachusetts."[18] In his State of the State address in January 2006, Romney hammered home his message that health care reform should be funded with federal Medicaid funds rather than a state tax increase, and that time was of the essence.

> Health insurance for all our citizens does not require new taxes. Some of you have your doubts about that. I know that the uncertainty could stall our progress, or even end it . . . [W[e have a once in a generation opportunity. Our citizens are counting on us. Federal funding depends on us.[19]

The Romney administration also solicited the help of health providers in pressuring state lawmakers, sending letters to dozens of hospitals warning that they faced cuts in federal Medicaid funding if the state failed to implement a plan in time.

As the deadline approached, transcripts of legislative proceedings revealed a growing sense of urgency among state lawmakers.

> Make no mistake, we're at a critical crossroads right now . . . if we don't do something soon, we're in jeopardy of losing $385 million. You've already heard how much that means to our hospitals. If that happens, we could also have to go into other accounts, and we don't want to do that.[20]

Other members warned that the health impasse was beginning to stunt progress on other state priorities, including an economic stimulus plan and capital projects.[21] As Speaker DiMasi later acknowledged, "The necessity of why we had to do something was very clear. The federal government had changed the rules on the waiver [and] we were going to lose it."[22]

In March 2006, the House and Senate cobbled together a compromise described by the news media as a "last-ditch effort," "an 11th-hour bid," and "a bill crafted to preserve $385 million in annual federal Medicaid funding."[23] As one state senator acknowledged, "The real thrust of this bill is to save the $385 million. Also, to expand access to health insurance."[24] Fearing that the federal government would not approve the plan unless it included strong incentives for uninsured individuals to purchase insurance, House and Senate leaders agreed to include the individual mandate favored by Governor Romney; individuals who chose not to purchase insurance would pay a penalty of up to $917 per year. They also included DiMasi's employer mandate, along with a relatively modest $295 per employee tax on businesses with more than 10 employees that did not offer insurance to their workers; a requirement that insurers offer low-cost plans; subsidies for low-income workers who could not afford to buy insurance on their own; and a clearinghouse (known as the "Connector") to help individuals purchase private health insurance.

The legislation—which Romney signed into law on April 12, 2006, as chapter 58 of the Acts of 2006: An Act Providing Access to Affordable, Quality, Accountable Health Care—included a number of important Medicaid-related provisions (Holahan and Blumberg 2006). It expanded eligibility for children up to 300 percent of the federal poverty level. Adults below the federal poverty level would continue to qualify; for adults between 100 and 300 percent of FPL, a new program called Commonwealth Care would provide coverage in Medicaid managed care programs—such as those operated by Boston Medical Center and Cambridge Health Alliance—at subsidized rates. To accommodate increased demand, the legislation raised provider reimbursement rates. In July, the Bush administration announced its approval of a new section 1115 waiver to support the state's reform plan.

The effects of the 2006 reform were dramatic. Within three years, the state's uninsured rate had dropped to 4 percent—by far the lowest in the country—despite the national recession (fig. 11). As with the earlier waves of reform, there has been little evidence of crowd-out; in fact, the share of employers offering coverage rose from 70 percent in 2006 to 76 percent in 2010. Fewer Massachusetts residents report significant out-of-pocket health expenses or unmet health-care needs. Health reform enjoys considerable public support, with 67 percent of nonelderly adults, 77 percent of employers, and 88 percent of physicians expressing favorable views of the reform.[25]

Leveraging Federal Medicaid Funds

Medicaid's federal-state cost-sharing structure played a critical role in health reform in Massachusetts. The potential loss of federal Medicaid funds created the impetus for the Republican governor and internally divided

Democrat-controlled legislature to break through a prolonged political impasse and reach a compromise. Securing approval to expand MassHealth through the federal waiver process brought additional federal funds into the state, reducing the need to rely on politically unpopular increases in state revenue.

Although the individual and employer mandates received most of the press and were the main source of public controversy in the state's health-reform debate, Medicaid actually accounts for the lion's share of the expansion. Within two years, more than 400,000 additional previously uninsured residents had health insurance; of these, more than half were enrolled in either MassHealth or Commonwealth Care—both supported by federal Medicaid funds (fig. 12). Overall, nearly 60 percent of the state's health-reform package was financed with federal Medicaid matching funds (fig. 13).

Paradoxically, Medicaid played a central role in health care reform in Massachusetts despite Governor Romney's professed antipathy toward the program. The Republican governor has railed against Medicaid as part of the United States' "political shell game" and "entitlement nightmare," and referred to the program as a "Pac-Man" that, during his governorship, "grew twice as fast as our state revenues, eating its way through everything else in the budget . . . crowd[ing] out spending on other priorities" (Romney 2010, 152–54). Yet Romney's desire to accomplish universal coverage without raising state taxes led him to advocate a reform package that took full advantage of federal Medicaid funding, thereby contributing to the program's growth. "RomneyCare" thus provides yet another example of policy feedback: the program's institutional structure creates irresistible incentives for political actors to promote its expansion—even when doing so is at odds with their ideology.

Massachusetts is not alone in leveraging federal Medicaid funds to solve the problem of the uninsured; several other states have adopted similar reforms. Aside from Massachusetts, the state that has gone the furthest toward comprehensive reform is Vermont. In 2006, Vermont's Republican Governor, Jim Douglas, signed legislation aimed at achieving near-universal coverage. This was a striking reversal from 2005, when Douglas had vetoed the Democrat-controlled legislature's proposal for a single-payer system funded by a payroll tax, which he called "inappropriate for a state with a high tax burden" (Maxwell 2007, w698). To win the governor's approval, the legislature switched gears and designed a reform program that built on the existing employer- and Medicaid-based system. In addition to an employer mandate

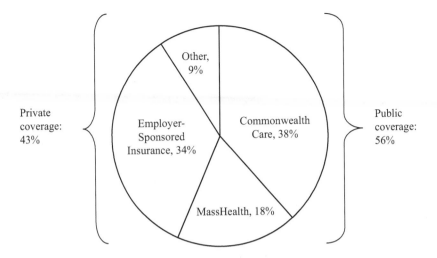

Fig. 12. Massachusetts health care reform plan: Distribution of newly insured. (Data from Kaiser Family Foundation.)

and premium assistance for low-income individuals, the legislation created Catamount Health—a private health-insurance plan for individuals who do not have access to employer-sponsored insurance—largely financed with federal Medicaid funds secured through a demonstration waiver. Residents with incomes up to 300 percent of the federal poverty level can enroll in Catamount Health and pay premiums on a sliding scale. By relying heavily on federal funds, the legislature minimized the need for new state taxes, which helped to neutralize the "politically charged and contentious issues of financing care for the uninsured" that had derailed the previous year's reform effort (Thorpe 2007, w705).

Between 2003 and 2009, a dozen other states including Maine, Colorado, Iowa, and New Mexico enacted smaller-scale health-reform initiatives extending Medicaid or its smaller companion program, the Children's Health Insurance Program, to tens of thousands of additional residents.[26] These expansions have been spearheaded by governors and state legislatures of both political parties and in diverse parts of the country, illustrating the universal appeal of leveraging federal Medicaid funding. However, the pace of state initiatives slowed considerably following the Great Recession due to a shortage of state funds. Moreover, after President Barack Obama took office in 2009 and began promoting an overhaul of the U.S. health-care system,

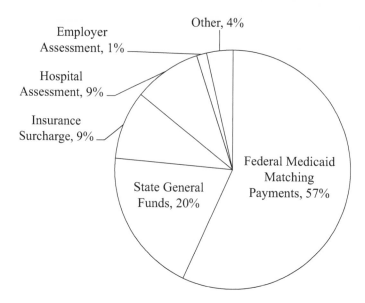

Fig. 13. Massachusetts health care reform plan: Revenue sources. (Data from Kaiser Family Foundation.)

many state leaders chose to wait for the dust to settle before pursuing further state-level reforms.

FEDERAL HEALTH CARE REFORM

The Patient Protection and Affordable Care Act of 2010 (ACA)—signed into law by President Barack Obama in March 2010—bears a strong resemblance to the Massachusetts reform. Among other provisions, the ACA features an individual mandate; an employer mandate; American Health Benefit Exchanges, through which individuals can purchase private insurance (much like Massachusetts's Connector); and a major expansion of Medicaid coverage. These similarities between "RomneyCare" and "ObamaCare" are no accident—national lawmakers explicitly used the Massachusetts model as the template for federal reform. According to one White House official, the Massachusetts reform "gave birth to" the Affordable Care Act; without it, it is unlikely that the ACA would have become law.[27]

Ironically, whereas conservatives had initially praised—or at least tolerated—Romney's reform as market-based and fostering personal responsibility, the Democratic president's reform became a lightning rod for conservative outrage over "socialized medicine" only a few years later. Thus, as Romney campaigned for president, he attempted to distance himself from the Affordable Care Act by claiming that while national reform involved "a huge entitlement, which is the federal government taking power away from the states," in Massachusetts, "we solved our problem at the state level."[28] Romney was attacked from both the left and right for this misrepresentation of his reform's financing mechanism. Jonathan Gruber, often described as the Democratic Party's most influential health-care expert, argued that it was misleading to claim that Massachusetts "did it on its own," observing: "Where are they getting the money?"[29] Conservative political commentator Bill O'Reilly lambasted Romney in a television interview: "You say you solved the problem in the state, but depending on 50 percent of your funding from the Feds . . . I don't know if you solved the problem or the people in Idaho solved it."[30]

In fact, Governor Romney's use of Medicaid's cost-sharing arrangement as a mechanism for achieving health reform on the cheap was yet another feature of the Massachusetts model emulated by national policy makers. The Affordable Care Act includes the single largest eligibility expansion in Medicaid's history, bringing in an estimated 17 million additional people—or half of the 34 million uninsured Americans who would be covered under the ACA—and revolutionizes Medicaid's structure by converting it into a program for all poor and near-poor Americans regardless of age, disability, or family status.[31] The story of how Medicaid became a centerpiece of the ACA is, in the words of health expert John Iglehart, "one of the largely untold sagas of health reform" (Iglehart 2010, 230). As I argue throughout the remainder of this chapter, Medicaid emerged as a central component of national health care reform largely as a means of cutting and shifting costs. However, the governors once again exerted tremendous influence over federal Medicaid policy, convincing Congress to provide states with supplemental funds for newly eligible enrollees and the Supreme Court to make the expansion optional rather than mandatory.

The Financing Challenge

One of the main reasons comprehensive health reform perennially fails in the United States is the difficulty of finding a politically palatable way to fund the expansion of coverage (Oberlander 2008, w544). Most recently, Bill Clinton's Health Security Plan had failed in 1994 largely because it became a foil for anti-tax and anti-government mobilization (Skocpol 1997). The Obama administration and Democratic leaders in Congress were painfully aware of this lesson, which had cost their party dearly in that year's midterm election; indeed, Clinton himself advised Democratic leaders in 2009 to come up with a reform plan that minimized the need for new revenues by finding savings in the existing health care system.[32]

The challenge of funding health reform was particularly acute in the economic and political climate of 2009. As the national economy struggled to recover from the Great Recession and the budget deficit approached a record $1.4 trillion or nearly 10 percent of GDP, health care reform had to compete with economic recovery and deficit reduction on the domestic policy agenda. Moreover, political resistance to the growth of government had reached a fever pitch with the emergence of the conservative Tea Party movement. Reformers were further constrained by two promises the president had made: that 95 percent of Americans would not see their taxes increase "by a single dime,"[33] and that health care reform would not "add one dime to the deficit, now or in the future, period."[34]

These economic and political constraints narrowed the already limited range of politically palatable financing mechanisms. When the Obama administration proposed to pay for reform by allowing the Bush tax cuts on the wealthiest Americans to expire as scheduled at the end of 2010, congressional Republicans and moderate Democrats vehemently rejected the proposal, arguing that it would hurt small businesses and hinder job creation. When the White House proposed limiting the value of tax deductions for mortgage interest and charitable donations, congressional Republicans accused the president of declaring "war against churches and charities," and interest groups representing the home-building and real estate industries protested that the measure would slow the pace of economic recovery.[35] An alternative favored by several congressional moderates was to eliminate the single largest tax break in the U.S. tax code: the exclusion of employer-sponsored health benefits. However, the idea was unpopular with organized labor— and thus many congressional Democrats—and conflicted with the president's promise not to raise taxes on 95 percent of Americans. Other tax proposals floated by an increasingly desperate congressional leadership throughout the spring of 2009—including a payroll tax, a value-added tax, and a surcharge on the wealthy—were shot down as well.

As the limitations on the revenue side of the health-reform equation became increasingly clear, congressional leaders began to focus on the expenditure side. And as they searched for ways to lower the cost of reform, they found themselves turning to Medicaid. Despite covering a population that is less healthy than average, Medicaid is quite inexpensive relative to private health insurance. According to Congressional Budget Office estimates, the per capita federal cost of providing coverage through Medicaid is roughly one-third that of coverage through a private insurance exchange: $1,826 compared to $5,926 in the year 2019 (Rosenbaum 2009).

Medicaid's relatively low federal cost reflects a variety of factors. First and foremost, the program's federal-state financing structure means that the federal government only pays for 57 percent of the cost of coverage, on average. (Whether states would actually contribute their customary 43 percent toward the expansion became the subject of heated debate, however, as discussed shortly.) Moreover, Medicaid's provider reimbursement rates are lower than what private insurance plans can get away with, the program contains no profit component, and it has lower administrative costs than private insurance firms (Rosenbaum 2009). Medicaid also provides a bigger bang for the buck since it includes benefits—such as home- and community-based care—not readily available in the private sector.

Medicaid expansion is also less politically costly than most alternatives. Hospitals and private insurers tend to support Medicaid expansion because the program provides funding for low-income populations that would otherwise have difficulty paying for care, while business leaders see Medicaid expansion as reducing pressure to provide employer-sponsored coverage for low-income workers (Sparer 2009). Moreover, as a fairly low-profile, state-administered program, Medicaid has the advantage of provoking less political outrage over the encroachment of federal government than many alternative platforms. But, political scientist Michael Sparer notes, the single most attractive feature of Medicaid expansion is arguably the potential for cost-shifting embedded the program's intergovernmental structure (Sparer 2009).

Thus, to the extent that there was disagreement among congressional leaders, it was not about whether to expand Medicaid, but rather by how much. Senate Finance Committee chairman Max Baucus (D-Montana) proposed a reform package that, among other measures, would provide every American living below the federal poverty level (FPL) with access to Medicaid, calling it "the quickest and most cost-effective way to cover every American living in poverty."[36] As the committee struggled to come up with a deficit-neutral plan, Medicaid's low cost relative to the exchange subsidies led him to propose expanding eligibility to 133 percent of FPL ($29,330 for a family of four). Similarly, the House tri-committee with jurisdiction over health care reform initially considered extending Medicaid eligibility to 133 percent of FPL, but when President Obama urged Congress to lower the reform package's federal cost, the committee proposed to expand eligibility to 150 percent of FPL ($31,804 for a family of four).

In addition to the question of how much to expand Medicaid, committee leaders had to decide how much of the cost to shift to the states. Requiring them to pay their customary average of 43 percent would clearly relieve pressure on Congress to raise taxes. On the other hand, the states were already struggling to balance their budgets in the wake of the Great Recession, and the stimulus funds for Medicaid under the American Recovery and Reinvestment Act of 2009 would soon expire. Since the states would be important partners in the implementation of any health-reform package, their buy-in was essential.

The two chambers took different positions on the issue of cost-sharing. An early draft of the Senate Finance Committee bill indicated that for the first five years of the expansion, the federal government would pick up between 77 and 95 percent of the cost of newly eligible enrollees instead of the usual 50 to 83 percent; thereafter, federal matching rates would return to their normal levels.[37] By contrast, the more liberal House tri-committee, led by Medicaid champion Henry Waxman (D-California), hoped to provide considerably more financial support to the states. Early drafts of the tri-committee's bill proposed that the federal government pay the full cost of the Medicaid expansion population indefinitely. However, pressure from fiscally conservative "Blue Dog" Democrats to pare back the federal cost ultimately led the House to instead propose full federal funding for the first several years, with the federal government paying 91 percent and the states paying 9 percent of the cost of the newly eligible thereafter.

The Governors' "Open Revolt"

As a general matter of principle, the nation's governors were divided on the issue of health reform. As congressional leaders struggled to hammer out the details of a deficit-neutral reform package, 22 of the nation's 28 Democratic governors signed a letter urging Congress to move forward, noting that "the status quo is no longer an option"—although the letter did not mention the proposed Medicaid expansion.[38] A handful of moderate Republican governors, such as Arnold Schwarzenegger of California, similarly saw reform as "noble" and "needed."[39] However, many Republican governors vehemently opposed the proposals being floated by the Democrat-controlled Congress and White House, and some threatened to sue the federal government if such reforms became law. As a result of their internal division, the governors repeatedly found themselves unable to achieve the two-thirds vote needed to issue policy resolutions on national health reform.

However, there was one area where the governors were in wholehearted agreement: if the federal government was going to require states to expand Medicaid coverage, the federal government should pick up the tab. Indeed, the National Governors Association's only letter to Congress throughout the health-reform debate—sent to the Senate Finance Committee on July 20, 2009—declared that the governors were "steadfastly opposed to unfunded federal mandates and reforms that simply shift costs to states" and cautioned that "any unfunded expansions would be particularly troubling given that states face budget shortfalls of over $200 billion over the next three years."[40] The NGA repeated this message to federal policy makers throughout the summer of 2009. Executive director Raymond Scheppach testified before Congress numerous times, warning that the states were in "dire financial straits" and that without full federal funding, health care reform would "overwhelm state budgets."[41] The NGA also formed a bipartisan 12-governor health care reform task force, which held numerous conference calls and meetings on Capitol Hill and at the White House to hammer home this message.

Individual governors also lobbied Congress and the White House and made media appearances defending the states' collective financial interests. Despite his support for other aspects of health reform, Governor Schwarzenegger warned that "If Congress thinks the Medicaid expansion is too expensive for the federal government, it is absolutely unaffordable for states."[42] Republican Haley Barbour of Mississippi—chairman of the Republican Governors Association and a staunch fiscal conservative—was among the most outspoken critics. In letters to his state's congressional delegation, he complained that "the debate in Congress has shifted to finding ways to . . . expand the Medicaid program at additional costs paid not by the federal government, but passed down to the states."[43] Barbour rallied his fellow Republican governors to join him in a "coordinated attack" on the Senate Finance Committee bill.[44] Most of the 22 Republican governors followed Barbour's lead by writing letters of concern to their states' congressional delegations, citing estimates of the bill's cost to their states' taxpayers.

Numerous Democratic governors, among them Tennessee governor Phil Bredesen, registered similar concerns.

> They've ruled out politically several of the sources of additional money . . . I mean, don't say, "Well, I can't pass a tax, I'm going to find some way to lay it off on somebody else." If you can't pass a tax; you can't do it, I guess. There's no free lunches in the world . . . The governors are obviously in open revolt about the notion of [Congress] just laying it on them, and rightly so.[45]

Even Brian Schweitzer—the Democratic governor of Max Baucus's home state of Montana, close ally of the Obama administration, and general advocate of health reform—warned that "if Congress wants to have a health care program, then they need to pay for it. They can't dump it back on the states."[46]

Apart from the issue of who would pay for newly eligible enrollees, governors had several concerns about the potential effects of Medicaid expansion on state budgets. First, governors were worried about the "woodwork effect," whereby millions of Americans who were already eligible for Medicaid under current law but not enrolled—due to enrollment barriers or lack of information—might sign up in response to the individual mandate, streamlined enrollment policies, and heavy media coverage that would likely accompany health reform. Governors feared that the states would be stuck paying their historic share of the cost of these woodwork enrollees. Second, governors worried that enhanced federal Medicaid funding would be accompanied by a maintenance-of-effort rule requiring states to retain their current eligibility criteria at a time when economic hardship made flexibility over enrollment particularly valuable. Third, the governors feared that a major expansion of Medicaid coverage would necessitate increases in provider reimbursement rates. As Scheppach explained in congressional testimony, "There simply are not enough providers willing to treat additional Medicaid enrollees . . . at current reimbursement rates." Scheppach told Congress that in the governors' view, "the federal government should only consider mandating significant expansions in Medicaid if they are prepared to pay for not only the expansion populations but . . . the short-run additional costs for the existing population."[47]

As congressional leaders debated the details of reform throughout the summer of 2009, Senate Finance Committee chairman Max Baucus initially refused to capitulate to the governors' demands, insisting, "We can't foot the entire bill for the states."[48] In an effort to convince the governors that state cost sharing could work, Baucus considered one particularly desperate measure that would have encouraged states to issue 30-year bonds to cover their share of the cost of expanded coverage. Expressing shock and disbelief, governors of both parties uniformly revolted. One governor compared the idea to "taking out a mortgage to pay the grocery bill."[49] Another pointed out that issuing bonds to fund ongoing programs was in fact illegal in 36 states.[50] A third simply stated: "We are not going to do that because it is going to hurt our bond rating."[51] After a flurry of phone calls from governors, Baucus dropped the idea.

By the end of the summer, state officials' opposition to sharing the cost of the proposed Medicaid expansion had become one of the biggest remaining obstacles to congressional negotiations. Deluged by letters and phone calls from their states' governors, a growing number of senators began to express grave concerns about the potential financial impact on their states. For example, Senator John Thune (R-South Dakota) noted that the proposed expansion "passes on an incredible new and costly mandate to State governments."

> My State of South Dakota is a good case in point. Our State legislature [and] Governor . . . have concluded it would cost South Dakota an additional $45 million a year in Medicaid costs, which may not sound like a lot of money in Washington, DC, but in a State such as South Dakota, where there is a requirement to balance the budget every year, that represents a lot of money.[52]

The White House grew increasing concerned about the governors' opposition. Worried that his major domestic policy initiative was in jeopardy, President Obama acknowledged that state leaders had a "legitimate concern" and urged Congress to pursue Medicaid expansion "in a way that is coordinated carefully with the governors." The White House also began reaching out to governors on a daily basis to convey the message: "we're working with you and we understand where you're coming from."[53]

Under pressure from state leaders, the White House, and his fellow senators, Chairman Baucus finally revised the bill to make the temporary increase in Medicaid matching rates permanent: the federal government would pay 77 to 95 percent of the cost of newly eligible enrollees indefinitely. The Senate

Finance Committee approved the revised bill in mid-October. Although the provision fell short of the governors' goal of full federal funding, the concession was a testament to state leaders' tremendous influence on Capitol Hill. As the *Washington Post* remarked, the governors had emerged as a "formidable lobbying force" in the national debate over health care reform.[54]

Sweetheart Deals

In addition to their "universal interest" in maximizing federal financial assistance for all states, many governors also pursued "particularistic interests" by seeking additional funds for their own states (Dinan 2011, 4). Four cases in particular stand out: "high-need states," "expansion states," the "Louisiana purchase," and Nebraska's infamous "cornhusker kickback."

First, the leaders of several states argued that their particularly dire economic situations qualified them as "high-need states" that deserved additional financial assistance. Under pressure from his state's Republican governor, Jim Gibbons, Senate majority leader Harry Reid (D-Nevada) proposed an amendment to provide 100 percent federal funding for the first five years for states with unemployment rates above 12 percent and lower-than-average Medicaid enrollment. Nevada was one of four states that fell into this category. The amendment caused an immediate uproar in the Senate. In addition to questioning Reid's use of his leadership position to cut a deal for his own state, many senators worried that—given the deficit-neutrality constraint—the resulting revision to the matching formula would come at their states' expense. Senator Lamar Alexander (R-Tennessee) was among those who expressed his concerns.

> [T]he majority leader had heard from his Governor . . . and he was deeply concerned about the legislation that is coming through because it would increase costs in Nevada . . . So the majority leader did exactly what I think a Senator would do. He . . . proposed an amendment . . . to the Senate Finance Committee and said: 'Take care of Nevada' . . . My guess is that [other senators] would be happy to cosponsor the Reid Amendment if it included [their states]. I certainly would be if it included Tennessee . . . The Governor of Arizona has written to Senator McCain [R-Arizona] and Senator Kyl [R-Arizona] to point out that 'Arizona is facing one of the worst financial deficits in the nation . . . ' If Arizona is facing one of the worst financial deficits in the Nation, why is it left out of the majority leader's amendment? It seems to me the citizens of Ari-

zona deserve just as much attention. I imagine their Senators would like to cosponsor it as well.[55]

Under pressure from senators and governors alike, Reid ultimately agreed to amend the bill to provide 100 percent federal funding for all states for the first three years of the expansion.

Second, the governors of so-called expansion states, which had already voluntarily expanded coverage to adults up to 100 percent or more of the federal poverty level, complained that since the enhanced match only applied to newly eligible enrollees, they would get less federal financial assistance than states with less generous eligibility criteria. As one expansion-state governor put it, "we are, in a sense, being punished for our own charity."[56] The governors of these states—Massachusetts, Vermont, Hawaii, and Minnesota, among others—lobbied their respective congressional delegations to remedy the situation. In mid-October, 14 senators from expansion states sent a letter to Senator Reid asking for an increase in federal matching funds. Senate leaders subsequently revised the bill to include a 2.2 percentage-point increase in the federal matching rate for expansion states that would not have any newly eligible Medicaid beneficiaries under the proposed reform because they already covered everyone up to 133 percent of the federal poverty level, at a cost of roughly $600 million over ten years.

Third, as the Senate approached a vote, concern mounted among Democratic leaders that they would fall short of the 60 votes needed to overcome a Republican filibuster. One of the last holdouts—Senator Mary Landrieu (D-Louisiana)—complained that her state was not receiving its fair share of Medicaid funds. The state's per-capita income had increased dramatically in the years following Hurricane Katrina due to a surge of federal recovery funds and the exodus of many poor residents. Since the FMAP formula is based on a state's relative per-capita income over the past three years, Louisiana's federal share was set to decline sharply in 2011. Although the state's conservative Republican governor, Bobby Jindal, was famous for criticizing "wasteful" federal grant programs, he pressed Landrieu to obtain additional federal Medicaid funds to make up for what he deemed a "flawed calculation" under the program's matching formula.[57] In late November, on the eve of a key vote on the health-reform bill, Senate leaders inserted an amendment, which came to be known as the "Louisiana Purchase," providing the state with $300 million in supplemental Medicaid funds.

Finally—and most infamously—the last Democratic holdout, Senator

Ben Nelson of Nebraska, leveraged his status as the sixtieth vote to secure full, permanent federal funding of the Medicaid expansion in his state. For months, the centrist senator had been under intense pressure from his state's Republican governor, Dave Heineman, not to vote for the Senate bill. In a July letter, Heineman cautioned Nelson that an "unfunded health care mandate would be unfair to state taxpayers." In September, he again warned that it would "result in higher taxes on Nebraskans or in cutting state aid to Nebraska's school districts as well as state appropriations to our universities, state colleges and community colleges." In a December letter, as the Senate vote neared, Heineman appealed to Nelson with heightened urgency.

> You are now the 60th vote, and as Governor of the State that we both represent, I urge you to vote against this bill . . . while the increased state costs for the initial three years of the Medicaid expansion would be covered, the program quickly becomes a substantial unfunded Medicaid mandate . . . passed on to citizens through direct or indirect taxes and fees . . . The bottom line is the current Senate bill is not in Nebraska's best interest.[58]

However, Nelson was also under intense pressure from Senate Democrats and the White House to vote for the bill. He negotiated a compromise that balanced these competing pressures: in exchange for his vote, he won an amendment—which came to be known as the "cornhusker kickback"—that would permanently provide full federal funding of the Medicaid expansion in Nebraska at a federal cost of roughly $100 million over ten years.

Thus, by the time the Senate passed the Patient Protection and Affordable Care Act on December 24, 2009, its Medicaid financing provisions had changed considerably. The Senate bill provided the states with 100 percent federal funding for newly eligible Medicaid enrollees in 2014 through 2016, and 80 to 95 percent thereafter with the exception of Nebraska, which was to continue receiving 100 percent federal funding indefinitely. Certain expansion states were to receive a temporary 2.2 percentage-point increase in the federal matching rate for already-eligible enrollees, and Louisiana was to receive $300 million in supplemental funding. The bill narrowly avoided a filibuster, with all 58 Democrats and two Independents voting for its passage, and all Republicans voting against it.

The Senate bill's sweetheart deals unleashed a tirade of criticism from around the nation, with the cornhusker kickback subject to the most scathing attacks. National newspaper headlines screamed of "vote selling" and "corruption"; numerous state leaders complained bitterly about Nebraska's special treatment, and fourteen states threatened to go to court over the provision. Governor Schwarzenegger (R-California) railed against the cornhusker kickback in his 2010 State of the State address.

> Health care reform, which started as noble and needed legislation, has become a trough of bribes, deals and loopholes . . . California's Congressional delegation should either vote against this bill that is a disaster for California or get in there and fight for the same sweetheart deal Senator Nelson of Nebraska got for the Cornhusker State. He got the corn; we got the husk.[59]

In his State of the Union address in January 2010, President Obama acknowledged that the special treatment afforded to certain states was undermining public support for reform, noting that "with all the lobbying and horse-trading, the process left most Americans wondering, 'What's in it for me?'"[60]

The sweetheart deals threatened to derail health reform, particularly following an unexpected political development: shortly after the Senate passed its bill, Republican Scott Brown won a special election to replace deceased Senator Edward Kennedy (D-Massachusetts). Having lost their 60-person, filibuster-proof majority in the Senate, congressional Democrats decided that the best way forward was to persuade the House to approve the Senate bill with the understanding that the Senate would then use the reconciliation process—which requires only 51 votes—to pass agreed-upon revisions. However, outrage over the sweetheart deals made the already-difficult task of convincing the House to pass the Senate bill even trickier. To secure passage, the White House asked the Senate to eliminate the cornhusker kickback. Senator Nelson subsequently withdrew his support, but due to use of reconciliation, the Senate no longer needed his vote.

Congressional leaders also considered trimming supplemental funding for expansion states from the reform package, but ultimately backed down under pressure from key representatives from Massachusetts.[61] The need for additional votes led them to instead level the field by increasing Medicaid funding for all states. The final bill provided 100 percent federal funding for the newly eligible in 2014 through 2016, phasing down gradually to 90 percent in 2020 and subsequent years. Moreover, it increased matching rates for already-eligible adults to 75 percent in 2014, phasing up gradually to 93 percent in 2019—yielding $8 billion in additional funding for a dozen expansion states. "State officials' success in securing this added funding can be attributed primarily to their direct lobbying of members of their congressional delegation who were in a position to cast a pivotal vote on the bill" (Dinan 2011, 17).

In late March, the House approved these and other proposed changes by a narrow margin of 220 to 211, with every Republican and a number of Democrats voting no. A few days later, the Senate approved the House's "fixes" by a vote of 56–43, and President Obama signed the bill into law.

Legal Action

Relative to early proposals considered by the Senate Finance Committee, the Affordable Care Act represented an enormous victory for the states. According to the Congressional Budget Office, the federal government will pick up roughly 93 percent of the tab in the first nine years.[62] In fact, this estimate, which takes into account the so-called woodwork effect, overestimates the cost to the states because it does not include the billions of dollars state and local governments will save on uncompensated care costs.[63] The governors' success in whittling down the state share of costs—despite intense political and economic pressures on congressional leaders to minimize the federal share of the burden—illustrates their tremendous influence in Washington.

Nonetheless, many cash-strapped governors were "exercised about having to contribute more in due course" (Jacobs and Skocpol 2010, 163). Republican governors in particular criticized the legislation, warning state residents that the law would "exact a huge cost on our state,"[64] which would be "paid through your state sales and income taxes."[65] Alan Weil, executive director of the National Academy for State Health Policy, compares the ACA's Medicaid provisions to a $200 pair of shoes on sale for $20. "If you like the $200 pair of shoes it's a great deal because you only have to pay 20 dollars." But, he says, "If you look in your wallet and you have a 10 and a couple of ones and some change and you're not sure you can come up with the 20 dollars, it doesn't really matter what a good deal it is."[66]

Following the ACA's passage, Florida's Republican attorney general, Bill McCollum—with the backing of the state's Republican governor, Charlie Crist—filed a lawsuit, which 25 other states subsequently joined, seeking to overturn the new law. Twenty-one of the plaintiff states had Republican governors; of the five Democrats, four publicly opposed their attorney general's decision to sue, while the fifth—Jay Nixon of Missouri—was deliberately evasive in an attempt to avoid riling his state's conservative voters. Many

Democratic governors spoke out against their Republican colleagues' legal action, while the Democratic Governors Association set up a website urging the public to "Tell the GOP: Stop the frivolous lawsuits."[67]

The lawsuit cited a variety of objections—among them, the Medicaid expansion's "unprecedented encroachment on the sovereignty of the states." In particular, the suit claimed that it was unduly coercive to require states to expand coverage as a condition of continuing to participate in the voluntary Medicaid program. Legal scholars cast doubt on the merits of this argument, since the funds are essentially a gift to the states for which the federal government is free to set the terms—as it does for countless other federal-state programs—and which the states are free to decline (Jacobs and Skocpol 2010). Nonetheless, the Supreme Court, while upholding the rest of the ACA, struck down the Medicaid provision as a "gun to the head of the states," suggesting that the states have grown so dependent on Medicaid funding that doing without it is not a real option.

The Supreme Court decision essentially makes the expansion of Medicaid coverage under the Affordable Care Act optional rather than mandatory. It remains to be seen how many states will voluntarily comply with the provision when it goes into effect in 2014. As of the time of writing, 25 governors have announced that they will expand coverage, while 14 Republican governors have publicly declared that they will not.[68]

Despite politically charged statements to the contrary, experience suggests that when given opportunities to expand Medicaid, states do so voluntarily—albeit to varying degrees. Nearly every state in the nation has already extended coverage for children well above the federal minimum level, and many have done the same for adults. Even the most conservative states cover services that are not required under federal law, such as eye exams and dental care; indeed, approximately 60 percent of current Medicaid spending is undertaken at the states' discretion—as discussed in the introduction.[69] And that is when the feds pick up only the customary 57 percent of costs—at 93 percent in the first decade, the incentives for expansion are even stronger under the ACA. In states where Republican governors are resisting, powerful stakeholders such as hospitals, for whom the Medicaid expansion will reduce charity care costs, and managed-care organizations, who see a growing Medicaid population as a profit opportunity, are already mounting lobbying campaigns to convince them to reconsider—as will be discussed in greater detail in the conclusion. Thus, if history is any indication, most states will opt to expand coverage.

CONCLUSION

Both the Affordable Care Act and the Massachusetts model on which it was based underscore two of this book's central arguments. First, state leaders have become a significant force in national health care policy making. Not only did the template for federal reform emerge from a state initiative, but the governors also exerted enormous influence over the final legislation. Second, the diffusion of responsibility for financing Medicaid has created incentives for both federal and state policymakers to use cost shifting as a vehicle for accomplishing health reform on the cheap.

Understanding how fiscal federalism contributed to Medicaid's central role in the ACA helps explain one of the central ironies of U.S. health care reform. When Medicaid and Medicare were created in 1965, progressives saw the universal Medicare program as a potential stepping stone to national health insurance, while the programs' fiscally conservative architect, Wilbur Mills, hoped that Medicaid—designed as a safety net for only the poorest, most vulnerable Americans—would serve as a firewall around Medicare to prevent such an eventuality. Yet ultimately it was Medicaid, not Medicare, that became the springboard for health care reform.

The debate over the so-called public option further underscores this irony. Early in the health-care debate, when President Obama proposed the creation of a public health-insurance plan modeled on Medicare—touted by supporters as "Medicare for all" —congressional Republicans and moderate Democrats rejected it as the "bugaboo" of "government-run health care." In eschewing the public option, these lawmakers were able to claim that they had prevented a "government takeover."[70] Yet the legislation Congress ultimately enacted includes an enormous expansion of an existing government-run health-care program—albeit one that is administered by the states, and tends to draw less public and media attention than the federal Medicare program.

As this chapter argued, when other avenues proved to be too costly or unpopular, national policy makers turned to Medicaid as a solution to the age-old problem of how to finance health care reform in a politically palatable way. As has been the case repeatedly throughout Medicaid's history, the financial incentives built into its federal-state cost-sharing arrangement, not to mention the political and practical ease of incrementalism relative to wholesale reform, proved to be irresistible.

Conclusion: The Future of Medicaid

REPUBLICAN GOVERNOR Rick Perry made headline news in November 2010 when he proposed that Texas opt out of the Medicaid program. In the wake of the Great Recession, Texas was, like many other states, struggling to close a massive budget shortfall. With the state's Medicaid program taking up 25 percent of the budget and growing at a rapid clip of 9 percent per year, it was a natural target for budget cuts. Although the Affordable Care Act's then-mandatory[1] expansion of Medicaid coverage would not go into effect until 2014, and would be almost entirely paid for by the federal government, the law's access regulations and maintenance-of-effort requirements—which limited the states' scope for cutting eligibility, services, and provider reimbursement rates—were already in place. Thus, despite the fact that federal Medicaid dollars covered 61 percent of Texas's health-care spending, Governor Perry—fresh off a big reelection victory, gearing up for a presidential bid, and touting his new book, *Fed Up! Our Fight to Save America from Washington*—announced that the best solution to Texas's budget woes was for the state to simply decline to participate in the voluntary federal program.

Governor Perry hoped that opting out of Medicaid would save the state billions of dollars each year. Indeed, a report circulated by the conservative Heritage Foundation the previous year had argued that virtually every state would be better off financially if it stopped participating in the program, and that Texas in particular stood to save nearly $10 billion per year. The report concluded that the potential "savings to state budgets are so enormous that failure to leave Medicaid might be viewed as irresponsible on the part of elected state officials."[2] To investigate the possibility further, Texas's Republican-controlled state legislature called for a study of the implications of shutting down the state's Medicaid plan.

The Texas Department of Insurance and Health and Human Services

Commission released a report, *Impact on Texas if Medicaid Is Eliminated,* in December 2010. Far from confirming the Heritage Foundation's savings estimates, the report found that opting out of Medicaid would in fact cost state taxpayers billions of dollars per year. The report estimated that if the state stopped participating in Medicaid, 2.6 million Texans would lose coverage. Since hospitals still would be required by federal law to treat the medical emergencies of the uninsured, their uncompensated care costs—already high due to Texas's 25 percent uninsured rate; the highest in the nation—would skyrocket, driving up insurance premiums. Even if the state preserved some form of coverage for Medicaid recipients using the state share of funding, the report warned that doing so without allocating any additional state funds would simply shift costs from the federal government to public hospitals and local governments—and thus to taxpayers in the form of higher property taxes. Meanwhile, the report noted that Texas residents and businesses would still have to pay federal taxes to support other states' Medicaid programs.

Moreover, the loss of federal Medicaid dollars would deal a crippling blow to the state's health-care infrastructure. Safety-net providers stood to lose billions in federal disproportionate-share hospital (DSH) and upper payment limit (UPL) payments, while teaching hospitals stood to lose federal graduate-medical-education payments. And, since Medicaid assists two-thirds of Texans in nursing homes, these institutions would take an enormous hit. The prospect of losing this lifeline of federal funding was inconceivable to the state's health-care providers. The CEO of the Dallas County Hospital called the opt-out proposal "so bizarre as to be unworthy of much consideration."[3]

Furthermore, by opting out of Medicaid, Texas would forgo an enormous inflow of federal funds under the Affordable Care Act starting in 2014. Ironically, Texas is poised to be one of the biggest winners under the health care reform legislation, as its large number of low-income, uninsured residents means the state will qualify for especially large federal subsidies for newly eligible Medicaid enrollees. According to one estimate, the ACA would increase Texas's Medicaid enrollment by 46 percent in the first five years, but would only increase state spending on Medicaid by about 3 percent—thereby relieving the state's hospitals of billions of dollars in uncompensated care costs almost entirely on the federal government's dime.[4]

After the report came out, Governor Perry quickly retracted his proposal. In a statement, he reiterated that "the current Medicaid system is financially unsustainable for states" but acknowledged that reducing the burden would ultimately require an act of Congress, not individual states acting in isolation. He implored federal policy makers to reform the program, warning that: "Without greater flexibility and the elimination of federal strings, Medicaid will strangle state budgets and taxpayers."[5] Perry's reversal was surprising to few; his proposal had been so impractical that many observers had questioned his sincerity, attacking him from both left and right for his "anti-Washington grandstanding"[6] and his "pistol-packing, Texas-sized rhetoric."[7]

Governor Perry was not alone, however. Whether motivated by politics or sheer desperation, half a dozen other states also considered opting out of Medicaid following enactment of the ACA, and all reached similar conclusions about its impracticality. Nevada's *Medicaid Opt-Out White Paper* concluded that ending participation in the program would cause the state's numbers of uninsured, and the resulting burden on providers and local governments, to explode.[8] Similarly, Wyoming's *Medicaid Opt-Out Impact Analysis* concluded that "the strain that will ensue should Wyoming determine to opt-out of participating in Medicaid without a solid plan to replace it is truly immeasurable."[9]

Since 1965, Medicaid's open-ended financing mechanism has provided enormous carrots—as well as some sticks—to encourage state participation, and the states have eagerly devoured them. Over time, these carrots have enticed the states into making ever-larger commitments which have increasingly strained state resources and proven extremely difficult to reverse. Political scientist Donald Kettl observes that, state leaders, like many of us, "have often complained about eating their veggies, but they've found them irresistible nonetheless." But now "the carrots have drawn states in so deep that there's no getting out."[10]

MEDICAID QUIETLY DODGES FEDERAL RETRENCHMENT

The governors are not the only ones who feel powerless to control Medicaid's ballooning costs. Throughout the program's history, federal policy makers of both parties—ranging from Wilbur Mills, Russell Long, and Richard Nixon in the late 1960s (chapter 2) to Ronald Reagan in 1981 (chapter 3) to George H. W. Bush in 1992 (chapter 5) to Newt Gingrich in 1995, Bill Clinton in 1997, and George W. Bush in 2003 (chapter 7)—have sought to rein in Medicaid's growth in one way or another, but have been blocked from doing so by the governors. Due to Medicaid's federal-state cost-sharing arrangement, state leaders of both parties have repeatedly rejected proposed reductions in the federal share as attempts to shift costs to the states.

More recently, in April 2011 the Obama administration proposed cutting federal Medicaid spending by $100 billion to help reduce the federal deficit, which, at 10 percent of GDP, was at its highest level since World War II. Instead of paying each state several different rates ranging from 50 to 100 percent for previously and newly eligible enrollees under Medicaid and CHIP, the president proposed to pay each state a single "blended" rate reflecting a weighted average of the varying rates, minus some factor designed to generate $65 billion in federal savings. He also proposed to limit states' use of provider taxes to help fund the nonfederal share of Medicaid costs, generating another $40 billion in federal savings.

Not surprisingly, the president's proposal caused an immediate uproar among the governors. NGA chair Christine Gregoire warned that "if blended rates is code for cutting benefits and cutting people, that is going to be a huge problem to the states."[11] The NGA sent a letter to congressional leaders urging them to reject the proposal on the grounds that "we do not believe spending reductions should be made disproportionately to state funds or result in merely shifting costs to the states."[12] The letter noted that the proposed $100 billion reduction was a nontrivial amount for the states—5 percent of state Medicaid spending in fiscal year 2012—and that in light of the ACA provisions limiting state flexibility over Medicaid policy, the likely outcome would be reductions in other important programs such as education, transportation, and public safety. Individual governors of both parties also lobbied their states' congressional delegations, who echoed the governors' concerns in letters and phone calls to the White House.

When the Obama administration released its final deficit-reduction proposal in the fall of 2011, the blended rate provision had been scaled back considerably. Instead of the original $65 billion target, the revised proposal included only $15 billion in federal savings. As one senior White House official explained, the administration had "refined" the blended-rate proposal as a result of "many conversations with governors."[13]

Meanwhile, on Capitol Hill, as the bipartisan Joint Select "Supercommittee" on Deficit Reduction—tasked by Congress with reducing the deficit by $1.2 trillion over 10 years—began to assemble its own deficit-reduction proposal in the fall of 2011, governors of both parties lobbied hard against Medicaid cuts. In a letter to the committee, a group of Republican governors, including Haley Barbour of Mississippi and Mitch Daniels of Indiana—ironically, two of Medicaid's most outspoken critics—warned the supercommittee that "Governors are opposed . . . to cost shifting as a way for the federal government to reduce Medicaid spending. Going to a new 'blended rate' for FMAP and reducing provider fees collected by states are unfair cost-shifting measures that increase the burden to states."[14]

Largely as a result of the governors' bipartisan opposition, the supercommittee reportedly had little appetite for Medicaid cuts, and chose to focus primarily on Medicare cuts instead. Ultimately the budget talks fell apart in November 2011, but since federal policy makers had exempted Medicaid from the across-the-board spending cuts that would be triggered if the supercommittee failed to meet its deficit-reduction target, Medicaid was spared. As a *Washington Post* headline observed, Medicaid had "quietly dodged the deficit reduction battle."[15] Once again, the governors' efforts to protect their states' financial interests served to protect Medicaid against retrenchment.

FISCALLY UNSUSTAINABLE, BUT POLITICALLY SELF-SUSTAINING

For decades, federal and state policy makers alike have warned that Medicaid is on a fiscally unsustainable trajectory. Almost immediately after the program's inception, members of Congress began complaining that Medicaid costs were "of a level totally inconsistent with the expectations of the Congress," while governors began protesting that the program threatened to "bankrupt" the states (as discussed in chapter 2). As the program has expanded over time, the burden on each level of government has only intensified. The Government Accountability Office recently warned that Medicaid's growth is contributing to the federal government's "imprudent and unsustainable" fiscal path, and that the program is "the primary driver of the fiscal challenges" facing state governments.[16]

Despite widespread agreement that Medicaid is on a fiscally unsustainable trajectory, federal and state efforts to alter its course have failed repeatedly throughout the program's history. As the preceding anecdotes illustrate—and as I have argued throughout this book—Medicaid's federal-state cost-sharing mechanism has caused the program to grow and persist largely by its own institutional logic and, through a policy-feedback process, has created societal commitments that have proven exceptionally difficult to reverse. Medicaid may be fiscally unsustainable, but it is politically self-sustaining.[17]

Efforts to control Medicaid spending have failed in large part because, under Medicaid's federal-state structure, the easiest form of cost control is not to cut costs at all, but rather to shift costs onto the other level of government—to "save a buck by passing the buck."[18] Such cost-shifting between federal and state governments has been compared to squeezing a balloon at one end, causing it to expand at the other end (Banting and Corbett 2002). This occurs, for example, when the federal government achieves national-policy objectives by mandating the expansion of Medicaid coverage, and requiring states to share the cost. For their part, state-policy entrepreneurs have found that it pays to be creative in exploiting open-ended matching grants through the use of waivers, creative financing mechanisms, and other vehicles that shift costs back to the federal government. The result is "catalytic federalism," whereby federal and state efforts to shift costs onto each other cause the program to grow incrementally over time (Brown and Sparer 2003, 38).

That Medicaid's federal-state structure is inherently expansionary and inhibitive to retrenchment is a good or bad thing, depending on whom you ask. For progressives who support the expansion of health coverage for low-income Americans, Medicaid's institutional design has undeniably helped fulfill this objective; for conservatives who wish to scale back the government's social role, it is a source of consternation. Whereas left-leaning think tanks defend Medicaid's financing arrangement as crucial to protecting the health of vulnerable populations,[19] right-leaning think tanks routinely lambast the "perverse incentives"[20] and "malign effects"[21] arising from fiscal decentralization.

This ideological divide underscores the irony of Medicaid's federalism-fueled growth. Conservatives have traditionally sought to augment the role of the states in the federal system, while liberals have viewed the states as less sympathetic than the national government to the interests of low-income citizens (Thompson and Fossett 2008). Yet by giving the states broad discretion and open-ended financial support, Medicaid has unexpectedly encouraged more government activity rather than less (Sparer, France, and Clinton 2011).

Despite their divergent views, liberals and conservatives can agree that Medicaid's growth is imposing an untenable burden on state budgets, crowding out other important priorities including education and public infrastructure (Hovey 1999; Holahan, Weil, and Weiner 2003; Marton and Wildasin 2007). To the extent that federal and state policy makers want to put

Medicaid on a more financially sustainable trajectory, as they frequently claim to, the key is to restructure the way in which the federal government and the states share responsibility for administering and financing health care for the poor. As Banting and Corbett (2002, 27) observe, efforts to constrain public-health spending in federations will be most effective when financial responsibility and policy control are "effectively lodged at one level of government."

Throughout the remainder of this chapter, I analyze two of the most widely discussed reform models: converting Medicaid's open-ended matching grants to block grants (thereby shifting greater responsibility and control to the states), and federalizing the program in whole or in part (thereby shifting greater responsibility and control to the federal government). Drawing on the lessons learned from Medicaid's historical evolution, I analyze the obstacles to, and likely implications of, each of these reform models.

BLOCK GRANTS

Since enactment of the Affordable Care Act, Republican governors have renewed calls for a Medicaid block grant. Just as the "mandate madness" of the late 1980s led conservative governors to espouse block grants in the 1990s (chapter 7), the expansion of coverage under the ACA impelled Governor Haley Barbour (R-Mississippi), among others, to request "a capped block grant in return for true flexibility to run the program in the best way."[22] And, as in the 1990s, congressional Republicans were happy to oblige. In April 2011, House Budget Committee chairman Paul Ryan (R-Wisconsin) drafted a proposal to convert Medicaid into a block grant that would grow roughly 3 percent per year, in line with inflation and population growth. Since Medicaid spending is projected to increase under existing law by more than 7 percent per year over the next decade (not including the ACA expansion), the plan would have generated $180 billion in federal savings over ten years—plus an additional $434 billion through repeal of the expansion of coverage under the ACA.[23]

Paul Ryan's block grant proposal, like its Medigrant predecessor in the mid-1990s, offered many advantages for the federal budget. In addition to slowing the growth of federal spending, a block grant would make that spending more predictable from year to year since it would no longer rise automatically during economic downturns. Moreover, since federal spending would no longer be a function of state eligibility and benefit policies, block grants would, as one proponent put it, eliminate "perverse incentives for states to bring as much into their Medicaid umbrella as possible."[24]

For state leaders interested in slashing Medicaid enrollment and benefits, block grants would provide the flexibility to do so. For those interested in retaining or expanding coverage, block grants are considerably less appealing. Thus, not surprisingly, Democratic governors opposed Ryan's proposal. As Governor Deval Patrick (D-Massachusetts) pointed out in testimony before the Senate Finance Committee in June 2011, for states to sustain current coverage under the proposed block grant, they would have to increase spending by 71 percent relative to current levels over the next decade—and "no state is fiscally prepared to deal with that." He concluded that a Medicaid block grant "is really a formula for limiting coverage, not sustaining the program."[25] Governor Dan Malloy (D-Connecticut) was more pointed in his criticism, remarking: "The reason people who don't support the program want block grants is they want to kill the program."[26]

Setting aside ideological debates over the desired scope of Medicaid coverage, block grants would impose enormous financial risks on state budgets—risks that tend to give even Republican governors pause (as discussed in chapter 7). Once the capped federal contribution is exhausted, states would be fully responsible for any cost growth arising from a host of factors including economic downturns, demographic changes, new diseases, and expensive new technologies. And since most states are legally required to balance their budgets, this means Medicaid coverage would likely swing wildly over the business cycle. Moreover, block grants would expose the states to increased political risk, since breaking the Medicaid entitlement would subject the program to the vagaries of the federal appropriations process.

For these reasons, congressional Democrats—as well as President Obama and some moderate Republicans—joined Democratic governors in rejecting Representative Ryan's proposal, referring to the block grant plan as "onerous and hardhearted," and warning that it would "inflict terrible harm on Americans."[27] Due to opposition from the Democrat-controlled Senate and White House, along with "warning cries" from state officials and a "firestorm of opposition" from the powerful hospital and nursing-home lobbies, House Republicans retreated, and by the end of the summer, the block grant proposal was considered dead.[28] Once again, federalism—along with another form of institutional fragmentation: separation of powers—prevented national policy makers from restructuring the Medicaid program.

Paul Ryan's unsuccessful Medicaid plan is only the latest in a series of failed block-grant proposals spanning three decades. History suggests that, in a political system characterized by multiple veto points, enacting a Medicaid block grant will likely require a perfect political and economic storm: Republican control of the White House, both chambers of Congress, and a majority of governors—plus a favorable economic and budgetary climate to increase governors' willingness to trade augmented flexibility for reduced funding and to decrease Congress's temptation to use block grants as a tool for slashing federal spending, which tends to raise governors' hackles. However, even if strong support for a block grant emerges at both levels of government, a formula fight like the one that erupted in the mid-1990s would make the task of reallocating funds among the states exceptionally difficult from a practical standpoint—not to mention potentially raising policy concerns about interstate equity (Lambrew 2005).

In short, the prospects for a Medicaid block grant appear dim in the foreseeable future. Despite the governors' dissatisfaction with the program's current structure, the states simply have too great a financial stake in the status quo. However, a more politically feasible approach would be to block grant a piece of the program as part of a broader reform package—as discussed later in this chapter.

FEDERALIZATION

Whereas converting Medicaid from matching grants to block grants would shift the locus of power to the states, an alternative reform model would take the opposite approach, shifting greater programmatic authority and financial responsibility to the national government. In a sense, this federalization process is already underway. First, in 2003 and again in 2009, the federal government temporarily assumed responsibility for a greater share of Medicaid costs to help the states cope with economic downturns—as discussed in chapter 7. Then, under the Affordable Care Act, the federal government agreed, under intense pressure from the governors, to pay 100 percent of the cost of newly eligible enrollees for the first several years, and 90 percent in the long run. In both cases, increased federal funding was accompanied by maintenance-of-effort requirements limiting state discretion over the scope of coverage provided.

The idea of federalizing Medicaid is not a new one. In a series of reports dating back to 1969, the U.S. Advisory Commission on Intergovernmental Relations (ACIR) recommended that the federal government assume full financial responsibility for public programs aimed at meeting basic human needs, including medical care. The commission argued that federalizing Medicaid would help realign an intergovernmental system that had grown "more pervasive, more intrusive, more unmanageable, more ineffective, more costly and above all, more unaccountable."[29] And in 1970, the U.S. Department of Health, Education, and Welfare's Task Force on Medicaid and Related Programs warned that the program was unsustainable in its current form because "the Federal-State grant structure on which it is based cannot, for the long run, stand the massive stresses of paying for quality services," particularly long-term care for the elderly and disabled. The report concluded that "Medicaid should be converted to a program with a uniform minimal level of health benefits financed 100 percent by Federal funds," and that federal-state matching should be retained only for benefits and individuals above and beyond the minimum plan, offered at the states' discretion.[30]

The National Governors Association has long supported federalization. Since Medicaid's inception, the NGA has issued a series of policy resolutions asking the federal government to assume full responsibility for administering and financing Medicaid—as well as other programs for the poor—leaving the states to specialize in funding education, local transportation, and public safety. Over time, as Medicaid has become more entrenched, the NGA has proposed more incremental, politically feasible varieties of federalization. For instance, in 2011, the NGA released a set of Medicaid reform principles that included federal assumption of "100 percent of the cost of any new mandates that implicate Medicaid" and "responsibility for some or all of the services required by dual eligibles" who are enrolled in both Medicaid and Medicare.[31]

The states' struggles to cope with the Great Recession and the Affordable Care Act have led a number of policy makers and scholars to resurrect the idea of federalization in recent years.[32] For instance, in a 2010 article, "Federalism and its Discontents," Greg Anrig, a scholar at the progressive Century Foundation, argued that "the states are drowning" and that "the best life-preserver that Washington can throw at them is to take over Medicaid." In addition to relieving the states of an unmanageable financial burden, he argues that federalization would reduce "unjust state-to-state disparities in coverage." Moreover, he conjectures that "because the federal government is not obligated to balance its budget, unlike states, economic downturns would be much less likely to lead to benefit cutbacks." In short, many progressive proponents of federalization hope that removing Medicaid from the states' hands would make health coverage for the poor more comprehensive and stable.

Although federalization does have the potential to minimize economically induced fluctuations in coverage, removing the states as veto players could in fact make the program considerably more vulnerable to retrenchment. One need only look back to Ronald Reagan's 1982 federalization proposal to understand why this is the case. In 1982, President Reagan—having failed to cap federal Medicaid contributions or convert the program to a block grant the prior year—shifted gears and sought to remove the program from the states' hands (as discussed in chapter 3). Internal White House memos and correspondence between the White House and the governors reveals that the Reagan administration planned to slash eligibility, particularly coverage for the medically needy, as well as covered services, most notably, long-term care. The governors ultimately rejected Reagan's proposal out of concern that this skimpy federalized program would leave the states holding the bag.

The Reagan experience suggests that federalization of Medicaid would—much like block grants—eliminate the incentive structure that has served to preserve and expand coverage throughout Medicaid's history. As noted earlier, virtually every president since the program's inception, not to mention numerous members of Congress, have proposed reducing federal spending on Medicaid, but the governors have repeatedly blocked these efforts. Federalizing Medicaid would effectively remove the program from the governors' purview, making it easier for a conservative national government to dramatically curtail coverage. Thus, contrary to progressives' arguments, federalization is not necessarily a recipe for programmatic stability.

At the same time, however, conservatives often oppose federalization—as many of Reagan's economic advisors did—out of concern that it would open the door for a liberal national government to merge Medicaid with Medicare, and perhaps even pave the way for a single-payer universal health-care system; indeed, progressive advocates often cite this possibility as one of the advantages of federalization (Anrig 2010). Other conservative national policy makers oppose federalization for the simple reason that taking over the states' share of costs would exacerbate the federal government's already-tenuous financial position. Recent efforts to reduce the nation's massive debt burden by cutting entitlement programs suggests that the federal government may not be ready to assume full financial responsibility for the enormous Medicaid program any time soon.

HYBRID REFORM MODEL

Despite the steep political and practical obstacles to replacing Medicaid with either a block grant or national program, it is possible to envision a more politically feasible hybrid approach. For instance, federalization of coverage for certain populations (such as the elderly and disabled) could be combined with a block grant for others (such as children and able-bodied, nonelderly adults). In fact, this very approach was advocated by a bipartisan NGA task-force in 2003, as discussed in chapter 7. This hybrid model has the potential to provide tremendous fiscal relief for the states and make federal health care spending more controllable, while also reducing inequitable state-by-state variations and improving the quality of care.

For years, the National Governors Association has urged the federal government to take over responsibility for dual eligibles—the poor elderly and disabled individuals who qualify for both Medicare and Medicaid—and many health-policy experts have made similar suggestions (see for example Holahan and Weil 2007). This expensive and rapidly growing demographic makes up only 15 percent of Medicaid enrollees, but 39 percent of the program's expenditures. Elderly and disabled Medicaid enrollees as a whole—including non-Medicare enrollees—account for 27 percent of Medicaid enrollees, and 66 percent of expenditures. The high cost of caring for these enrollees is largely due to nursing-home and home-based care—expensive services that are covered by Medicaid, but not Medicare. In fact, 70 percent of Medicaid spending on dual eligibles goes to long-term care.[33]

In addition to relieving the states of the most expensive and fastest-growing component of Medicaid spending, federal assumption of full responsibility for the elderly and disabled has a compelling logic to it. As the National Governors Association has argued, "it is a well-accepted general rule that the federal government administers programs for the elderly [and disabled] as reflected in Social Security and Medicare . . . There is no need for any state role."[34] The NGA has also noted that federalization has the potential to improve the quality of care through better coordination between Medicaid and Medicare, and would also increase interstate equity since dual eligibles are not equally distributed among states.

For the federal government, federalization of coverage for the elderly and disabled—while costly—has the advantage of greatly increasing control over Medicaid expenditures. Fully 85 percent of spending on optional Medicaid populations—those covered at states' discretion—goes to the elderly and disabled. Nursing-home care is the single largest service for optional populations, accounting for nearly 60 percent of such spending.[35]

Of course, the main federal objection to taking full responsibility for the elderly and disabled is the price tag; when the NGA task force proposed such a federal takeover in 2003, the Bush administration balked at the cost. Thus, to compensate the federal government, the states would need to take on significantly more responsibility for children and nonelderly, able-bodied adults. This might take the form of a block grant, which would both limit the federal contribution and make it more predictable from year to year, as noted earlier.

Breaking the Medicaid program in two, and giving each level of government greater control and financial responsibility over its own piece, would reduce the scope for intergovernmental cost-shifting, potentially putting health-care spending on a more fiscally sustainable trajectory—albeit at the cost of potential reductions in coverage. Whether or not the federal government and the states could actually agree on the terms of such a swap remains to be seen. However, history suggests that such a hybrid approach is more likely to win broad support at both levels of government than would either reform in isolation.

CONCLUSION

Medicaid's evolution over the past five decades has been nothing short of remarkable. This humble program for the poor has dramatically reshaped state officials' incentives and resources in ways that have, unexpectedly and against all odds, served to protect the program against retrenchment and promote its incremental expansion. In a classic case of policy feedback, seemingly small decisions about Medicaid's institutional design—open-ended matching grants combined with broad state discretion over eligibility and benefits—caused state leaders to emerge as a supportive constituency, constraining policy makers' subsequent ability to reverse course. Despite repeated efforts to restructure the program, its original institutional design remains firmly in place.

Medicaid's experience yields several broad lessons for the study of political science and public policy. First, the role of federal funding in promoting Medicaid's growth underscores the importance of following the money in future research on politics and policy. Second, it suggests the need for more research on the conditions under which policy feedback occurs—and does not occur. Patashnik and Zelizer's (2010) theory emphasizing policy design, timing, and institutional support provides a useful foundation upon which other scholars might develop theoretical refinements and applications. Finally, Medicaid's profound impact on the governors' incentives, resources, and political organization points to the potential importance of feedback effects on not only a policy's proximate targets, but also other political actors—such as government elites.

Notes

Introduction

1. "One Man Veto on Medicare," *New York Times,* June 24, 1964.

2. Medicaid was, in fact, an extension of a small preexisting program—the Kerr-Mills Program of Medical Assistance to the Aged—which is explained in chapter 1.

3. Lewis E. Weeks, *Wilbur J. Cohen, In First Person: An Oral History,* Hospital Administration Oral History Collection, 1984 http://www.aha.org/research/rc/chhah/oral-histories.shtml.

4. Eve Edstrom, "U.S. Medicaid Bill Tops Billion," *Washington Post,* November 16, 1966.

5. Natalie Jaffe, "State is Called Medicaid Leader," *New York Times,* August 7, 1966.

6. Thompson and DiIulio 1998, 3; Michael Cannon, "Welfare Reform's Unfinished Business Medicaid Has to Be Reined In," *National Review,* May 17, 2005; Robert Kuttner, "Taming the Medicaid Monster," *Boston Globe,* February 16, 2005; Jennifer Steinhauer, "New York, Which Made Medicaid Big, Looks to Cut it Back," *New York Times,* March 3, 2003; Myers 1970, 267; Weil 2003, 13.

7. This is the average number of enrollees throughout the year; the total number of people covered by Medicaid during the year is considerably higher at 70 million. Medicaid and CHIP Payment and Access Commission (MACPAC). Report to the Congress on Medicaid and CHIP, March 2012. Washington, DC.

8. Henry J. Kaiser Family Foundation, *Medicaid: A Primer,* 2010. http://www.kff.org/medicaid/upload/7334-4.pdf.

9. U.S. Department of Health and Human Services, *2011 Actuarial Report on the Financial Outlook for Medicaid,* Washington, DC, March 2012.

10. The Affordable Care Act also includes a special deduction to income that effectively raises the eligibility level to 138 percent. Douglas W. Elmendorf, "CBO's Analysis of the Major Health Care Legislation Enacted in March 2010," Testimony before the Subcommittee on Health, Committee on Energy and Commerce, U.S. House of Representatives, March 30, 2011.

11. Anna Sommers, Arunabh Ghosh, and David Rousseau, *Medicaid Enrollment*

and Spending by 'Mandatory' and 'Optional' Eligibility and Benefit Categories, Report of the Kaiser Commission on Medicaid and the Uninsured, June 2005. http://www.kff.org/medicaid/upload/Medicaid-Enrollment-and-Spending-by-Mandatory-and-Optional-Eligibility-and-Benefit-Categories-Report.pdf.

12. The formula is:

$$Federal\ Share\ (FMAP) = 1 - 0.45 \times (State\ Per\ Capita\ Income\ / \\ U.S.\ Per\ Capita\ Income)^2;$$

$$State\ Share = 0.45 \times (State\ Per\ Capita\ Income\ /\ U.S.\ Per\ Capita\ Income)^2$$

Each state's FMAP is determined annually based on the average annual per capita income in the three previous years. Thus, a state's FMAP may fluctuate somewhat from year to year. The history of the FMAP is discussed in chapter 1.

13. However, some research suggests that lump-sum grants stimulate spending on the targeted good to a greater extent than predicted by economic theory due to the so-called flypaper effect; see for example Hines and Thaler 1995.

14. See also John Holahan, Joshua M. Wiener, Randall R. Bovbjerg, Barbara A. Ormond, and Stephen Zuckerman, *The State Fiscal Crisis and Medicaid: Will Health Programs be Major Budget Targets? Overview and Case Studies,* Washington, DC: Kaiser Commission on Medicaid and the Uninsured, 2003; James W. Fossett and Courtney E. Burke, *Medicaid and State Budgets in FY2004: Why Medicaid Is So Hard to Cut* (Albany, NY: Rockefeller Institute of Government Federalism Research Group, 2004).

15. At the time, the program was known as Aid to Dependent Children (ADC). Although Congress subsequently increased the AFDC matching rate, it was not until Medicaid's creation in 1965 that policy makers allowed states that adopted Medicaid programs to receive open-ended matching grants for AFDC at the higher Medicaid matching rate, as is discussed in chapter 1.

16. Robert Pear, "Governors Resist Bush Plan to Slow Costs of Medicaid," *New York Times,* May 25, 2003; "Experimental States," *Newsweek,* May 17, 1993, 38; National Governors' Conference, *Proceedings of the 1969 Mid-Year Meeting,* Washington, DC, February 26–27, 1969, 55.

17. Kaiser Commission on Medicaid and the Uninsured, *The Role of Medicaid in State Economies: A Look at the Research,* January 2009. http://www.kff.org/medicaid/upload/7075_02.pdf.

18. Henry J. Kaiser Family Foundation, *Kaiser Health Tracking Poll,* Washington, DC, May 2011, http://www.kff.org/kaiserpolls/8190.cfm.

19. See chapter 2, at note 13.

20. Robert H. Finch and Roger O. Egeberg, *The Health of the Nation's Health Care System,* Washington, DC, July 10, 1969.

Chapter 1

1. Frank Prial, "And Now 'Medicaid,'" *Wall Street Journal,* July 11, 1966.

2. Norman Miller, "Wilbur Mills, Enigma," *Wall Street Journal,* August 14, 1967.

3. Transcript, Wilbur Mills oral history interview II, 3/25/87, by Michael L. Gillette, Internet Copy, LBJ Library, 2, http://www.lbjlib.utexas.edu/johnson/ar chives.hom/oralhistory.hom/Mills-w/mills2.pdf.

4. U.S. Social Security Administration, Oral History Collection, Robert Ball interview no. 3, April 3, 2001, http://www.ssa.gov/history/orals/ball3.html.

5. Marjorie Hunter, "Wilbur Cohen Picked for Gardner's Cabinet Post," *New York Times,* March 23, 1968, 1.

6. Peter A. Corning, *The Evolution of Medicare: From Idea to Law,* Department of Health, Education, and Welfare, Office of Research and Statistics, Research Report no. 29 (GPO, 1969), http://www.ssa.gov/history/corningchap4.html.

7. "The Administration: The Salami Slicer," *Time,* April 5, 1968.

8. U.S. Social Security Administration, Oral History Collection, Robert Ball interview no. 3, April 3, 2001, http://www.ssa.gov/history/orals/ball3.html.

9. U.S. Advisory Commission on Intergovernmental Relations, *Intergovern- mental Problems in Medicaid,* September 1968, 4.

10. U.S. Department of Health, Education, and Welfare, *Medical Resources Available to Meet the Needs of Public Assistance Recipients,* H.R. Report No. 1799, 87th Congress, 1st session, 1961, 31.

11. Transcript, Wilbur J. Cohen, December 8, 1968, interview with David G. McComb, tape no. 1, Oral History Collection, Lyndon Baines Johnson Library.

12. Lewis E. Weeks, *Wilbur J. Cohen, In First Person: An Oral History,* Hospital Administration Oral History Collection, 1984, http://www.aha.org/research/rc/ chhah/oral-histories.shtml.

13. "Public Assistance: Number of Recipients and Average Payments, by Program and State," table XIV, *Social Security Bulletin,* vol. 28, December 1965, 46–47.

14. "One Man Veto on Medicare," *New York Times,* June 24, 1964.

15. Transcript, Lawrence F. O'Brien oral history interview XI, 7/24/86, by Michael L. Gillette, Internet Copy, LBJ Library, 30, http://www.lbjlib.utexas.edu/ johnson/archives.hom/oralhistory.hom/obrienl/OBRIEN11.PDF.

16. Transcript, Wilbur Mills oral history interview II, 3.

17. Transcript, Clinton P. Anderson, Oral History Collection, Lyndon Baines Johnson Library, May 20, 1969, http://web2.millercenter.org/lbj/oralhistory/ anderson_clinton_1969_0520.pdf.

18. Congressional Quarterly Almanac, 88th Congress, 2nd session, 1964, 231–32.

19. Arlen Large, "Mills and Medicine," *Wall Street Journal,* August 2, 1965.

20. Transcript, Wilbur Mills oral history interview II, 2–3.

21. Arlen Large, "Mills and Medicine."

22. Austin Wehrwein, "A.M.A. Consults States Societies," *New York Times,* December 14, 1964.

23. Arlen Large, "Mills and Medicine."

24. U.S. Social Security Administration, Oral History Collection, Robert Ball interview no. 3.

25. Congressional Record 7213 (daily ed. April 1, 1965) (statement of Representative Mills).

26. Congressional Record 7213 (daily ed. April 1, 1965) (statement of Representative Mills).

27. Arlen Large, "Mills and Medicine."

28. Lewis E. Weeks, *Nelson H. Cruikshank, In First Person: An Oral History,* Hospital Administration Oral History Collection, 1984, http://www.aha.org/research/rc/chhah/oral-histories.shtml.

29. Richard Harris, "Medicare: A Sacred Trust (Part IV)," *New Yorker,* July 23, 1966, 40.

30. Memo, Wilbur J. Cohen to the President, March 2, 1965, EX LE/IS1, White House Central File, Box 75, LBJ Library.

31. "Medicoup," *Newsweek,* April 5, 1965, 28.

32. Robert J. Myers, interview with Peter Corning, March 8, 1967, Columbia Center for Oral History, 90–91.

33. Richard Harris, "Medicare: A Sacred Trust (Part IV)," *New Yorker,* July 23, 1966, 40.

34. For an account of the Johnson administration's secret role in developing the Medicare legislation, see Blumenthal and Morone (2009).

35. Transcript, Wilbur Mills oral history interview II, 2, 15.

36. Recording of telephone conversation between Lyndon B. Johnson and Lawrence [Larry] O'Brien [Other Speakers: Wilbur Mills], June 11, 1964, 3:55 p.m., citation no. 3686, Recordings and Transcripts of Conversations, LBJ Library.

37. Recording of telephone conversation between Lyndon B. Johnson and Wilbur Mills, June 9, 1964, 9:55 a.m., citation no. 3642, Recordings and Transcripts of Conversations, LBJ Library.

38. Recording of telephone conversation between Lyndon B. Johnson and Wilbur Cohen, March 21, 1964, 6:04 p.m., citation no. 2612, Recordings and Transcripts of Conversations, LBJ Library.

39. Memo, Wilbur J. Cohen to Mike Manatos and Harry Wilson, September 10, 1964, EX LE/WE, Box 164, White House Central File, LBJ Library.

40. Memo, Lawrence F. O'Brien to the President, January 27, 1964, EX LE/IS1, Box 75, White House Central File, LBJ Library.

41. Recording of telephone conversation between Lyndon B. Johnson and Lawrence [Larry] O'Brien [Other Speakers: Wilbur Mills], June 11, 1964, 3:55 p.m., citation no. 3686, Recordings and Transcripts of Conversations, LBJ Library.

42. Recording of telephone conversation between Lyndon B. Johnson and Lawrence [Larry] O'Brien, June 22, 1964, 5:10 p.m., citation no. 3804, Recordings and Transcripts of Conversations, LBJ Library.

43. U.S. Social Security Administration, Oral History Collection: Robert Ball interview no. 3.

44. Transcript, Lawrence F. O'Brien oral history interview XI, 22–23. Emphasis added.

45. Transcript, Douglass Cater oral history interview III, 5/26/74, by Joe B. Frantz, Internet Copy, LBJ Library, 14, http://www.lbjlib.utexas.edu/johnson/archives.hom/oralhistory.hom/cater/cater03.pdf.

46. U.S. Social Security Administration, Oral History Collection: Robert Ball interview no. 3.

47. Arlen Large, "Mills and Medicine."

48. Recording of telephone conversation between Lyndon B. Johnson and Wilbur Cohen [Other Speakers: Wilbur Mills], March 23, 1965, 5:00 p.m., citation no. 7142, Recordings and Transcripts of Conversations, LBJ Library.

49. Recording of telephone conversation between Lyndon B. Johnson and John McCormack [Other Speakers: Wilbur Mills, Wilbur Cohen, Carl Albert], March 23, 1965, 4:54 p.m., citation no. 7141, Recordings and Transcripts of Conversations, LBJ Library.

50. U.S. Social Security Administration, *Legislative History: Vote Tallies for Passage of Medicare in 1965,* http://www.ssa.gov/history/tally65.html.

51. "Medicare," *New York Times,* July 3, 1966.

52. Memo, Theodore C. Sorenson to Wilbur Mills, June 14, 1966, Folder 580, Box 51, Series 10.3, Record Group 15, Nelson A. Rockefeller Papers, Gubernatorial, Rockefeller Family Archives, Rockefeller Archive Center, Sleepy Hollow, New York.

53. President Lyndon B. Johnson, "Remarks With President Truman at the Signing in Independence of the Medicare Bill," July 30, 1965, http://www.lbjlib.utexas.edu/johnson/archives.hom/speeches.hom/650730.asp.

54. Lewis E. Weeks, *Wilbur J. Cohen, In First Person: An Oral History.*

55. Memo, Wilbur J. Cohen to the President, February 25, 1965, EX LE/IS1, Box 75, White House Central File, LBJ Library.

Chapter 2

1. "Medical Economics Revolution," *New York Times,* May 4, 1970.

2. Robert H. Finch and Roger O. Egeberg, *The Health of the Nation's Health Care System,* Washington, DC, July 10, 1969.

3. Martin Tolchin, "Javits, Governor Split on Medicaid," *New York Times,* September 3, 1966.

4. "Excerpts of Remarks by Governor Rockefeller Prepared for Delivery to Celebrate Start of Medicare and Medical Assistance, Mount Sinai Hospital, New York, New York, Friday, July 1, 1966, 2:30 p.m." Folder 1575, Box 43, Series 33, Record Group 15. Nelson A. Rockefeller Papers, Gubernatorial, Rockefeller Family Archives, Rockefeller Archive Center, Sleepy Hollow, New York.

5. "Health Care for the Aged: A Program and a Workable Approach: Presented at the Governors' Conference, Glacier National Park, Montana, June 29, 1960." Folder 105, Box 18, Series 46, Record Group 15. Nelson A. Rockefeller Papers, Gubernatorial, Rockefeller Family Archives, Rockefeller Archive Center, Sleepy Hollow, New York.

6. "Medical Care for the Aged: Social Security and Freedom of Choice: An Address Delivered by Governor Nelson A. Rockefeller at the Statewide Conference on Aging Held in New York City, May 1, 1962." Folder 76, Box 2, Series 27, Record Group 15. Nelson A. Rockefeller Papers, Gubernatorial, Rockefeller Family Archives, Rockefeller Archive Center, Sleepy Hollow, New York.

7. "Statement to the Legislature, March 9, 1966." Folder 577, Box 50, Series 10.3, Record Group 15. Nelson A. Rockefeller Papers, Gubernatorial, Rockefeller Family Archives, Rockefeller Archive Center, Sleepy Hollow, New York.

8. U.S. House of Representatives, March 29, 1965, *Social Security Amendments of 1965: Report of the Committee on Ways and Means on H.R. 6675.* House Report No. 213, 89-1, 75.

9. "Statement of Governor Nelson A. Rockefeller before the Joint Legislative Committee on Problems of Public Health and Medicare, Albany, New York, Tuesday, May 24, 1966, 10 a.m.," 3-4. Folder 515, Box 22, Series 34, Record Group 15. Nelson A. Rockefeller Papers, Gubernatorial, Rockefeller Family Archives, Rockefeller Archive Center, Sleepy Hollow, New York.

10. "Statement to the Legislature, March 9, 1966." Folder 577, Box 50, Series 10.3, Record Group 15. Nelson A. Rockefeller Papers, Gubernatorial, Rockefeller Family Archives, Rockefeller Archive Center, Sleepy Hollow, New York.

11. T. N. Hurd to Earl W. Brydges. Folder 585, Box 51, Series 10.3, Record Group 15. Nelson A. Rockefeller Papers, Gubernatorial, Rockefeller Family Archives, Rockefeller Archive Center, Sleepy Hollow, New York.

12. *Journal of the Assembly of the State of New York,* 1966, vol. 2, 2883.

13. "Excerpts of Remarks by Governor Rockefeller Prepared for Delivery to Celebrate Start of Medicare and Medical Assistance, Mount Sinai Hospital, New York, New York, Friday, July 1, 1966, 2:30 p.m." Folder 1575, Box 43, Series 33, Record Group 15. Nelson A. Rockefeller Papers, Gubernatorial, Rockefeller Family Archives, Rockefeller Archive Center, Sleepy Hollow, New York.

14. Frank Prial, "And Now 'Medicaid,'" *Wall Street Journal,* July 11, 1966.

15. Natalie Jaffe, "State is Called Medicaid Leader," *New York Times,* August 7, 1966.

16. "Rush-Hour Lawmaking," *New York Times,* May 21, 1966.

17. John Sibley, "Medical Care Furor: The Confusion and Sudden Opposition Indicate Little Understanding of Plan," *New York Times,* May 21, 1966.

18. Eve Edstrom, "U.S. Medicaid Bill Tops Billion," *Washington Post,* November 16, 1966; Richard Reeves, "Travia, In Reversal, To Ask Tightening of Medicaid Rules," *New York Times,* July 1, 1966.

19. Sibley, "Medical Care Furor."

20. Association of New York State Physicians and Dentists to Appropriations Committee members, July 21, 1966. Folder 580, Box 51, Series 10.3, Record

Group 15. Nelson A. Rockefeller Papers, Gubernatorial, Rockefeller Family Archives, Rockefeller Archive Center, Sleepy Hollow, New York.

21. Memo, Theodore C. Sorenson to Wilbur Mills, June 14, 1966. Folder 580, Box 51, Series 10.3, Record Group 15. Nelson A. Rockefeller Papers, Gubernatorial, Rockefeller Family Archives, Rockefeller Archive Center, Sleepy Hollow, New York.

22. Norman Miller, "Medicaid Mistake," *Wall Street Journal,* October 20, 1966.

23. Miller, "Medicaid Mistake."

24. Miller, "Medicaid Mistake."

25. Miller, "Medicaid Mistake."

26. Sydney Schanberg, "House Committee Agrees on New Plan to Cut U.S. Funds for Medicaid," *New York Times,* October 6, 1966.

27. Tolchin, "Javits, Governor Split on Medicaid."

28. Miller, "Medicaid Mistake."

29. Nan Robinson, "Senate Puts Off Early Increase in Social Security," *New York Times,* October 15, 1966.

30. U.S. Senate, Committee on Finance, *Social Security Amendments of 1967, Part 1.* 90th Congress, 1st session, August 22-24, 1967, 280.

31. U.S. Senate, Committee on Finance, *Social Security Amendments of 1967, Part 3.* 90th Congress, 1st session, September 20-22 and 26, 1967, p. 1551.

32. Report of the Committee on Finance, United States Senate, on H.R. 12080 (Social Security Amendments of 1967), 176.

33. Nelson A. Rockefeller, "Testimony on Creative Federalism before the Senate Committee on Government Operations, Subcommittee on Intergovernmental Relations," February 1, 1967.

34. Senate Committee on Finance, SSA 1967, S. Report No. 744 to accompany HR 12080, 90th Congress, 1st session, 1967, 197-98.

35. Hulett Smith, "Testimony on Creative Federalism before the Senate Committee on Government Operations, Subcommittee on Intergovernmental Relations," February 2, 1967.

36. Richard Madden, "State's Medicaid Program Faces Cut of Up to $90-Million in Federal Funds," *New York Times,* September 26, 1968. Long had introduced this measure once before, as part of the Social Security Amendments of 1967, but it had been rejected in the House.

37. "Assails Medicaid Cut," *New York Times,* November 18, 1967.

38. John Morris, "Senate Affirms Medicaid Reductions in Federal Payments to the States," *New York Times,* November 21, 1967.

39. "Appeal on Medicaid Is Sent to Johnson," *New York Times,* December 13, 1967.

40. Nelson A. Rockefeller, "Testimony on Health Care in America before the Senate Committee on Government Operations, Subcommittee on Executive Reorganization," February 24, 1968, 411.

41. "Volpe Protests to Conferees on Proposed Medicaid Cuts," *New York Times,* December 10, 1967.

42. Eve Edstrom, "Cut in Medicaid Funds Shocks Welfare Chiefs," *Washington Post,* September 26, 1968.

43. Murray Illson, "Governor Scores Medicaid Attack," *New York Times,* September 29, 1968.

44. Richard L. Madden, "Javits and Goodell Stop Medicaid Cut with a 'Minibuster,'" *New York Times,* October 12, 1968.

45. Carroll Kilpatrick, "$2.5 Billion Spending Cut Proposed by Nixon," *Los Angeles Times,* February 27, 1970.

46. Norbett Tiemann, "Testimony on the Social Security Amendments of 1970 before the Senate Finance Committee," September 21, 1970, 813.

47. William Cahill, "Testimony on the Social Security Amendments of 1970 before the Senate Finance Committee," September 16, 1970, 564.

48. Marvin Mandel, "Testimony on the Social Security Amendments of 1970 before the Senate Finance Committee," September 17, 1970, 705.

49. Bill Kovach, "States Grow Wary of Cost-Sharing Aid," *New York Times,* November 28, 1971.

50. "A Predictable 'Disaster,'" *Chicago Tribune,* January 12, 1968.

51. Nelson A. Rockefeller, "Testimony on Health Care in America before the Senate Committee on Government Operations, Subcommittee on Executive Reorganization," February 24, 1968, 417, 429.

52. Richard L. Madden, "States to Weigh Cuts in Medicaid," *New York Times,* June 8, 1969.

53. Madden, "States to Weigh Cuts in Medicaid."

54. Congressional Record 17703 (daily ed. June 30, 1969) (statement of Senator Anderson).

55. Madden, "States to Weigh Cuts in Medicaid."

56. "Senate Liberals Fight Cutting Medicaid," *Washington Post,* June 19, 1969.

57. William Robbins, "Senate and Finch Act to Put Federal and State Controls on Medicaid Costs," *New York Times,* July 1, 1969.

58. National Governors' Conference, *Proceedings of the Sixty-First Annual Meeting,* Colorado Springs, CO, August 31–September 3, 1969, 75.

59. National Governors' Conference, *Proceedings of the Sixty-First Annual Meeting,* 15.

60. James Naughton, "Governors," *New York Times,* September 7, 1969.

61. Bill Kovach, "Governors Urge U.S. to Take Over All Relief Costs," *New York Times,* September 3, 1969.

62. Richard Lyons, "U.S. Unit to Study Wider Health Aid," *New York Times,* September 19, 1969.

63. U.S. Department of Health, Education, and Welfare, *Report of the Task Force on Medicaid and Related Programs,* Washington, DC, 1970, 128.

64. Carroll Kilpatrick, "Welfare Revisions Sent to Hill," *Washington Post,* June 11, 1970.

65. "Excerpts from the President's Message Urging 'a New National Health Strategy,'" *New York Times,* February 19, 1971.

66. Advisory Commission on Intergovernmental Relations (ACIR), *Significant Features of Fiscal Federalism,* 1981–1982 edition, M-135, Washington, DC, 1983, 66.

67. Nancy Hicks, "Governors Will Vote on Medicaid Reform," *New York Times,* February 27, 1977.

68. James Reston, "Big Problems and Little Men in State Capitals," *New York Times,* October 5, 1962.

69. David Broder, "The Rise of the Governors," *Washington Post,* June 12, 1974.

70. Advisory Commission on Intergovernmental Relations (ACIR), *The Question of State Government Capability,* Washington, DC, 1985, 140.

71. ACIR, *The Question of State Government Capability,* 140.

72. Warren Weaver, "Governors Plan Office in Capital," *New York Times,* December 18, 1966.

73. Broder, "The Rise of the Governors."

74. Broder, "The Rise of the Governors."

75. National Governors Association, *Proceedings of the Sixty-Ninth Annual Meeting,* Detroit, MI, September 7–9, 1977, 35.

76. David Broder, "Governor Unit Meets in Colo.," *Washington Post,* August 31, 1969.

77. Warren Weaver, "Governors: They Talk but Does Anybody Listen?" *New York Times,* August 16, 1970.

78. National Governors Association, *A Governor's Guide to NGA,* 2010, http://www.nga.org/files/live/sites/NGA/files/pdf/1010GOVSGUIDENGA.PDF.

79. See for example Robert Pear, "Regions Fight over the Way Health Money is Distributed," *New York Times,* September 21, 1995.

Chapter 3

1. B. Drummond Ayers Jr., "Reagan Plans Welfare Shift to States," *New York Times,* August 14, 1981.

2. Interview with *LA Times* Reporters, January 20, 1982, Ronald Reagan Presidential Library, http://www.reagan.utexas.edu/archives/speeches/1982/12082e.htm.

3. Tom Goff, "Reagan Calls for Cuts in Welfare, Medicaid," *Washington Post,* January 13, 1971.

4. Ronald Reagan, "Address before a Joint Session of the Congress on the Program for Economic Recovery," Washington, DC, February 18, 1981, Ronald Reagan Presidential Library, http://www.reagan.utexas.edu/archives/speeches/1981/21881a.htm.

5. Kenneth Bacon and Timothy Schelhardt, "Reagan Promises His Tax, Spending Cuts Will Reduce Inflation and Increase Growth," *Wall Street Journal,* February 19, 1981.

6. David Broder, "Reagan Runs into Resistance in Transferring Program to States," *Washington Post,* March 2, 1981.

7. Ronald Reagan, "Address to the Nation on the Economy," Washington, DC, February 5, 1981, Ronald Reagan Presidential Library, http://www.reagan.utexas.edu/archives/speeches/1981/20581c.htm.

8. "White House Report on the Program for Economic Recovery," February 18, 1981, Ronald Reagan Presidential Library, http://www.reagan.utexas.edu/archives/speeches/1981/21881c.htm.

9. Ronald Reagan, "Remarks During a White House Briefing on the Program for Economic Recovery," February 24, 1981, Ronald Reagan Presidential Library, http://www.reagan.utexas.edu/archives/speeches/1981/22481a.htm.

10. Letter, Richard A. Snelling to the president, December 16, 1981, File 12/14/81–4/5/82, Box 2, Handwriting II: Records, Ronald Reagan Library.

11. David Broder, "Reagan Runs into Resistance in Transferring Program to States," *Washington Post,* March 2, 1981.

12. Adam Clymer, "Governors Warned of Effect on States of Reagan's Budget," *New York Times,* February 22, 1981.

13. National Governors Association, "Policy Positions 1980–81," November 1980, 13.

14. Ronald Reagan, "Toasts at a Dinner Honoring the Nation's Governors," February 24, 1981, Ronald Reagan Presidential Library, http://www.reagan.utexas.edu/archives/speeches/1981/22481h.htm.

15. National Governors Association, "Policy Positions 1980–81," November 1980, 15.

16. Advisory Commission on Intergovernmental Relations. *The Federal Role in the Federal System: The Dynamics of Growth,* June 1980, 28, http://www.library.unt.edu/gpo/acir/Reports/policy/a-84.pdf.

17. John T. Woolley and Gerhard Peters, "Democratic Party Platform of 1980," *The American Presidency Project,* August 11, 1980, http://www.presidency.ucsb.edu/ws/index.php?pid=29607.

18. Congressional Record S6102 (daily ed. April 1, 1981) (statement of Senator Moynihan).

19. David Broder, "Reagan Runs into Resistance in Transferring Program to States," *Washington Post,* March 2, 1981.

20. Broder, "Reagan Runs Into Resistance on Transferring Programs to States."

21. National Governors Association, "Policy Positions 1980–81," November 1980, 38.

22. "New Federalism, Bad Bargain," *New York Times,* August 14, 1982.

23. Bernard Weinraub, "U.S. Limit on Medicaid Would Shift Burden to States," *New York Times,* April 6, 1981.

24. Robin Herman, "Carey Sees 'Regional Bias' in Reagan Plan," *New York Times,* February 25, 1981.

25. David Broder and Herbert Denton, "Governors Opposing Reagan on Medicaid, Welfare Plans," *Washington Post,* February 24, 1981.

26. Memo, Jim Medas to Robert Carleson, March 4, 1981, Folder Medicaid (2 of 6), Box OA 9587, Robert Carleson Files, Ronald Reagan Library.

27. Broder and Denton, "Governors Opposing Regan on Medicaid, Welfare Plans."

28. National Governors Association, "Transcript of Proceedings, National Governors Association Winter Meeting," 59.

29. National Governors Association, "Transcript of Proceedings, National Governors Association Winter Meeting," 62–63.

30. Irvin Molotsky, "Tristate Governors Assail Reagan Plan," *New York Times,* February 23, 1981.

31. U.S. House, Subcommittee on Health and the Environment of the Committee on Energy and Commerce, *Statement of Stephen B. Farber,* HRG-1981-HEC-0013, March 10, 1981, 343.

32. U.S. House, Subcommittee on Health and the Environment of the Committee on Energy and Commerce, *Statement of James B. Hunt, Jr., Chairman, Human Resources Committee, National Governors Association,* HRG-1981-HEC-0013, March 10, 1981, 9–10.

33. Congressional Record H14139–40 (daily ed. June 25, 1981) (statement of Representative Waxman).

34. David G. Smith and Judith D. Moore, Interview with Henry Waxman, CMS oral history project, 2003–2006, January 25, 2005, 746, https://www.cms.gov/History/Downloads/cmsoralhistory.pdf.

35. Congressional Record S13841 (daily ed. June 25, 1981) (statement of Senator Dole).

36. David G. Smith and Judith D. Moore, Interview with Sheila Burke, CMS oral history project, 2003–2006, June 20, 2003, 102, https://www.cms.gov/History/Downloads/cmsoralhistory.pdf.

37. Helen Dewar, "Spending Cuts Make 97th Congress Unique," *Washington Post,* June 14, 1981.

38. Ellen Hume and Paul Houston, "$10 Billion in Welfare Cuts Voted," *Los Angeles Times,* May 6, 1981.

39. Steven Weismann, "President Meets a Snag in Drive for Economic Program," *New York Times,* June 24, 1981.

40. Congressional Record S13922 (daily ed. June 25, 1981) (statement of Senator Kennedy).

41. Congressional Record S14065 (daily ed. June 25, 1981) (statement of Representative Crockett).

42. Spencer Rich and Joanne Omang, "Amid Friday's Budget Pandemonium, One Victory Denied Reagan," *Washington Post,* June 30, 1981.

43. Dennis Farney, "Budget Conferees Agree on Ground Rules, Confident of Passage Before August Recess," *Wall Street Journal,* July 15, 1981.

44. Smith and Moore, Interview with Henry Waxman, 746.

45. A 3 percent cut meant that, for example, the minimum matching rate of 50 percent would become 48.5 percent.

46. The effects of OBRA 1981 on state Medicaid programs will be discussed in chapter 4.

47. "They Ain't Seen Nothing Yet," *Washington Post,* August 16, 1981.

48. Herbert H. Denton, "Only Pieces of Reagan Block Grant Plan Remain in Budget Bills," *Washington Post,* July 13, 1981.

49. National Governors Association, "Proceedings of the National Governors Association Annual Meeting 1981," August 9–11, 1981, 39.

50. B. Drummond Ayres Jr., "Governors Warn on Welfare Cuts," *New York Times,* August 12, 1981.

51. Bruce Babbit, "The Governors Will Fight," *Washington Post,* July 14, 1981.

52. National Governors Association, "Proceedings of the National Governors Association Annual Meeting 1981," 21.

53. "The Counterrevolution," *Washington Post,* October 3, 1981.

54. National Governors Association, "Proceedings of the National Governors Association Annual Meeting 1981," 30.

55. David S. Broder, "States Offer Reagan a Deal on Aid Cuts," *Washington Post,* August 12, 1981.

56. National Governors Association, "Proceedings of the National Governors Association Annual Meeting 1981," 21.

57. Ayers, "Reagan Plans Welfare Shift to States."

58. Letters, Ronald Reagan to various governors, August 18, 1981, Folder Entitlements (2 of 3), Box OA 5665, Richard Williamson Files, Ronald Reagan Library.

59. Memo, Richard S. Williamson to James A. Baker, October 16, 1981, Folder Entitlements (2 of 3), Box OA 5665, Richard Williamson Files, Ronald Reagan Library.

60. Meeting notes, Richard S. Williamson and Richard Snelling, December 15, 1981, Folder Richard Snelling, Box OA 5665, Richard Williamson Files, Ronald Reagan Library.

61. Letter, Richard A. Snelling to the president, December 4, 1981, Folder 12/17/90–12/13/81, Box 1, Handwriting II: Records, Ronald Reagan Library.

62. Meeting notes, Richard S. Williamson and Richard Snelling, December 15, 1981, Folder Richard Snelling, Box OA 5665, Richard Williamson Files, Ronald Reagan Library.

63. Memo, Richard S. Williamson to Kenneth Cribb, October 23, 1981, Folder Entitlements (2 of 3), Box OA 5665, Richard Williamson Files, Ronald Reagan Library.

64. Ronald Reagan, "Address Before a Joint Session of the Congress Reporting on the State of the Union," Washington, DC, January 26, 1982, Ronald Reagan Presidential Library, http://www.reagan.utexas.edu/archives/speeches/1982/12682c.htm.

65. Interview with Local Reporters in Bloomington, Minnesota, on Budget Issues and the Federalism Initiative, Bloomington, MN, February 8, 1982, Ronald Reagan Presidential Library, http://www.reagan.utexas.edu/archives/speeches/1982/20882e.htm.

66. Ronald Reagan, "Address before a Joint Session of the Congress Reporting on the State of the Union," January 26, 1982, Ronald Reagan Presidential Library, http://www.reagan.utexas.edu/archives/speeches/1982/12682c.htm.

67. David Broder and Herbert Denton, "Hill Prospects Remain Clouded," *Washington Post,* January 29, 1982.

68. David Broder and Herbert Denton, "Huge 'Sorting-Out' of Federal Role: By Decade's End, States Would Fund, Run Most Major Programs," *Washington Post,* January 27, 1982.

69. David Broder and Herbert Denton, "Hill Prospects Remain Clouded," *Washington Post,* January 29, 1982.

70. David Broder and Herbert Denton, "Baker Wants Action, But O'Neill Cautious," *Washington Post,* February 24, 1982.

71. "The New Old Deal," *New York Times,* January 28, 1982.

72. Michael Barone, "New Federalism and American Poverty," *Newsday,* February 21, 1982.

73. Telephone call to Richard Snelling, recommended to the president by Richard S. Williamson, January 29, 1982, Folder 1/1/82–8/5/82, Box 2, Handwriting IV: Calls, Ronald Reagan Library.

74. The White House Office of the Press Secretary, "Background and Status Report on Federalism Initiative," July 13, 1982. FG PR016, WHORM: Subject File, Ronald Reagan Library.

75. Lou Cannon and David Broder, "Reagan Says 'Federalism' Is Flexible, Reagan Says Federalism is a 2-Way Street," *Washington Post,* February 2, 1982.

76. Interview with Jeremiah O'Leary of the *Washington Times* on Federal Tax and Budget Reconciliation Legislation, Washington, DC, August 13, 1982, Ronald Reagan Presidential Library, http://www.reagan.utexas.edu/archives/speeches/1982/81382f.htm.

77. Suggested Remarks, Meeting with Nation's Governors, February 22, 1982, Folder 1/1/82–3/16/82, Box 3, Handwriting III: Speeches, Ronald Reagan Library.

78. Letter, Richard A. Snelling to the president, March 3, 1982, Folder MC001: Governors Conferences, Box 6, Ronald Reagan Library.

79. Ronald Reagan, "Toasts at a Dinner Honoring the Nation's Governors," Washington, DC, February 23, 1982, Ronald Reagan Presidential Library, http://www.reagan.utexas.edu/archives/speeches/1982/22382b.htm.

80. Memo, Don W. Moran to Richard S. Williamson, May 11, 1982, IS-IS001, WHORM: Subject File, Ronald Reagan Library.

81. Memo, Don W. Moran to Richard S. Williamson, May 11, 1982, IS-IS001, WHORM: Subject File, Ronald Reagan Library.

82. Memo, Richard S. Schweiker to Edwin Meese, February 26, 1982, FG IS001, WHORM: Subject File, Ronald Reagan Library.

83. Memo, Robert Carlson and James Dwight to Edwin Meese III, February 18, 1982, Folder Medicaid (6 of 6), Box OA 9587, Robert Carlson Files, Ronald Reagan Library.

84. Memo, Robert Carlson and James Dwight to Edwin Meese III, February 18, 1982, Folder Medicaid (6 of 6), Box OA 9587, Robert Carlson Files, Ronald Reagan Library.

85. Memo, Don W. Moran to Richard S. Williamson, May 11, 1982, IS-IS001, WHORM: Subject File, Ronald Reagan Library.

86. Memo, Robert B. Carleson to Edwin Meese III, July 21, 1982, FG LG ST MC, WHORM: Subject File, Ronald Reagan Library.

87. Memo, Don W. Moran to Richard S. Williamson, May 11, 1982, IS-IS001, WHORM: Subject File, Ronald Reagan Library.

88. Memo, Richard S. Williamson to Edwin Meese et al., May 21, 1982, FG LG ST MC, WHORM: Subject File, Ronald Reagan Library.

89. Memo, Alan F. Holmer to David B. Swoap et al., June 24, 1982, IS-IS001, WHORM: Subject File, Ronald Reagan Library.

90. Joanne Omang, "Newest Version of New Federalism Leaves Gate as Trojan Horse," *Washington Post,* July 25, 1982.

91. Irvin Molotsky, "White House Revises 'New Federalism' Proposals," *New York Times,* June 24, 1982.

92. Letter, Richard A. Snelling to the president, July 14, 1982, Folder 1/1/82–8/5/82, Box 2, Handwriting IV: Calls, Ronald Reagan Library.

93. Letter, Richard A. Snelling to the president, August 2, 1982, FG 072820–88399, Box 5, WHORM: Subject File, Ronald Reagan Library.

94. David S. Broder, "Reagan Isn't Kidding," *Washington Post,* July 7, 1982.

95. Congressional Record S12682 (daily ed. May 17, 1984) (statement of Senator Sarbanes).

96. National Governors Association, "Transcript of Proceedings, National Governors Association, Opening Plenary Session," August 5, 1985, 139.

97. Smith and Moore, Interview with Henry Waxman, 762.

Chapter 4

1. However, by the late 1980s, governors unanimously opposed additional mandates for reasons that will be explained in this chapter.

2. "Equal Rights for Infants," *New York Times,* January 17, 1984.

3. Southern Regional Task Force on Infant Mortality (SRTFIM), *A Fiscal Imperative* (Washington, DC, February 1985), 8.

4. Southern Regional Task Force on Infant Mortality (SRTFIM), *An Investment in the Future: Legislative Strategies for Maternal and Infant Health* (Washington, DC, July 1985), 21.

5. Richard Riley, "Southern and Poor," *Washington Post,* April 29, 1985.

6. Peter Applebome, "3 Governors in the South Seek to Lift Their States," *New York Times,* February 12, 1989.

7. U.S. House of Representatives, Subcommittee on Oversight and Investigations and the Subcommittee on Health and the Environment of the Committee On Energy and Commerce, *Infant Mortality Rates: Failure to Close the Black-White Gap: Testimony of Jeffery R. Taylor,* HRG-1984-HEC-0071, March 16, 1984, 266.

8. David G. Smith and Judith D. Moore, Interview with Vern Smith, CMS Oral History Project, 2003–2006, June 5, 2003, 670, https://www.cms.gov/History/Downloads/cmsoralhistory.pdf.

9. Robert Pear, "States are Found More Responsive on Social Issues," *New York Times,* May 19, 1985.

10. "The Governors and Poor Children," *New York Times,* July 1, 1988.

11. See for example U.S. Office of Technology Assessment, "The Implications of Cost Effectiveness: Analysis of Medical Technology: Background Paper 2: Case Studies of Medical Technologies: Case Study 10: The Costs and Effectiveness of Neonatal Intensive Care," August 1981.

12. This problem was compounded in 1986 when Congress passed the Emergency Medical Treatment and Active Labor Act (EMTALA), requiring hospitals to provide care to anyone needing emergency treatment, regardless of ability to pay.

13. Gilbert Omenn, "Let Federalism Work in Medicaid," *Wall Street Journal,* April 26, 1985.

14. "'Welfare Queen' Loses Her Cadillac Limousine," *New York Times,* February 29, 1976.

15. David G. Smith and Judith D. Moore, Interview with Sarah Shuptrine, CMS Oral History Project, 2003–2006, July 16, 2003, 585, https://www.cms.gov/History/Downloads/cmsoralhistory.pdf.

16. SRTFIM, *An Investment in the Future* (Washington, DC, July 1985), 26.

17. Applebome, "3 Governors in the South."

18. Jack Bass, Interview with Ann 'Tunky' Yarborough Riley, South Carolina Political Collections Oral History Project, University Libraries University of South Carolina, January 22, 1987, http://www.sc.edu/library/scpc/ohariley.pdf.

19. David G. Smith and Judith D. Moore, Interview with Henry Waxman, CMS Oral History Project, 2003–2006, January 25, 2005, 745, https://www.cms.gov/History/Downloads/cmsoralhistory.pdf.

20. Smith and Moore, Interview with Henry Waxman, 752. Additional support for the bill came from an unexpected source: pro-life conservatives such as Henry Hyde of Illinois and Thomas Bliley of Virginia, who had grown increasingly concerned about the infant mortality problem and wanted to expand access to prenatal care on the grounds that, from a moral standpoint, a child is just as deserving of care before birth as after.

21. Helen Dewar, "House Rejects Medicare Cost-Cut Plan," *Washington Post,* April 13, 1984.

22. "Deficit Reduction Act of 1984: Provisions Related the Medicare and Medicaid Programs," *Social Security Bulletin* 47, no. 11 (November 1984).

23. SRTFIM, *An Investment in the Future,* 20–21.

24. Julie Kosterlitz, "Watch Out for Waxman," *National Journal,* March 11, 1989, 577.

25. SRTFIM, *A Fiscal Imperative,* 15.

26. SRTFIM, *A Fiscal Imperative,* 16.

27. SRTFIM, *An Investment in the Future,* 18.

28. Southern Regional Task Force on Infant Mortality (SRTFIM), *Final Report: For the Children of Tomorrow* (Washington, DC, November 1985), 24.

29. Congressional Record H11826 (daily ed. May 21, 2986) (statement of Governor Riley).

30. Smith and Moore, Interview with Sarah Shuptrine, 589.

31. Smith and Moore, Interview with Sarah Shuptrine, 590.

32. Smith and Moore, Interview with Sarah Shuptrine, 591.

33. U.S. Senate Committee on Labor and Human Resources, *Barriers to Health Care/Children's Health: Testimony of Edward Kennedy*, HRG-1986-LHR-0033, July 16, 1986, 7.

34. Congressional Record S7991 (daily ed. April 17, 1986) (statement of Senator Bentsen).

35. U.S. Senate Subcommittee on Intergovernmental Relations of the Committee on Governmental Affairs, *Access to Health Insurance and Health Care*, HRG-1986-SGA-0004, June 26, 1986.

36. Smith and Moore, Interview with Sarah Shuptrine, 586.

37. Smith and Moore, Interview with Sarah Shuptrine, 586.

38. Smith and Moore, Interview with Sarah Shuptrine, 591.

39. Robert Pear, "States Act to Provide Health Care Benefits to Uninsured People," *New York Times,* November 22, 1987; Pear, "Expanded Right to Medicaid."

40. Ian T. Hill, "Broadening Medicaid Coverage of Pregnant Women and Children: State Policy Responses," Washington, DC: State Medicaid Information Center, Health Policy Studies, Center for Policy Research, National Governors Association, 1987, 14.

41. Hill, "Broadening Medicaid Coverage," A-3.

42. Pear, "States Act to Provide Health Care Benefits to Uninsured People," 1.

43. National Governors Association, "Transcript of Proceedings, National Governors Association, First Plenary Session," August 24, 1986, 81, http://www.nga.org/Files/pdf/1986NGAAnnualMeeting.pdf.

44. U.S. Senate Committee on Finance, *Health Care Coverage for Children: Testimony of Raymond C. Scheppach*, HRG-1989-FNS-0032, June 20, 1989, 38–39.

45. Smith and Moore, Interview with Vern Smith, 669.

46. National Governors Association, "Transcript of Proceedings, National Governors Association Winter Meeting, First Plenary Session," February 25, 1990, 23–25, http://www.nga.org/Files/pdf/1990NGAWinterMeeting.pdf.

47. Smith and Moore, Interview with Sarah Shuptrine, 591.

48. Martin Tolchin, "Cuts After Decade of Cuts: Governors Grim at Meeting," *New York Times,* February 4, 1991.

49. Interview with Raymond Scheppach, July 14, 2011.

50. Smith and Moore, Interview with Henry Waxman, 745.

51. Julie Rovner, "Reagan Sides with Bowen on Medicare Plan," *Congressional Quarterly,* February 14, 1988, 115.

52. "Address Before a Joint Session of Congress on the State of the Union," Washington, DC, February 4, 1986, Ronald Reagan Presidential Library, http://www.reagan.utexas.edu/archives/speeches/1986/20486a.htm.

53. David G. Smith and Judith D. Moore, Interview with Robert Helms, CMS oral history project, 2003–2006, July 31, 2003, 238, https://www.cms.gov/History/Downloads/cmsoralhistory.pdf.

54. Smith and Moore, Interview with Henry Waxman, 755.

55. "How a Modest Idea Evolved into a Watershed Bill," *AARP Bulletin,* Febru-

ary 1988; "Catastrophic Bill Nears Final OK as Senate Approves," *AARP Bulletin,* December 1987.

56. "Remarks on Signing the Medicare Catastrophic Coverage Act of 1988," Washington, DC, July 1, 1988, Ronald Reagan Presidential Library, http://www. reagan.utexas.edu/archives/speeches/1988/070188d.htm.

57. Mark Hosenball, "Letters Sealed with Fear: Direct-Mail Moguls and the Catastrophic-Care Bill," *Washington Post,* October 22, 1989.

58. Susan F. Rasky, "Stage Set for Congressional Battle With Elderly on Tax for Medicare," *New York Times,* January 12, 1989.

59. Martin Tolchin, "16 States Failing to Pay Medicare Costs of the Poor," *New York Times,* March 9, 1989.

60. U.S. Senate Committee on Finance, *Health Care Coverage for Children: Testimony of Raymond C. Scheppach,* HRG-1989-FNS-0032, June 20, 1989, 38–39.

61. Smith and Moore, Interview with Henry Waxman, 757.

62. Interview with Raymond Scheppach, July 14, 2011.

63. National Association of State Budget Officers (NASBO), *State Expenditure Report 1990* (Washington, DC). Another factor was the states' use of creative financing mechanisms (the subject of chapter 5).

64. NASBO, *State Expenditure Report 1990.*

65. National Governors Association, "Proceedings of the 1991 Annual Meeting," Seattle, WA, August 20, 1991, 17.

66. National Governors Association, "National Governors Association Annual Conference," August 1, 1989, http://www.nga.org/Files/pdf/1989NGAAnnual Meeting.pdf.

67. Dan Morgan, "Henry Waxman and the Medicaid Time Bomb," *Washington Post,* January 20, 1994.

68. Kosterlitz, "Watch Out for Waxman," 577.

69. Robert Pear, "Deficit or No Deficit, Unlikely Allies Bring About Expansion in Medicaid," *New York Times,* November 4, 1990.

70. Pear, "Deficit or No Deficit."

71. David G. Smith and Judith D. Moore, Interview with Don Moran, CMS oral history project, 2003–2006, October 16, 2003, 404, https://www.cms.gov/His tory/Downloads/cmsoralhistory.pdf.

72. National Governors Association, "Transcript of Proceedings, National Governors Association Winter Meeting, First Plenary Session," February 25, 1990, 23–24, http://www.nga.org/Files/pdf/1990NGAWinterMeeting.pdf.

73. National Governors Association, "Transcript of Proceedings, National Governors Association Winter Meeting, First Plenary Session," 25.

74. U.S. House Subcommittee on Health and the Environment, *Medicaid Budget Initiatives,* September 10, 14, 1990, 112–14.

75. U.S. House Subcommittee on Human Resources and Intergovernmental Relations of the Committee on Government Operations, *Medicaid Funding Crisis,* HRG-1990-OPH-0022, December 7, 1990, 67–69.

76. National Governors Association, "Transcript of Proceedings, National

Governors Association 1991 Winter Meeting, Plenary Session," February 5, 1991, 52, http://www.nga.org/Files/pdf/1991NGAWinterMeeting.pdf.

77. Martin Tolchin, "White House Reassures Hard-Pressed Governors," *New York Times,* February 3, 1991.

78. David G. Smith and Judith D. Moore, Interview with Michael Fogarty, CMS oral history project, 2003–2006, August 11, 2003, 183, https://www.cms.gov/History/Downloads/cmsoralhistory.pdf.

Chapter 5

1. Richard Grimes, "Moore's Medicaid Plan Was Innovative," *Charleston Daily Mail,* August 18, 1987.

2. Federal legislation known as the Boren Amendment in 1980 had required the states to provide "reasonable and adequate" payments to "efficiently and economically operated" hospitals, nursing facilities, and intermediate-care facilities. The intent of the law was to help states control costs by paying providers for services based on predetermined reimbursement rates rather than the providers' reported actual costs, but the main result was a flurry of litigation. As Edward Miller explains, "while the Boren Amendment was enacted as a way to enhance state discretion, the way it was implemented served to constrict state flexibility by transferring federal oversight from the executive to the judiciary" (2008).

3. David G. Smith and Judith D. Moore, Interview with Patricia MacTaggart, CMS oral history project, 2003–2006, June 5, 2003, 672, https://www.cms.gov/History/Downloads/cmsoralhistory.pdf.

4. "An Analysis of the Impacts of a DRG-Specific Price Blending Option for Medicare's Prospective Payment System." Congressional Budget Office, December 20, 1984.

5. David G. Smith and Judith D. Moore, Interview with Vern Smith, CMS oral history project, 2003–2006, June 5, 2003, 672, https://www.cms.gov/History/Downloads/cmsoralhistory.pdf.

6. Mark Merlis, "Medicaid: Provider Donations and Provider-Specific Taxes." Congressional Research Service, October 2, 1991.

7. Chris Knap, "Deal Reduces State's Medicaid Payments," *Charleston Gazette,* December 13, 1986.

8. Trina Kleist, "Moore's Promises to Hospitals on Tape," *Charleston Gazette,* August 9, 1987.

9. Chris Knap, "Hospitals to Get Better Return on Medicaid Bills," *Charleston Gazette,* December 16, 1986.

10. Kleist, "Moore's Promises to Hospitals on Tape."

11. Phil Kabler, "Medicaid Ruling Called Partial Victory," *Charleston Gazette,* December 8, 1987.

12. Kleist, "Moore's Promises to Hospitals on Tape."

13. Patty Vandergrift, "Protection Extended in Medicaid Funds Fight," *Charleston Gazette,* April 10, 1987.

14. "Federal Officials Reject Moore's Medicaid Plan," *Charleston Daily Mail,* March 27, 1987.

15. Fanny Seller, "Rules Allowed Medicaid Donations, State Says," *Charleston Gazette,* August 20, 1987.

16. Ronald Sutter, "Round One in Medicaid Funding Bout: Defining 'Donation,'" *Healthcare Financial Management,* January 1991, 99.

17. Michael Cass, "Ned McWherter, 'A Man of the People,' Dies," *Tennessean,* April 5, 2011.

18. Gordon Bonnyman, "Tennessee's Use of Provider Donations and Taxes to Finance Its Medicaid Program," in *Medicaid Provider Tax and Donation Issues* (Washington, DC: Health Policy Alternatives, Inc., 1992), 3.

19. David G. Smith and Judith D. Moore, Interview with Gerald Radke, CMS Oral History Project, 2003–2006, June 5, 2003, 463, https://www.cms.gov/History/Downloads/cmsoralhistory.pdf; Carole R. Myers, "A Critical Case Study of Program Fidelity in TennCare," *Trace: Tennessee Research and Creative Exchange,* January 8, 2006, http://trace.tennessee.edu/cgi/viewcontent.cgi?article=1095&context=utk_nurspubs.

20. Gordon Bonnyman, "Tennessee's Use of Provider Donations and Taxes to Finance Its Medicaid Program," in *Medicaid Provider Tax and Donation Issues* (Washington, DC. Health Policy Alternatives, Inc., 1992), 4.

21. Departmental Appeals Board, U.S. Department of Health and Human Services, "Tennessee Department of Health and Environment Docket Nos. 88–137, 88–194 and 89–32, Decision No. 1047," May 4, 1989, http://www.hhs.gov/dab/decisions/dab1060.htm.

22. Dan Morgan, "Tennessee Medicaid Crunch Mirrors a National Ill," *Washington Post,* March 29, 1993; Morgan, "Small Provision Turns into a Golden Goose."

23. Departmental Appeals Board, U.S. Department of Health and Human Services, "Tennessee Department of Health and Environment Docket Nos. 88–137, 88–194 and 89–32, Decision No. 1047," May 4, 1989, http://www.hhs.gov/dab/decisions/dab1060.htm.

24. Rebecca Ferrar, "Legislature Plan Averts State, Federal Cuts in Medicaid," *Knoxville News Sentinel,* May 20, 1991.

25. National Association of State Budget Officers, State Expenditure Report, various years, http://nasbo.org/Publications/StateExpenditureReport/StateExpenditureReportArchives/tabid/107/Default.aspx.

26. Dan Morgan, "Louisiana Took 'Every Federal Dollar We Could Get Our Hands On,'" *Washington Post,* January 31, 1994.

27. Sandy Lutz, "LA. Ponders Novel Way to Plug Its 'Dispro Hole,'" *Modern Healthcare,* June 27, 1994, 62.

28. Morgan, "Louisiana Took 'Every Federal Dollar We Could Get Our Hands On.'"

29. Morgan, "Louisiana Took 'Every Federal Dollar We Could Get Our Hands On.'"

30. "Louisiana's Medicaid Program: Annual Report 1997/1998," Bureau of Health Service Financing, Louisiana Department of Health and Hospitals, November 2, 1998, 5.

31. Chris Adams, "LA. Duped Feds Over Medicaid: Washington Not Eager to Bail State Out of Crisis," *Times Picayune,* February 12, 1995.

32. Adams, "LA. Duped Feds Over Medicaid."

33. Medicaid and CHIP Payment and Access Commission (MACPAC), "Report to the Congress on Medicaid and CHIP," March 2012, http://www.macpac.gov/reports/.

34. Social Security Act § 1902, 42 U.S.C § 1396a, "State Plans for Medical Assistance," http://www.ssa.gov/OP_Home/ssact/title19/1902.htm.

35. Andy Schneider and David Rousseau, "Medicaid Financing," in *The Medicaid Resource Book* (Washington, DC: Kaiser Commission on Medicaid and the Uninsured, 2002), http://www.kff.org/medicaid/loader.cfm?url=/commonspot/se curity/getfile.cfm&pageID=14261.

36. Texas Senate Finance Interim Subcommittee on Graduate Medical Education, "Final Report on Medicaid Disproportionate Share Hospital Funding," Senate Finance Committee, May 15, 2000, 7–8.

37. Gary Martin, "Medicaid Plan Will Hurt Texas," *San Antonio Express-News,* November 20, 1990.

38. "Magazine Recognizes Six State Hospitals," *San Antonio Express-News,* January 1, 1992.

39. Robin Herman, "The Architect of Alabama's Turnaround," *Washington Post,* August 6, 1991; Morgan, "Small Provision Turns into a Golden Goose."

40. Diane Stewart, "Texas' Use of Intergovernmental Transfers and Provider Taxes in its Medicaid Disproportionate Share Program," in *Medicaid Provider Tax and Donation Issues* (Washington, DC: Health Policy Alternatives, Inc., 1992), 4.

41. David G. Smith and Judith D. Moore, Interview with Don Moran, CMS oral history project, 2003–2006, October 16, 2003, 405, https://www.cms.gov/History/Downloads/cmsoralhistory.pdf.

42. David G. Smith and Judith D. Moore, Interview with Gerald Radke, CMS oral history project, 2003–2006, June 17, 2003, 455, https://www.cms.gov/History/Downloads/cmsoralhistory.pdf.

43. Congressional Record H35856 (daily ed. November 26, 1991) (statement of Representative Ritter).

44. David G. Smith and Judith D. Moore, Interview with Bruce Vladeck, CMS oral history project, 2003–2006, July 7, 2003, 732, https://www.cms.gov/History/Downloads/cmsoralhistory.pdf.

45. Smith and Moore, Interview with Don Moran, 410.

46. Gordon Bonnyman, "Tennessee's Use of Provider Donations and Taxes to Finance Its Medicaid Program," in *Medicaid Provider Tax and Donation Issues* (Washington, DC: Health Policy Alternatives, Inc., 1992), 8.

47. Bonnyman, "Tennessee's Use of Provider Donations and Taxes," 9.

48. David G. Smith and Judith D. Moore, Interview with Thomas E. Hoyer,

CMS, at the National Health Policy Forum, CMS oral history project, 2003–2006, January 14, 2003, 288, https://www.cms.gov/History/Downloads/cmsoralhistory.pdf.

49. Morgan, "Small Provision Turns into a Golden Goose."

50. Martha Shirk, "Hospitals' Donation to State Would Profit Both," *St. Louis Post-Dispatch,* February 25, 1991.

51. David G. Smith and Judith D. Moore, Interview with Mark Reynolds, CMS oral history project, 2003–2006, August 23, 2003, 487, https://www.cms.gov/History/Downloads/cmsoralhistory.pdf.

52. Dan Morgan, "Medicaid Windfall Cut N.H. Deficit; State Officials Used Loophole While Bloating U.S. Budget," *Washington Post,* February 28, 1993.

53. Morgan, "Medicaid Windfall Cut N.H. Deficit."

54. Marylynne Pitz, "Pa. 'Schemes' for Medicaid Funds," *Pittsburgh Post-Gazette,* May 31, 1991.

55. Smith and Moore, Interview with Gerald Radke.

56. Centers for Medicare and Medicaid Services, National Health Expenditures, https://www.cms.gov/nationalhealthexpenddata/02_nationalhealthaccountshistorical.asp.

57. Website of Covington & Burling, LLP, http://www.cov.com/practice/federal_state_programs/.

58. Interview with Donna Checkett, former director of the Missouri Division of Medical Services, July 24, 2012.

59. Martha Shirk, "Missouri to Fight Bush on Medicaid," *St. Louis Post-Dispatch,* July 12, 1991.

60. Spencer Rich, "Task Force Says Medicaid Costs May Reach $200 Billion in 1996," *Washington Post,* July 11, 1991.

61. Morgan, "Small Provision Turns into a Golden Goose."

62. Richard Kusserow, Inspector General, U.S. Department of Health and Human Services, "States Increase Their Use of Revenues Generated by Provider Tax and Donation Programs as the States' Share of Medicaid Expenditures," May 10, 1991; "The Use of Medicaid Provider Tax and Donation Programs Needs to be Controlled," July 25, 1991.

63. U.S. Senate Committee on Finance, HCFA Regulation Restricting Use of Medicaid Provider Donations and Taxes, HRG-1991-FNS-0045, Nov 19, 1991, 41.

64. U.S. Senate Committee on Finance, HCFA Regulation Restricting Use of Medicaid Provider Donations and Taxes, HRG-1991-FNS-0045, Nov 19, 1991, 35.

65. National Governors Association, "National Governors Association Plenary Session," August 20, 1991, 42, http://www.nga.org/Files/pdf/1991NGAAnnualMeeting.pdf.

66. National Governors Association, "National Governors Association Plenary Session," 37.

67. Pear, "U.S. Moves to Curb Medicaid Payments for Many States."

68. National Governors Association, fax to all governors, October 4, 1991.

69. David G. Smith and Judith D. Moore, Interview with Julie James, CMS oral history project, 2003–2006, May 13, 2003, 314–15, https://www.cms.gov/History/Downloads/cmsoralhistory.pdf.

70. Interview with Raymond Scheppach, July 14, 2011.

71. "Medicaid Provider Tax and Donation Issues: The Federal Debate."

72. "Medicaid Provider Tax and Donation Issues: The Federal Debate."

73. David G. Smith and Judith D. Moore, Interview with Sheila Burke, CMS oral history project, 2003–2006, June 20, 2003, 110, https://www.cms.gov/History/Downloads/cmsoralhistory.pdf.

74. Morgan, "Small Provision Turns into a Golden Goose."

75. Victor J. Miller, "Medicaid Financing Mechanisms and Federal Limits: A State Perspective," in *Medicaid Provider Tax and Donation Issues* (Washington, DC: Health Policy Alternatives, Inc., 1992), 29.

76. "Medicaid Provider Tax and Donation Issues: The Federal Debate," 19. Ultimately, one state—Alabama—did file suit against the federal government. However, the state ultimately shelved its lawsuit after the White House and NGA announced that they had reached an agreement.

77. Interview with Raymond Scheppach, July 14, 2011.

78. "Medicaid Provider Tax and Donation Issues: The Federal Debate," 24–25.

79. U.S. Senate Committee on Finance, HCFA Regulation Restricting Use of Medicaid Provider Donations and Taxes, HRG-1991-FNS-0045, Nov 19, 1991, 12.

80. David G. Smith and Judith D. Moore, Interview with Sheila Burke, CMS oral history project, 2003–2006, June 20, 2003, 109, https://www.cms.gov/History/Downloads/cmsoralhistory.pdf.

81. Dan Morgan, "Medicaid Windfall Cut N.H. Deficit," *Washington Post,* February 28, 1993.

82. Morgan, "Medicaid Windfall Cut N.H. Deficit."

83. National Governors Association, fax to all governors, November 19, 1991.

84. Interview with Raymond Scheppach, July 14, 2011.

85. Social Security Act § 1903, 42 U.S.C § 1396b, "Payment to States," http://www.ssa.gov/OP_Home/ssact/title19/1903.htm.

86. "Medicaid Provider Tax and Donation Issues: The Federal Debate."

87. Congressional Record H35854 (daily ed. November 26, 1991) (statement of Representative Waxman).

88. Mary K. Reinhart, "State's Expected Medicaid Funds Cut in Half," *Arizona Daily Star,* March 18, 1992.

89. Morgan, "Small Provision Turns into a Golden Goose."

90. Dan Morgan, "Medicaid Funds Release Adds to Deficit; States Line Up to Collect Millions in Payments Withheld Under Bush," *Washington Post,* February 13, 1993.

91. George Anders, "Health-Care Fund Fight Erupts Over States' Use of the Federal 'Disproportionate Share' Clause," *Wall Street Journal,* June 3, 1993.

92. Morgan, "Are Cash-Starved States 'Looting' Medicaid Coffers?; N. Carolina May Use Windfall For a Construction Project."

93. Smith and Moore, Interview with Vern Smith, 673.

94. Jean Hearne, "Medicaid Disproportionate Share Payments," Congressional Research Service, January 10, 2005.

95. Interview with Bruce Vladeck, July 7, 2011.

96. Social Security Act § 1903, 42 U.S.C § 1396b, "Payment to States."

97. Karen Matherlee, "The Federal-State Medicaid Match: An Ongoing Tug-of-War over Practice and Policy," National Health Policy Forum, December 15, 2000, 1.

98. "Department of Health and Human Services Budget for Fiscal Year 2005," Office of Management and Budget, January 24, 2004, http://www.gpoaccess .gov/usbudget/fy05/pdf/budget/hhs.pdf.

99. David G. Smith and Judith D. Moore, Interview with Andreas Schneider, CMS oral history project, 2003–2006, May 13, 2003, 314–15, https://www.cms .gov/History/Downloads/cmsoralhistory.pdf.

Chapter 6

1. John F. Kennedy, "Special Message to Congress on Public Welfare Programs," Washington, DC, February 1, 1962, Social Security online history pages, http://www.ssa.gov/history/jfkstmts.html.

2. Social Security Act § 1115, 42 U.S.C § 1315, "Demonstration Projects," http://www.socialsecurity.gov/OP_Home/ssact/title11/1115.htm.

3. Kennedy, "Special Message to Congress on Public Welfare Programs."

4. For a more detailed history of the Arizona waiver, see Charles Brecher, "Medicaid Comes to Arizona: A First-Year Report on AHCCCS," *Journal of Health Politics, Policy and Law* 9, no. 3 (Fall 1984): 411–25.

5. David G. Smith and Judith D. Moore, Interview with Andreas Schneider, CMS oral history project, 2003–2006, May 22, 2003, 577, https://www.cms .gov/History/Downloads/cmsoralhistory.pdf.

6. Arthur H. Rotstein, "ACCESS Resulted from State Refusal to Fund Medicaid," *Kingman (AZ) Daily Miner,* September 28, 1983.

7. Rotstein, "ACCESS Resulted from State Refusal to Fund Medicaid."

8. Arthur H. Rotstein, "Arizona's Answer to Medicaid Has Controversial Anniversary," *Kingman (AZ) Daily Miner,* September 27, 1983.

9. AHCCCS Member News, February 17, 2011, http://www.azahcccs.gov/ members/membernews.aspx.

10. Smith and Moore, Interview with Andreas Schneider, 579.

11. National Governors Association, "National Governors Association Plenary Session," August 20, 1991, 60, http://www.nga.org/Files/pdf/1991NGAAnnualMe eting.pdf.

12. National Governors Association, "Transcript of Proceedings, National Governors Association Winter Meeting, First Plenary Session," February 21,

1988, 66, http://www.nga.org/files/live/sites/NGA/files/pdf/1988NGAWinter Meeting.pdf.

13. Smith and Moore, Interview with Joseph Antos, 44.

14. Frank J. Murray and Karen Riley, "Clinton Gives States a Break on Medicaid," *Washington Times*, February 2, 1993.

15. Knickerbocker, "Clinton Pushes Limits in Bid to Expand Scope of National Health Care," 1.

16. Judi Hasson, "Governors Applaud 'Do-Something' Policy," *USA Today*, February 2, 1993.

17. National Governors Association, "Transcript of Proceedings, National Governors Association 1993 Winter Meeting, Plenary Session," February 1, 1993, 21–26, http://www.nga.org/Files/pdf/1993NGAWinterMeeting.pdf.

18. Murray and Riley, "Clinton Gives States a Break on Medicaid."

19. Letter, John Monahan to Raymond Scheppach, August 11, 1993, DPC-Carol Rasco Subject Files, Box 27, Folder 7, William J. Clinton Presidential Library.

20. National Governors Association, "Transcript of Proceedings, National Governors Association 1993 Winter Meeting," 4.

21. Linda Darnell Williams, "John Kitzhaber: Reforming Oregon's Health System Long Before National Debate Began," *Los Angeles Times*, January 19, 1992. See also Oregon Senate President John Kitzhaber, Testimony Before the Oregon House Committee on Human Resources, April 19, 1989.

22. Brad Knickerbocker, "Clinton Pushes Limits In Bid to Expand Scope Of National Health Care," *Christian Science Monitor*, February 18, 1993.

23. Alan K. Ota, "Oregon Health Proposal Reaches Cabinet Level," *Oregonian* (Portland, OR), February 27, 1992.

24. Smith and Moore, Interview with Thomas E. Hoyer, 285.

25. Chris Lydgate, "In Sickness and in Health," *Willamette Week*, 1993.

26. Oregon Department of Human Services, "The Oregon Health Plan: An Historical Overview," July 2006, http://www.oregon.gov/OHA/healthplan/data_pubs/eligibles/main.shtml.

27. Smith and Moore, Interview with Joseph Antos, 43.

28. David G. Smith and Judith D. Moore, Interview with Patricia MacTaggart, CMS oral history project, 2003–2006, July 15, 2003, 368, https://www.cms.gov/History/Downloads/cmsoralhistory.pdf.

29. However, this changed somewhat in the 2000s, as discussed at the end of the chapter.

30. United States General Accounting Office, "Medicaid: Spending Pressures Drive States toward Program Reinvention," Report to the Chairman, Committee on the Budget, House of Representatives, April 4, 1995, 2.

31. Smith and Moore, Interview with Patricia MacTaggart, 356.

32. David G. Smith and Judith D. Moore, Interview with Bruce Vladeck, CMS oral history project, 2003–2006, July 7, 2003, 722, https://www.cms.gov/History/Downloads/cmsoralhistory.pdf.

33. David G. Smith and Judith D. Moore, Interview of Jack Ebeler, Alliance of Community Health Plans, CMS oral history project, 2003–2006, January 22, 2003, 146, https://www.cms.gov/History/Downloads/cmsoralhistory.pdf.

34. Smith and Moore, Interview with Bruce Vladeck, 722.

35. Smith and Moore, Interview with Thomas E. Hoyer, 286.

36. United States General Accounting Office, "States Turn to Managed Care to Improve Access and Control Costs: Statement of Janet L. Shikles, Director, Health Financing and Policy Issues, Human Resources Division," Testimony Before the Subcommittee on Oversight and Investigations, Committee on Energy and Commerce, House of Representatives, March 17, 1993.

37. However, in a few cases a state accepted an "aggregate" cap in exchange for other concessions, thereby taking on the full financial risk of unexpected enrollment growth.

38. United States General Accounting Office, "Medicaid: Spending Pressures Drive States toward Program Reinvention."

39. Jeff Nesbit, "Medicaid Waivers a Cash Cow for States," Washington Times, April 7, 1995.

40. Memo, Nancy-Ann Min and Kathi Way to Carol Rasco, September 7, 1994, DPC-Carol Rasco Subject Files, Box 32, Folder 11, William J. Clinton Presidential Library.

41. United States General Accounting Office, "Medicaid: Spending Pressures Drive States toward Program Reinvention," 53–54.

42. United States General Accounting Office, "Statewide Section 1115 Demonstrations' Impact on Eligibility, Service Delivery, and Program Cost: Statement of William J. Scanlon, Associate Director, Health Financing and Policy Issues, Health, Education, and Human Services Division," Testimony Before the Subcommittee on Health and Environment, Committee on Commerce, House of Representatives, June 21, 1995, 5.

43. Smith and Moore, Interview with Andreas Schneider, 578.

44. Dan Morgan, "Medicaid Loopholes Closing for Strapped States; Facing Loss of Billions in Matching Money, Governors Revise Tax and Budget Plans," Washington Post, February 7, 1993.

45. David Brown, "Tennessee's Economy of Care: TennCare's First Three Years," Washington Post, June 9, 1996.

46. Rebecca Ferrar, "Hospital Tax to Help Struggling Facilities," Knoxville News Sentinel, April 11, 1992.

47. Dan Morgan, "Tennessee Medicaid Crunch Mirrors a National Ill," Washington Post, March 29, 1993.

48. Rebecca Ferrar, "$505 Million Hospital Tax Package Approved," Knoxville News Sentinel, April 29, 1992.

49. Joe Klein, "How Tennessee Has Managed Care," Newsweek, February 21, 1994, 23.

50. Klein, "How Tennessee Has Managed Care," 23.

51. Interview with Bruce Vladeck, July 7, 2011.

52. David L. Manning, "A Proposal for Health Care Reform in Tennessee," March 23, 1993, Chris Jennings Files, Box 16, Folder 5, William J. Clinton Presidential Library.

53. Memo, Kevin Thurm to Carol Rasco and Marcia Hale, September 10, 1993, DPC-Carol Rasco Subject Files, Box 27, Folder 3, William J. Clinton Presidential Library.

54. "The Tennessee Medicaid Waiver (TennCare): A Background Paper," Chris Jennings Files, Box 16, Folder 4, William J. Clinton Presidential Library.

55. Letter, Tennessee Medical Association to Carol Rasco, October 22, 1993, DPC-Carol Rasco Subject Files, Box 27, Folder 6, William J. Clinton Presidential Library.

56. Smith and Moore, Interview with Joseph Antos, 44.

57. Smith and Moore, Interview with Joseph Antos, 44–45.

58. David G. Smith and Judith D. Moore, Interview with Mark Reynolds, CMS oral history project, 2003–2006, August 21, 2003, 498, https://www.cms.gov/History/Downloads/cmsoralhistory.pdf.

59. Friar, "Tennessee's Medicaid Revolution: TennCare," 8.

60. Smith and Moore, Interview with Mark Reynolds, 498.

61. Smith and Moore, Interview with Bruce Vladeck, 723.

62. Memo, Kevin Thurm to Carol Rasco and Marcia Hale, September 10, 1993, DPC-Carol Rasco Subject Files, Box 27, Folder 3, William J. Clinton Presidential Library.

63. Tennessee Waiver Request, September 21, 1993, DPC-Carol Rasco Subject Files, Box 27, Folder 3, William J. Clinton Presidential Library.

64. Brown, "Tennessee's Economy of Care: TennCare's First Three Years."

65. "What is TennCare?," Tennessee Justice Center, http://www.tnjustice.org/resources/tenncare/.

66. "Medicaid Enrollment as a % of Pop, FY07," Kaiser Family Foundation, http://www.statehealthfacts.org/comparemaptable.jsp?typ=2&ind=199&cat=4&sub=52&sortc=1&o=a.

67. Smith and Moore, Interview with Mark Reynolds, 500–502.

68. Memo, HCFA Administrator to HHS Secretary, May 26, 1993, DPC-Carol Rasco Subject Files, Box 32, Folder 11, William J. Clinton Presidential Library.

69. Memo, Nancy-Ann Min and Kathi Way to Carol Rasco, September 7, 1994, DPC-Carol Rasco Subject Files, Box 32, Folder 11, William J. Clinton Presidential Library.

70. Klein, "How Tennessee Has Managed Care," 23.

71. Frank J. Murray and Karen Riley, "Clinton Gives States a Break on Medicaid," Washington Times, February 2, 1993.

72. Richard L. Berke, "In Remarks for Governors, Clinton Presses Health Plan," New York Times, August 16, 1993.

73. Richard L. Berke, "Clinton is Facing State Resistance on Health Plan," New York Times, August 15, 1993.

74. National Governors Association, "Health Care Reform: A Call to Action," January 31, 1994, DPC-Carol Rasco Subject Files, Box 27, Folder 7, William J. Clinton Presidential Library.

75. Berke, "Clinton is Facing State Resistance on Health Plan"; Dan Balz and William Claiborne, "Health Care Flexibility and Additional Costs Concern the States," *Washington Post,* August 16, 1993.

76. Balz and Claiborne, "Health Care Flexibility and Additional Costs Concern the States."

77. Balz and Claiborne, "Health Care Flexibility and Additional Costs Concern the States."

78. William Claiborne, "Health Reform on the Go, State by State; Hawaii Launched the Movement in 1974; It's Gaining Momentum as Others Get in Step," *Washington Post,* November 26, 1993.

79. Berke, "Clinton is Facing State Resistance on Health Plan"; Peter G. Gosselin, "Governors Spar Gingerly on Health Sides Appear Reluctant for Big Fight," *Boston Globe,* July 17, 1994.

80. Berke, "In Remarks for Governors, Clinton Presses Health Plan."

81. Robert Pear, "The Health Care Debate: The States; Governors Oppose Key Dole Proposal on a Health Plan," *New York Times,* July 17, 1994.

82. William Neikirk, "Reform Shortcut: Waiver System Lets Clinton Use States as Labs," *Chicago Tribune,* May 8, 1994.

83. United States General Accounting Office, "Medicaid and SCHIP: Recent HHS Approvals of Demonstration Waiver Projects Raise Concerns," Report to the Committee on Finance, U.S. Senate, July 12, 2002.

Chapter 7

1. Dan Balz, "GOP Leaders Tell Governors Hard Choices Follow Power," *Washington Post,* November 23, 1994.

2. However, the Contract did include a few relatively small Medicaid reforms such as denial of coverage to legal aliens.

3. David G. Smith and Judith D. Moore, Interview with Alan Weil, CMS oral history project, 2003–2006, August 13, 2003, 774, https://www.cms.gov/History/Downloads/cmsoralhistory.pdf

4. Smith and Moore, Interview with Alan Weil, 776.

5. Smith and Moore, Interview with Alan Weil, 778.

6. Interview with Raymond Scheppach, July 14, 2011.

7. "The Unanimous Bipartisan National Governors Association Agreement on Medicaid: Hearings before the Committee on Commerce," House of Representatives, 104th Cong., 2nd sess., February 21 and March 6, 1996, vol. 4, February 21, 1996, 28, 44.

8. National Association of State Budget Officers, *Fiscal Survey of States,* Fall 1995, 9.

9. Carl M. Cannon and Karen Hosler, "Medicaid Entitlement at Center of Impasse; GOP, White House Show Little Movement in Budget Negotiations," *Baltimore Sun,* December 13, 1995.

10. Interview with Raymond Scheppach, July 14, 2011.

11. Judith Havemann and Barbara Vobejda, "Governors Ask Control of Medicaid," *Washington Post,* April 1, 1995.

12. National Governors Association, "Block Grants: Issues for Consideration," January 26, 1995, Bruce Reed Files, Box 25, Folder NGA [4], William J. Clinton Presidential Library.

13. Robert Pear, "Republicans Want to Give States Vast New Powers Over Medicaid," *New York Times,* April 1, 1995.

14. Robert Pear, "Attention is Turning Governors' Heads," *New York Times,* January 30, 1995.

15. Robert Pear, "Battle Over the Budget: Welfare; G.O.P. Bills to Overhaul Welfare Worry City and County Officials," *New York Times,* May 18, 1995.

16. National Governors Association, "Transcript of Proceedings, National Governors Association Winter Meeting, First Plenary Session," January 29, 1995, 104.

17. National Governors Association, "Block Grants: Issues for Consideration," January 26, 1995, Bruce Reed Files, Box 25, Folder NGA [4], William J. Clinton Presidential Library.

18. Interview with Raymond Scheppach, July 14, 2011.

19. "Medicaid Issues and Perspectives: Hearings before the Committee on Finance," United States Senate, 104th Cong., 1st sess., June 28, 1995, 12.

20. National Governors Association, "Principles to Guide the Restructuring of the Federal-State Relationship," Bruce Reed Files, Box 25, Folder NGA [3], William J. Clinton Presidential Library.

21. Interview with Raymond Scheppach, July 14, 2011.

22. Judith Havemann and Eric Pianin, "Medicaid Plan Divides House, Senate GOP; Governors Also at Odds," *Washington Post,* September 13, 1995.

23. Interview with Raymond Scheppach, July 14, 2011.

24. Robert Pear, "Congress Preparing a Major Overhaul of Medicaid," *New York Times,* June 12, 1995.

25. David G. Smith and Judith D. Moore, Interview with Sheila Burke, CMS oral history project, 2003–2006, June 20, 2003, 115, https://www.cms.gov/History/Downloads/cmsoralhistory.pdf.

26. Pear, "Battle Over the Budget."

27. Kurt Shillinger, "Welfare Reform in Central as Clinton, Dole Jockey for '96," *Christian Science Monitor,* August 1, 1995.

28. National Governors Association, "National Governors Association 87th Annual Meeting, Closing Plenary Session," August 1, 1995, 24.

29. William M. Welch, "Governors in Search of a Consensus," *USA Today,* August 2, 1995.

30. Judith Havemann, "House GOP Amends Medicaid Plan; Move Made to

Bolster Support Among Governors for Cutting Costs," *Washington Post,* September 19, 1995.

31. Congressional Record S15157 (daily ed. October 13, 1995) (statement of Senator Harkin).

32. Smith and Moore, Interview with Sheila Burke, 115.

33. Judith Havemann and Helen Dewar, "Senate GOP Took an Old Road to Budget Revolution; Support for Medicaid Provisions Required Last-Minute Deal Making State by State," *Washington Post,* October 31, 1995.

34. Havemann and Dewar, "Senate GOP Took an Old Road to Budget Revolution."

35. Smith and Moore, Interview with Sheila Burke, 113.

36. "Clinton Plan Does Little to End Major Medicaid Disputes," *Congressional Quarterly Weekly,* December 9, 1995, 3447.

37. William J. Clinton, Presidential Radio Address, December 9, 1995, American Presidency Project, http://www.presidency.ucsb.edu/ws/index.php?pid=50874#axzz1fxsGZjKe.

38. National Governors Association, "Transcript of Proceedings, National Governors Association Winter Meeting, Plenary Session and Executive Committee," February 4, 1996, 14.

39. Smith and Moore, Interview with Alan Weil, 777.

40. Judith Havemann and David S. Broder, "Governors Offer Deal on Medicaid," *Washington Post,* February 6, 1996.

41. National Governors Association, "Restructuring Medicaid," February 6, 1996, Bruce Reed Files, Box 25, NGA [1], William J. Clinton Presidential Library.

42. National Governors Association, "Transcript of Proceedings, National Governors Association Winter Meeting, Plenary Session and Executive Committee," February 4, 1996, 98.

43. National Governors Association, "Restructuring Medicaid," February 6, 1996, Bruce Reed Files, Box 25, Folder NGA [1], William J. Clinton Presidential Library.

44. Havemann and Broder, "Governors Offer Deal on Medicaid"; David S. Broder and Judith Havemann, "Governors Seeking Deal on Medicaid; State Leaders Warn of Impact of Impasse," *Washington Post,* February 4, 1996.

45. National Governors Association, "Transcript of Proceedings, National Governors Association Winter Meeting, Plenary Session and Executive Committee," February 4, 1996, 94–95.

46. Robert Pear, "Partisan Split is Obstructing Medicaid Plan by Governors."

47. National Governors Association, "Transcript of Proceedings, National Governors Association Winter Meeting, Plenary Session and Executive Committee," February 4, 1996, 114.

48. Linda Feldmann, "America's Governors Emerge as 'Third House of Congress,'" *Christian Science Monitor,* February 8, 1996.

49. National Governors Association, "Transcript of Proceedings, National

Governors Association Winter Meeting, Plenary Session and Executive Committee," February 4, 1996, 102.

50. National Governors Association, "Transcript of Proceedings, National Governors Association Winter Meeting, Plenary Session and Executive Committee," February 4, 1996, 113.

51. Smith and Moore, Interview with Alan Weil, 779.

52. George Rodriguez and Wayne Slater, "Party Chiefs Laud Governors' Pact; They Hope Compromise Puts Budget Process Back on Track," *Dallas Morning News,* February 7, 1996.

53. John F. Harris and Anne Devroy, "Governors Agree on Entitlement Overhaul; Clinton, Hill Leaders Offer Qualified Praise for Welfare and Medicaid Plans; Overhaul Could Help Budget Talks," *Washington Post,* February 7, 1996.

54. Memo, Chris Jennings and Jennifer Klein to Distribution, February 6, 1996, Carol Rasco Subject Files, Box 20, Folder 19, William J. Clinton Presidential Library.

55. David G. Smith and Judith D. Moore, Interview with Bruce Vladeck, CMS oral history project, 2003–2006, July 7, 2003, 728, https://www.cms.gov/History/Downloads/cmsoralhistory.pdf.

56. Smith and Moore, Interview with Bruce Vladeck, 728.

57. Smith and Moore, Interview with Bruce Vladeck, 729.

58. Smith and Moore, Interview with Alan Weil, 780.

59. Letter from Governors Miller, Romer, Chiles, and Carper, May 28, 1996, Bruce Reed–Welfare, Box 8, Folder Democratic Governors Association, William J. Clinton Presidential Library.

60. Governors Miller, Romer, Chiles, and Carper, "Testimony Submitted to the Senate Committee on Finance," June 13, 1996, Bruce Reed, Box 25, Folder NGA [1], William J. Clinton Presidential Library.

61. Democratic Governors Association conference call with Tom Daschle and Leon Panetta, May 1, 1996, Bruce Reed, Files, Box 25, Folder NGA [1], William J. Clinton Presidential Library.

62. Smith and Moore, Interview with Alan Weil, 782.

63. Letter from Governors Miller, Romer, Chiles, and Carper, May 28, 1996, Bruce Reed–Welfare, Box 8, Folder Democratic Governors Association, William J. Clinton Presidential Library.

64. David G. Smith and Judith D. Moore, Interview with Jack Ebeler, CMS oral history project, 2003–2006, January 22, 2003, 142, https://www.cms.gov/History/Downloads/cmsoralhistory.pdf.

65. Robert Pear, "Hatch Joins Kennedy to Back a Health Program," *New York Times,* March 14, 1997.

66. Robert Pear, "Governors Oppose Clinton Proposal for Medicaid Cap," *New York Times,* January 31, 1997.

67. Robert Pear, "Senate Panel Rebuffs Clinton on Child Health Plan," *New York Times,* June 18, 1997.

68. Roughly equal numbers of states have selected each of the three ap-

proaches; some states have found that the lower administrative burden associated with the Medicaid approach outweighs the cost of reduced discretion over the benefit package.

69. "Governors Hail Plan on Children's Health," *Reuters*, July 30, 1997.

70. National Governors Association, "Transcript of Proceedings, National Governors Association Annual Meeting, Plenary Session," July 28, 1997, 109.

71. Kaiser Commission on Medicaid and the Uninsured, "Health Coverage of Children: The Role of Medicaid and CHIP," February 2011, http://www.kff.org/uninsured/upload/7698-5.pdf; Genevieve Kenney, Allison Cook, and Lisa Dubay, "Progress Enrolling Children in Medicaid/CHIP," *Urban Institute Real Time Analysis*, November 2009.

72. Robert Dodge, "Fiscal Ills Hurting Medicaid; States Struggle to Raise Revenue, Meet Demand Propelled by Slowdown," *Dallas Morning News*, May 12, 2002.

73. Robert Pear, "Governors Resist Bush Plan to Slow Costs of Medicaid," *New York Times*, May 25, 2003; Ceci Connolly, "Governors Efforts to Revise Medicaid Stalls; GOP Group Looks to White House," *Washington Post*, June 13, 2003.

74. Pear, "Governors Resist Bush Plan to Slow Costs of Medicaid."

75. Amy Goldstein, "Governors Finalizing Proposal to Revamp Medicaid; Some Congressional Democrats and Health Care Groups Oppose Plan, Which May go to Bush this Week," *Washington Post*, June 3, 2003.

76. Pam Belluck, "A Nation Challenged: State Finances; First Round of Budget Cuts Aren't Enough, States Find," *New York Times*, October 12, 2001.

77. Dan Balz, "Governors Make Plea for Money from Washington," *Washington Post*, July 14, 2002.

78. Joe Mahoney, "Gov Vows Push on Medicaid," *Daily News*, January 18, 2002.

79. Dale Russakoff and Mike Allen, "Governors' Meeting Verges on Partisan Warfare; Usually Harmonious Group Argues Over Bush's Responsibility for States' Fiscal Crisis," *Washington Post*, February 24, 2003.

80. Louis Jacobson and Shawn Zeller, "Struggling States Send a Bailout Message," *National Journal*, February 22, 2003, 594.

81. Raymond Hernandez, "States Calling for More Help with Medicaid," *New York Times*, December 10, 2001.

82. Evelyne P. Baumrucker, *Medicaid: The Federal Medical Assistance Percentage (FMAP)*, Congressional Research Service, September 24, 2010.

Chapter 8

1. Robert W. Seifert, "The Uncompensated Care Pool: Saving the Safety Net," Massachusetts Health Policy Forum Issue Brief, October 23, 2002, http://masshealthpolicyforum.brandeis.edu/publications/pdfs/16-Oct02/IB%20UncompCarePool%2016.pdf.

2. Irene M. Wielawski, "Forging Consensus: The Path to Health Reform in Massachusetts," Blue Cross Foundation, July 2007, 11, http://bluecrossfoundation.org/foundationroot/en_US/documents/ForgingConsensus.pdf.

3. Wielawski, "Forging Consensus," 11.

4. Mary B. W. Tabor, "State Worker's Budget Coup: A Windfall for Massachusetts," *New York Times*, June 8, 1991.

5. Richard A. Knox, "Governor is Leaning toward a New Stance on Health Care," *Boston Globe*, October 26, 1993.

6. Richard A. Knox, "2 State Health Reform Plans Share Philosophy and Limits," *Boston Globe*, April 13, 1994.

7. Stephanie Anthony, Robert W. Seifert, and Jean C. Sullivan, "The MassHealth Waiver: 2009–2011 . . . and Beyond," Center for Health Law and Economics, University of Massachusetts Medical School, February 2009, http://www.massmedicaid.org/~/media/MMPI/Files/MassHealth%20Waiver%20 2009%20to%202011%20and%20Beyond.pdf.

8. See chapter 6 for a more detailed discussion of budget neutrality.

9. Randall R. Bovbjerg, "State Responses to Budget Crisis in 2004: Massachusetts," Washington, DC, Urban Institute, 2004, http://www.urban.org/publica tions/410951.html.

10. U.S. Department of Health and Human Services, Office of the Assistant Secretary for Planning and Evaluation, "Overview of the Uninsured in the United States: An Analysis of the 2007 Current Population Survey," September 2007, http://aspe.hhs.gov/health/reports/07/uninsured/index.htm.

11. Alice Dembner, "US Threatens to Cut $600M in Medicaid," *Boston Globe*, November 11, 2004.

12. Wielawski, "Forging Consensus," 19.

13. Jim O'Sullivan, "Kennedy Vows to Shepherd 'Singular' Health Bill in Washington," State House News Service, March 22, 2006.

14. Wielawski, "Forging Consensus," 19.

15. Wielawski, "Forging Consensus," 19.

16. Ryan Lizza, "Romney's Dilemma," *New Yorker*, June 6, 2011.

17. Scott S. Greenberger, "Romney Plan Would Expand Healthcare," *Boston Globe*, November 21, 2004.

18. Amy Lambiaso, "Federal Health Chief Urges Conferees to Finish Work on Insurance Bill," State House News Service, January 25, 2006.

19. Mitt Romney, "Massachusetts State of the Commonwealth Address 2006," January 18, 2006.

20. "Senate Session," State House News Service, February 28, 2006.

21. Jim O'Sullivan, "Caucus Consensus: House Shouldn't Budge on Health Care," State House News Service, March 2, 2006.

22. Wielawski, "Forging Consensus," 19.

23. Scott Helman, "Senate OK's Scaled Down Health Bill; The Uninsured Could Still Pay Costs or Penalties," *Boston Globe*, March 1, 2006; Scott Helman and Scott S. Greenberger, "New Senate Bill Would Cover Half of State Uninsured," *Boston Globe*, February 28, 2006; Scott Helman, "Leaders Look to Bridge Gap on Health Bill; Meeting Today; DiMasi Balks at Senate Plan," *Boston Globe*, March 3, 2006.

24. "Senate Session," State House News Service, February 28, 2006.

25. "Health Reform in Massachusetts: Expanding Access to Health Insurance Coverage: Assessing the Results," Blue Cross Blue Shield of Massachusetts Foundation, April 2011, http://bluecrossfoundation.org/HealthReform/~/media/DoDDA3D667BE49D58539821F74C723C7.pdf.

26. Kaiser Commission on Medicaid and the Uninsured, "States Moving Toward Comprehensive Health Care Reform," 2009, http://www.kff.org/uninsured/kcmu_statehealthreform.cfm.

27. Jennifer Rubin, "Exclusive Interview: RomneyCare Author Jonathan Gruber," *Washington Post: Right Turn,* March 4, 2011, http://www.washingtonpost.com/blogs/right-turn/post/exclusive-interview-romneycare-author-jonathan-gruber/2011/03/04/AF2WJorB_blog.html.

28. Igor Volsky, "Romney Says He Solved Health Care 'at the State Level,' but Admits 'the Feds Fund Half of It,'" Think Progress, April 13, 2010, http://thinkprogress.org/politics/2010/04/13/91392/romney-federal-funds/.

29. Rubin, "Exclusive Interview."

30. Volsky, "Romney Says."

31. After the Supreme Court's decision in June 2012, which made the mandatory expansion of Medicaid eligibility optional, the Congressional Budget Office estimated that 6 million fewer people would be covered under the law's Medicaid provision, but acknowledged that this estimate is imprecise given that the extent of state participation is "highly uncertain." Congressional Budget Office, "Estimates for the Insurance Coverage Provisions of the Affordable Care Act Updated for the Recent Supreme Court Decision," July 2012.

32. "What to Tax to Pay for Health Care?" Associated Press, May 18, 2009.

33. White House Office of the Press Secretary, "Remarks by the President on Taxes," April 15, 2009, http://www.whitehouse.gov/the_press_office/Remarks-by-the-President-on-Taxes-4-15-9/.

34. White House Office of the Press Secretary, "Remarks by the President to a Joint Session of Congress on Health Care," September 9, 2009, http://www.whitehouse.gov/the_press_office/Remarks-by-the-President-to-a-Joint-Session-of-Congress-on-Health-Care/.

35. Doyle McManus, "Obama's Tax Deduction Miscalculation," *Los Angeles Times,* April 19, 2009.

36. Max Baucus, "Reforming America's Health Care System: A Call to Action," November 12, 2008, http://asatest.asahq.org/news/Baucusfinalwhitepaper.pdf.

37. Chairman's Mark of the Finance Committee health care reform bill, The America's Healthy Future Act, September 16, 2009, http://finance.senate.gov/download/?id=a2b7dd18-544f-4798-917e-2b1251f92abb.

38. Democratic Governors Association, "Democratic Governors write Congress to Urge Health Reform," October 2, 2009, http://www.democraticgovernors.org/news/press_releases?id=0288.

39. Devin Dwyer, "Schwarzenegger Withdraws Support for Democrats' Health Care Reform," *ABC News: Political Punch,* January 6, 2010, http://abcnews.go.

com/blogs/politics/2010/01/schwarzenegger-withdraws-support-for-democrats-health-care-reform/.

40. James H. Douglas and Joe Manchin III, "July 20, 2009 Letter—Senate Medicaid," July 20, 2009, http://www.nga.org/cms/home/federal-relations/nga-letters/executive-committee-letters/col2-content/main-content-list/title_july-20-2009-l.html.

41. "Healthcare Reform Roundtable (Part I)," S. Hrg. 111–974, June 11, 2009.

42. "Blue-Dog Deal Dogs Health Overhaul Effort," Kaiser Health News, July 31, 2009, http://www.kaiserhealthnews.org/Stories/2009/July/31/states.aspx.

43. 155: 145 Congressional Record E2473–E2474 (daily ed. October 8, 2009) (statement of Representative Rogers).

44. Molly K. Hooper, "Republican Govs. Blast Baucus bill," *The Hill*, September 28, 2009.

45. Andy Sher, "Governors Leery of Health Proposal," *Chattanooga (TN) Times Free Press*, July 21, 2009.

46. Sam Stein, "Obama Ally Throws Cold Water on Health Care Plan," Huffington Post, July 19, 2009, http://www.huffingtonpost.com/2009/07/19/obama-ally-throws-cold-wa_n_239869.html.

47. United States Senate Committee on Finance, "Roundtable Discussion on Expanding Health Care Coverage," May 5, 2009, http://finance.senate.gov/hearings/hearing/?id=d8c677d4-fa54–11f2–1c31–64fbd9076f32.

48. Jeffrey Young, "Medicaid Costs Fueling Dispute between States, Senate," *The Hill*, August 6, 2009.

49. Sack and Pear, "Governors Fear Medicaid Cost in Health Plan."

50. Andy Sher, "Governors Leery of Health Proposal," *Chattanooga (TN)Times Free Press*, July 21, 2009.

51. Sam Stein, "Obama Ally Throws Cold Water on Health Care Plan," Huffington Post, July 19, 2009, http://www.huffingtonpost.com/2009/07/19/obama-ally-throws-cold-wa_n_239869.html.

52. 155: 115 Congressional Record S 8157 (daily ed. July 28, 2009) (statement of Senator Thune).

53. Young, "Medicaid Costs Fueling Dispute."

54. Shailagh Murray, "States Resist Medicaid Growth," *Washington Post*, October 5, 2009.

55. Johnny Isakson, "Colloquy on Health Care Reform," Remarks delivered on the Senate Floor, United States Congress, October 1, 2009, http://isakson.senate.gov/floor/2009/100109healthcare.htm.

56. Kate Zernike, "States With Expanded Health Coverage Fight Bill," *New York Times*, December 27, 2009.

57. Jordan Fabian, "Obama's Healthcare Plan Nixes Ben Nelson's 'Cornhusker Kickback' Deal," *The Hill*, February 22, 2010; J. Taylor Rushing, "Sen. Landrieu Defends 'Louisiana Purchase,' Says Jindal Asked For It," *The Hill*, February 4, 2010.

58. Christina Bellantoni, "Nebraska Governor Urges Nelson to Oppose Health

Care," Talking Points Memo, December 16, 2009, http://tpmdc.talkingpoints memo.com/2009/12/nebraska-governor-urges-nelson-to-oppose-health-care. php.

59. Arnold Schwarzenegger, "2010 State of the State Address," January 6, 2010, http://gov.ca.gov/news.php?id=14118.

60. "The State of the Union & the State of Health Reform," *The White House Blog,* January 27, 2010, http://m.whitehouse.gov/blog/2010/01/27/state-union-state-health-reform.

61. Susan Milligan, "Bay State Seeks Fair Shake in Health Bill," *Boston Globe,* March 12, 2010.

62. Congressional Budget Office, "Updated Estimates for the Insurance Coverage Provisions of the Affordable Care Act," March 2012, http://www.cbo.gov/sites/default/files/cbofiles/attachments/03-13-Coverage%20Estimates.pdf.

63. January Angeles, "How Health Reform's Medicaid Expansion Will Impact State Budgets," Center on Budget and Policy Priorities, July 12, 2012, http://www.cbpp.org/cms/index.cfm?fa=view&id=3801.

64. "Georgia Joins Lawsuit against Health Overhaul," *Chattanooga (TN) Times Free Press,* May 15, 2010.

65. Eric Bradner, "State Fears Fiscal Tsunami," *Courier Press (Evansville, IN),* March 23, 2010.

66. Julie Rovner, "Medicaid Pain Might Be Less than Governors Claim," *Shots: NPR's Health Blog,* http://www.npr.org/blogs/health/2010/05/26/127168826/medicaid-pain-might-be-less-than-governors-claim.

67. Democratic Governors Association, "Tell the GOP: Stop the Frivolous Lawsuits," n.d., http://action.democraticgovernors.org/page/s/barbourpetd.

68. Advisory Board Company, "Where Each State Stands on ACA's Medicaid Expansion," July 5, 2012, http://www.advisory.com/Daily-Briefing/2012/07/05/Where-each-state-stands-of-the-Medicaid-expansion.

69. Brigette Courtot, Emily Lawton, and Samantha Artiga, "Medicaid Enrollment and Expenditures by Federal Core Requirements and State Options," Kaiser Commission on Medicaid and the Uninsured, January 2012, http://www.kff.org/medicaid/upload/8239.pdf.

70. Paul Starr, "Sacrificing the Public Option," *American Prospect,* August 19, 2009.

Conclusion

1. The Supreme Court later struck down the mandatory Medicaid expansion, as discussed in chapter 8.

2. Dennis Smith and Edmund Haislmaier, *Medicaid Meltdown: Dropping Medicaid Could Save States $1 Trillion,* Washington, DC: Heritage Foundation, December 1, 2009, http://www.heritage.org/research/reports/2009/11/medicaid-meltdown-dropping-medicaid-could-save-states-1-trillion. One of the study's main assumptions was that Medicaid enrollees who lost coverage could join the health

exchanges created by the ACA. However, the study was written before the ACA legislation was finalized with language excluding the Medicaid-eligible population from the exchanges.

3. Corrie MacLaggan, "Is Texas really thinking of opting out of Medicaid?," *Austin American Statesman,* November 13, 2010.

4. John Holahan and Irene Headen, "Medicaid Coverage and Spending in Health Reform: National and State-by-State Results for Adults at or Below 133% FPL," Washington, DC: Kaiser Commission on Medicaid and the Uninsured, 2010.

5. State of Texas: Office of the Governor, "Statement by Gov. Rick Perry on Future of Medicaid in Texas," December 3, 2010, http://governor.state.tx.us/news/press-release/15439/.

6. Emily Ramshaw and Marilyn Serafini, "Battle Lines Drawn over Medicaid in Texas," *New York Times,* November 12, 2010.

7. Peter Suderman, "Rick Perry's Superficial Extremism," *Reason,* August 19, 2011.

8. Nevada Department of Health and Human Services and the Division of Health Care Financing and Policy, *Medicaid Opt Out White Paper,* January 22, 2011, http://media.lasvegassun.com/media/pdfs/blogs/documents/2010/01/28/medcaid0128.pdf.

9. Wyoming Department of Health, *Medicaid Opt-Out Impact Analysis,* September 1, 2010, www.health.wyo.gov/Media.aspx?mediaId=9529.

10. Donald Kettl, "Medicaid, Incentives and the Future of Federalism," *Governing,* February 2011.

11. Sam Baker, "Dem Governor: Obama Medicaid Plan Could Pose 'Huge Problem,'" *The Hill,* July 8, 2011.

12. National Governors Association, "July 9, 2011 Letter—Medicaid Reductions," July 9, 2011, http://www.nga.org/cms/home/federal-relations/nga-letters/executive-committee-letters/col2-content/main-content-list/july-9-2011-letter---medicaid-re.html.

13. Sarah Kliff, "Medicaid Quietly Dodges Deficit Reduction Battle," *Washington Post,* September 20, 2011.

14. Republican Governors' Public Policy Committee, Letter to Patty Murray and Jeb Hensarling, October 24, 2011, http://www.aucd.org/docs/policy/medicaid/debt%20RGA%20letter%20to%20super%20commt.pdf.

15. Kliff, "Medicaid Quietly Dodges Deficit Reduction Battle."

16. United States Government Accountability Office, "State and Local Governments: Growing Fiscal Challenges Will Emerge during the Next 10 Years," 2008.

17. Michael S. Greve and Philip Wallach, "As Arizona Goes, So Goes the Nation: How Medicaid Ruins the States' Fiscal Health," Washington, DC: American Enterprise Institute, 2008.

18. National Governors Association, "Proceedings of the National Governors Association Annual Meeting 1981," 21.

19. See for example Leighton Ku, Matt Broaddus, and Victoria Wachino, "Med-

icaid and SCHIP Protected Insurance Coverage for Millions of Low-Income Americans," Center on Budget and Policy Priorities, 2005.

20. James Frogue, "Medicaid's Perverse Incentives, The State Factor," American Legislative Exchange Council, 2004.

21. Greve and Wallach, "As Arizona Goes, So Goes the Nation."

22. Sarah Kliff and J. Lester Feder, "GOP Governors Want Medicaid Block Grants," *Politico,* February 27, 2011.

23. Robert Pear, "GOP Blueprint Would Remake Health Policy," *New York Times,* April 5, 2011.

24. Mary Agnes Carey and Marilyn Werber Serafini, "GOP Governors Revive Historic Call for Medicaid Block Grants," National Public Radio, March 8, 2011.

25. Testimony of Massachusetts Governor Deval L. Patrick before the Senate Finance Committee, United States Congress, Washington, DC, June 23, 2011, 13.

26. Kliff and Feder, "GOP Governors Want Medicaid Block Grants."

27. Representative John Garamendi, floor remarks delivered April 13, 2011; Representative Henry Waxman, Statement on H.Con.Res. 34, the Fiscal Year 2012 Budget Resolution, April 15, 2011.

28. Julian Pecquet, "Medicaid Advocates Breathe Easy on Ryan's Entitlement Reform Proposal," *The Hill,* July 8, 2011.

29. Advisory Commission on Intergovernmental Relations, "The Federal Role in the Federal System: The Dynamics of Growth," 1980.

30. U.S. Department of Health, Education, and Welfare, "Report of the Task Force on Medicaid and Related Programs," 1970.

31. National Governors Association, *HHS-27: Medicaid Reform Principles,* July 17, 2011.

32. See for example Robert J. Samuelson, "It's Time to Federalize Medicaid," *Columbus (OH) Dispatch,* July 23, 2012.

33. Kaiser Commission on Medicaid and the Uninsured, "Dual Eligibles: Medicaid's Role for Low-Income Medicare Beneficiaries," May 2011.

34. National Governors Association, "Dual Eligibles: Making the Case for Federalization," February 2005.

35. Kaiser Commission on Medicaid and the Uninsured, "Medicaid: An Overview of Spending on 'Mandatory' vs. 'Optional' Populations and Services," June 2005.

Bibliography

Adams, E. Kathleen, and Martcia Wade. 2001. "Fiscal Response to a Matching Grant: Medicaid Expenditures and Enrollments, 1984–1992." *Public Finance Review* 29 (1): 26–48.

Allen, Robert S., ed. 1949. *Our Sovereign State.* New York: Vanguard Press.

Andersen, Elizabeth. 1994. "Administering Health Care: Lessons from the Health Care Financing Administration's Waiver Policy-Making." *Journal of Law and Politics* 10 (2): 215–62.

Anrig, Greg. 2010. "Federalism and Its Discontents." *Democracy: A Journal of Ideas* 15 (Winter).

Arthur, W. Brian. 1994. *Increasing Returns and Path Dependence in the Economy.* Ann Arbor: University of Michigan Press.

Baicker, Katherine, and Douglas Staiger. 2005. "Fiscal Shenanigans, Targeted Federal Health Care Funds, and Patient Mortality." *Quarterly Journal of Economics* 120 (1): 345–86.

Balla, Steven J. 2001. "Interstate Professional Associations and the Diffusion of Policy Innovations." *American Politics Research* 29 (3): 221–45.

Banting, Keith, and Stanley Corbett. 2002. *Health Policy and Federalism: A Comparative Perspective on Multi-Level Governance.* Montreal: Queens University.

Barrilleaux, Charles J., and Mark E. Miller. 1988. "The Political Economy of State Medicaid Policy." *American Political Science Review* 82 (4): 1089–1107.

Berkowitz, Edward. 1995. *Mr. Social Security: The Life of Wilbur J. Cohen.* Lawrence: University Press of Kansas.

Berkowitz, Edward. 1996. "Social Security and the Financing of the American State." In *Funding the Modern American State, 1941–1995: The Rise and Fall of the Era of Easy Finance,* edited by W. Edward Brownlee. Cambridge: Cambridge University Press.

Berry, Jeffrey M., and David F. Arons. 2003. *A Voice for Nonprofits.* Washington, DC: Brookings Institution Press.

Blumenthal, David, and James A. Morone. 2009. *The Heart of Power: Health and Politics in the Oval Office.* Berkeley and Los Angeles: University of California Press.

Bodenheimer, Thomas. 1997. "The Oregon Health Plan—Lessons for the Nation." *New England Journal of Medicine* 337 (9): 651–56.

Bovbjerg, Randall, and John Holahan. 1982. *Medicaid in the Reagan Era.* Washington, DC: Urban Institute Press.

Brecher, Charles. 1984. "Medicaid Comes to Arizona: A First-Year Report on AHCCCS." *Journal of Health Politics, Policy and Law* 9 (3): 411–25.

Brown, Lawrence D. 1990. "The New Activism: Federal Health Politics Revisited." *Bulletin of the New York Academy of Medicine* 66 (4): 293–318.

Brown, Lawrence D. 2010. "Pedestrian Paths: Why Path-Dependence Theory Leaves Health Policy Analysis Lost in Space." *Journal of Health Politics, Policy and Law* 35 (4): 643–61.

Brown, Lawrence D., and Michael S. Sparer. 2003. "Poor Program's Progress: The Unanticipated Politics of Medicaid Policy." *Health Affairs* 22 (1): 31–44.

Buchanan, James M. 1975. *The Limits of Liberty: Between Anarchy and Leviathan.* Chicago: University of Chicago Press.

Bulman-Pozen, Jessica, and Heather K. Gerken. 2009. "Uncooperative Federalism." *Yale Law Journal* 118: 1256–1310.

Cammisa, Anne Marie. 1995. *Governments as Interest Groups: Intergovernmental Lobbying and the Federal System.* Westport, CT: Praeger.

Campbell, Andrea. 2003. *How Policies Make Citizens: Senior Citizen Activism and the American Welfare State.* Princeton: Princeton University Press.

Caro, Robert A. 2002. *Master of the Senate: The Years of Lyndon Johnson.* New York: Knopf.

Castles, Francis G. 1999. *Comparative Public Policy: Patterns of Postwar Transformation.* Cheltenham, UK: Edward Elgar.

Chernick, Howard. 1999. "State Fiscal Substitution between the Food Stamp Program and AFDC, Medicaid, and SSI." Unpublished manuscript.

Chernick, Howard. 2000. "Federal Grants and Social Welfare Spending: Do State Responses Matter?" *National Tax Journal* 53 (1): 143–52.

Cohen, Sally. 1990. "The Politics of Medicaid: 1980–89." *Nursing Outlook* 38 (5): 229–33.

Cohen, Wilbur J. 1983. "Reflections on the Enactment of Medicare and Medicaid." *Health Care Financing Review,* 1983 annual supplement: 3–11.

Cohen, Wilbur J., and Robert M. Ball. 1965. "Social Security Amendments of 1965: Summary and Legislative History." *Social Security Bulletin* (September): 3–21.

Cohen, Wilbur J., and Milton Friedman. 1972. *Social Security: Universal or Selective?* Washington, DC: American Enterprise Institute.

Conlan, Timothy J. 1986. "Federalism and Competing Values in the Reagan Administration." *Publius: The Journal of Federalism* 16 (1): 29–47.

Conlan, Timothy J. 1991. "And the Beat Goes On: Intergovernmental Mandates and Preemption in an Era of Deregulation." *Publius: The Journal of Federalism* 21 (3): 43–57.

Conlan, Timothy J. 1998. *From New Federalism to Devolution: Twenty-Five Years of Intergovernmental Reform.* Washington, DC: Brookings Institution Press.

Conlan, Timothy J. 2006. "From Cooperative to Opportunistic Federalism: Reflections on the Half-Century Anniversary of the Commission on Intergovernmental Relations." *Public Administration Review* 66 (5): 663–76.

Conover, Christopher J., and Hester H. Davies. 2000. "The Role of TennCare in Health Policy for Low-Income People in Tennessee." Urban Institute Occasional Paper 33.

Cook, Fay L., and Edith J. Barrett. 1992. *Support for the American Welfare State: The Views of Congress and the Public.* New York: Columbia University Press.

Corwin, Edward S. 1950. "The Passing of Dual Federalism." *Virginia Law Review* 36 (1): 1–22.

Coughlin, Theresa A., Leighton Ku, and John Holahan. 1994. *Medicaid since 1980: Costs, Coverage, and the Shifting Alliance between the Federal Government and the States.* Washington, DC: Urban Institute Press.

Coughlin, Teresa A., and Stephen Zuckerman. 2002. "States' Use of Medicaid Maximization Strategies to Tap Federal Revenues: Program Implications and Consequences." In *Assessing the New Federalism Discussion Papers.* Washington, DC: Urban Institute Press.

Coughlin, Theresa A., Stephen Zuckerman, and Joshua McFeeters. 2007. "Restoring Fiscal Integrity to Medicaid Financing?" *Health Affairs* 26 (5): 1469–80.

Coughlin, Teresa A., Stephen Zuckerman, Susan Wallin, and John Holahan. 1999. "A Conflict of Strategies: Medicaid Managed Care and Medicaid Maximization." *Health Services Research* 34 (1): 281–93.

Crotty, William J. 1983. *Party Reform.* New York: Longman Publishing Group.

Crouser, Brad. 2006. *Arch: The Life of Governor Arch A. Moore, Jr.* Chapmanville, WV: Woodland Press.

Currie, Janet, and Jonathan Gruber. 1996. "Saving Babies: The Efficacy and Cost of Recent Changes in the Medicaid Eligibility of Pregnant Women." *Journal of Political Economy* 104 (6): 1263–96.

Davis, S. Rufus. 1978. *The Federal Principle: A Journey through Time in Quest of Meaning.* Berkeley and Los Angeles: University of California Press.

Derthick, Martha. 1979. *Policymaking for Social Security.* Washington, DC: Brookings Institution Press.

Derthick, Martha. 1987. "American Federalism: Madison's Middle Ground in the 1980s." *Public Administration Review* 47 (1): 66–74.

Derthick, Martha. 1996. "New Players: The Governors and Welfare Reform." *Brookings Review* 14 (2): 43–45.

Derthick, Martha. 2001. *Keeping the Compound Republic: Essays on American Federalism.* Washington, DC: Brookings Institution Press.

Dinan, John. 2011. "Shaping Health Reform: State Government Influence in the Patient Protection and Affordable Care Act," *Publius: The Journal of Federalism* 41 (3): 395–420.

Dobson, Allen, Donald Moran, and Gary Young. 1992. "The Role of Federal Waivers in the Health Policy Process." *Health Affairs* 11 (4): 72–94.

Drew, Elizabeth. 1997. *Showdown: The Struggle between the Gingrich Congress and the Clinton White House.* New York: Touchstone.

Elazar, Daniel J. 1962. *The American Partnership: Intergovernmental Cooperation in the Nineteenth Century United States*. Chicago: University of Chicago Press.

Engel, Jonathan. 2006. *Poor People's Medicine: Medicaid and American Charity Care since 1965*. Durham: Duke University Press.

Erskine, Hazel. 1975. "The Polls: Health Insurance." *Public Opinion Quarterly* 39 (1): 128–43.

Farber, Stephen B. 1983. "The 1982 New Federalism Negotiations: A View from the States." *Publius: The Journal of Federalism* 13 (2): 33–38.

Finkelstein, Amy, Sarah Taubman, Bill Wright, Mira Bernstein, Jonathan Gruber, Joseph P. Newhouse, Heidi Allen, and Katherine Baicker. 2011. The Oregon Health Study Group, "The Oregon Health Insurance Experiment: Evidence from the First Year." National Bureau of Economic Research working paper no. 17190.

Fossett, James W., and Frank J. Thompson. 1999. "Back-Off Not Backlash in Medicaid Managed Care." *Journal of Health Politics, Policy and Law* 24 (5): 1159–72.

Fraser, Irene. 1991. "Health Policy and Access to Care." In *Health Politics and Policy*, edited by Theodor J. Litman and Leonard S. Robins. New York: Delmar.

Friar, Monica. 1999. "Financing the Expansion of Missouri's Medicaid Program: 1987-1992." *John F. Kennedy School of Government Case Program*.

Friedman, Emily. 1995. "The Compromise and the Afterthought: Medicare and Medicaid after 30 Years." *Journal of the American Medical Association* 274 (3): 278–82.

Gais, Thomas, and James Fossett. 2005. "Federalism and the Executive Branch." In *Institutions of American Democracy: The Executive Branch*, edited by Joel D. Aberbach and Mark A. Peterson. New York: Oxford University Press.

Gamkhar, Shama. 2003. "The Role of Federal Budget and Trust Fund Institutions in Measuring the Effect of Federal Highway Grants on State and Local Government Highway Expenditure." *Public Budgeting and Finance* 23 (1): 1–21.

Gilens, Martin. 1999. *Why Americans Hate Welfare: Race, Media, and the Politics of Antipoverty Policy*. Chicago: University of Chicago Press.

Gilman, Jean Donovan. 1998. *Medicaid and the Costs of Federalism, 1984-1992*. New York: Routledge.

Gormley, William T. 2006. "Money and Mandates: The Politics of Intergovernmental Conflict." *Publius: The Journal of Federalism* 36 (4): 523–40.

Gordon, Colin. 2003. *Dead on Arrival: The Politics of Health Care in Twentieth-Century America*. Princeton: Princeton University Press.

Granneman, Thomas W., and Mark V. Pauly. 1983. *Controlling Medicaid Costs: Federalism, Competition, and Choice*. Washington, DC: AEI Press.

Granneman, Thomas W., and Mark V. Pauly. 2010. *Medicaid Everyone Can Count On: Public Choices for Equity and Efficiency*. Washington, DC: AEI Press.

Greenberg, Joshua, and Barry Zuckerman. 1997. "State Health Care Reform in Massachusetts: How One State Expanded Health Insurance for Children." *Health Affairs* 16 (4): 188–93.

Gray, Virginia. 1994. "Competition, Emulation, and Policy Innovation." In *New*

Perspectives on American Politics, edited by Lawrence C. Dodd and Calvin Jillson. Washington, DC: CQ Press.

Greenfield, Margaret. 1968. *Medicare and Medicaid: The 1965 and 1967 Social Security Amendments.* Berkeley, CA: Greenwood Press.

Grodzins, Morton. 1966. *The American System: A New View of the Government of the United States.* New York: Rand McNally.

Grogan, Colleen M. 1994. "Political-Economic Factors Influencing State Medicaid Policy." *Political Research Quarterly* 47 (3): 589–622. See also "Correction Note." 49 (3): 673–75.

Grogan, Colleen M. 1999. "The Influence of Federal Mandates on State Medicaid and AFDC Decision-Making." *Publius: The Journal of Federalism* 29 (3): 1–30.

Grogan, Colleen M. 2006. "A Marriage of Convenience: The History of Nursing Home Coverage and Medicaid." In *Putting the Past Back In: History and Health Policy in the United States,* edited by Rosemary A. Stevens, Charles E. Rosenberg, and Lawton R. Burns. New Brunswick, NJ: Rutgers University Press.

Grogan, Colleen M. 2008. "Medicaid: Health Care for You and Me?" In *Health Politics and Policy,* edited by James A. Morone, Theodor J. Litman, and Leonard S. Robins. New York: Delmar.

Grogan, Colleen M. 2008. "Medicalization of Long-Term Care: Weighing the Risks." In *Handbook of Long-Term Care Administration and Policy,* edited by Cynthia Massie Mara and Laura Katz Olson. New York: CRC Press.

Grogan, Colleen M., and Christina Andrews. 2011. "The Politics of Aging within Medicaid." In *The New Politics of Old Age Policy.* 2nd ed., edited by Robert B. Hudson. Baltimore: Johns Hopkins University Press.

Grogan, Colleen M., and Michael K. Gusmano. 2007. *Healthy Voices, Unhealthy Silence: Advocacy and Health Policy for the Poor.* Washington, DC: Georgetown University Press.

Grogan, Colleen, and Eric Patashnik. 2003. "Between Welfare Medicine and Mainstream Entitlement: Medicaid at the Political Crossroads." *Journal of Health Policy, Politics, and Law* 28 (5): 821–58.

Grogan, Colleen M., and Eric M. Patashnik. 2003. "Universalism within Targeting: Nursing Home Care, the Middle Class, and the Politics of the Medicaid Program." *Social Service Review* 77 (1): 51–71.

Grogan, Colleen M., and Vernon Smith. 2008. "From Charity Care to Medicaid: Governors, States, and the Transformation of American Health Care." In *A Legacy of Innovation: Governors and Public Policy,* edited by Ethan Sribnick. Philadelphia: University of Pennsylvania Press.

Gruber, Jonathan. 2006. "The Massachusetts Health Care Revolution: A Local Start for Universal Access." *Hastings Center Report* 36 (5): 14–19.

Gruber, Jonathan. 2008. "Incremental Universalism for the United States: The States Move First." *Journal of Economic Perspectives* 22 (4): 51–68.

Grupp, Fred W., Jr., and Alan R. Richards. 1975. "Variations in Elite Perceptions of American States as Referents for Public Policy Making." *American Political Science Review* 69 (3): 850–58.

Hacker, Jacob S. 1998. "The Historical Logic of National Health Insurance: Structure and Sequence in the Development of British, Canadian, and U.S. Medical Policy." *Studies in American Political Development* 12 (Spring): 57–130.

Hacker, Jacob S. 2002. *The Divided Welfare State: The Battle over Public and Private Social Benefits in the United States.* New York: Cambridge University Press.

Haider, Donald H. 1974. *When Governments Come to Washington: Governors, Mayors, and Intergovernmental Lobbying.* Washington, DC: Free Press.

Harris, Richard. 1969. *A Sacred Trust: The Story of America's Most Powerful Lobby—Organized Medicine.* Baltimore: New American Library.

Hill, Ian. 1990. "Improving State Medicaid Programs for Pregnant Women and Children," *Health Care Financing Review* annual supplement: 75–87.

Himmelfarb, Richard. 1995. *Catastrophic Politics: The Rise and Fall of the Medicare Catastrophic Coverage Act of 1988.* University Park: Penn State University Press.

Hines, James R., Jr., and Richard H. Thaler. 1995. "Anomalies: The Flypaper Effect." *Journal of Economic Perspectives* 9 (4): 217–26.

Holahan, John, and Linda Blumberg. 2006. "Massachusetts Health Care Reform: A Look at the Issues." *Health Affairs* 25 (6): w432–w443.

Holahan, John, Teresa Coughlin, Leighton Ku, Debra J. Lipson, and Shruti Rajan. 1995. "Insuring the Poor through Section 1115 Medicaid Waivers." *Health Affairs* 14 (1): 199–216.

Holahan, John, Alan Weil, and Joshua M. Wiener. 2003. "Which Way for Federalism and Health Policy?" *Health Affairs Web Exclusive* July (W3): 317–33.

Holahan, John, and Alan Weil. 2007. "Toward Real Medicaid Reform." *Health Affairs* 26 (2): w254–70.

Hovey, Harold A. 1999. *Can the States Afford Devolution? The Fiscal Implications of Shifting Federal Responsibilities to State and Local Governments.* New York: Century Foundation.

Hurley, Robert E. 2006. "TennCare—A Failure of Politics, Not Policy: A Conversation with Gordon Bonnyman." *Health Affairs* 25(3): w217–w225.

Iglehart, John K. 1981. "The New Role of the Federal Government." *Journal of Health Politics, Policy and Law* 6 (1): 179–83.

Iglehart, John K. 2010. "Medicaid Expansion Offers Solutions, Challenges." *Health Affairs* 29 (2): 230–32.

Ikenberry, G. John. 1994. "History's Heavy Hand: Institutions and the Politics of the State." Unpublished manuscript.

Jacobs, Lawrence R. 1993. "Health Reform Impasse: The Politics of American Ambivalence toward Government." *Journal of Health Politics, Policy and Law* 18 (3): 629–55.

Jacobs, Lawrence R., Theodore Marmor, and Jonathan Oberlander. 1999. "The Oregon Health Plan and the Political Paradox of Rationing: What Advocates and Critics Have Claimed and What Oregon Did." *Journal of Health Politics, Policy and Law* 24 (1): 161–80.

Jacobs, Lawrence R., and Theda Skocpol. 2010. *Health Care Reform and American Politics: What Everyone Needs to Know.* New York: Oxford University Press.

Johnston, Jocelyn M. 1997. "The Medicaid Mandates of the 1980s: An Intergovernmental Perspective." *Public Budgeting and Finance* 17 (1): 3–34.

Kane, Thomas J., Peter R. Orszag, and Emil Apostolov. 2005. "Higher Education Appropriations and Public Universities: The Role of Medicaid and the Business Cycle." Brookings-Wharton Papers on Urban Affairs, 99–127.

Katz, Michael B. 2008. *The Price of Citizenship: Redefining the American Welfare State*. Philadelphia: University of Pennsylvania Press.

Kincaid, John. 1990. "From Cooperative to Coercive Federalism." *Annals of the American Academy* 509 (May): 139–52.

Kingdon, John W. 1984. *Agendas, Alternatives, and Public Policies*. Boston: Little, Brown.

Kooijman, Jaap. 1999. *And the Pursuit of National Health: The Incremental Strategy toward National Health Insurance in the United States of America*. Amsterdam: Rodopi.

Kornai, Janos. 1979. "Resource-Constrained versus Demand-Constrained Systems." *Econometrica* 47 (4): 801–19.

Kousser, Thad. 2002. "The Politics of Discretionary Medicaid Spending, 1980–1993." *Journal of Health Politics, Policy and Law* 27 (4): 639–71.

Kramer, Lucy M. 1959. "Highlights of the Social Security Amendments of 1958." *Public Health Reports* 74 (1): 67–76.

Kronebusch, Karl. 1997. "Medicaid and the Politics of Groups: Recipients, Providers, and Policymaking." *Journal of Health Politics, Policy, and Law* 22 (3): 839–78.

Kronebusch, Karl. 2001. "Children's Medicaid Enrollment: The Impacts of Mandates, Welfare Reform, and Policy Delinking." *Journal of Health Politics, Policy, and Law* 26 (6): 1223–60.

Kronebusch, Karl. 2004. "Matching Rates and Mandates: Federalism and Children's Medicaid Enrollment." *Policy Studies Journal* 32 (3): 317–39.

Ku, Leighton, and Teresa A. Coughlin. 1995. "Medicaid Disproportionate Share and Other Special Financing Programs." *Health Care Financing Review* 16 (3): 27–54.

Lambrew, Jeanne M. 2005. "Making Medicaid a Block Grant Program: An Analysis of the Implications of Past Proposals." *Milbank Quarterly* 83 (1): 1–23.

Leichter, Howard M. 1999. "Oregon's Bold Experiment: Whatever Happened to Rationing?" *Journal of Health Politics, Policy and Law* 24 (1): 147–60.

Lowi, Theodore. 1964. "American Business, Public Policy, Case Studies and Political Theory." *World Politics* 16 (4): 677–715.

Lykens, Kristine A., and Paul A. Jargowsky. 2002. "Medicaid Matters: Children's Health and Medicaid Eligibility Expansions." *Journal of Policy Analysis and Management* 21 (2): 219–38.

Mahoney, James, and Daniel Schensul. 2006. "Historical Context and Path Dependence." In *Oxford Handbook of Contextual Political Analysis*, edited by Robert E. Goodin and Charles Tilly. Oxford: Oxford University Press.

Marmor, Theodore. 1973. *The Politics of Medicare*. Hawthorne, NY: Aldine de Gruyter.

Marton, James, and David E. Wildasin. 2007. "Medicaid Expenditures and State Budgets: Past, Present, and Future." *National Tax Journal* 60 (2): 279–304.

Maxwell, James. 2007. "Comprehensive Health Care Reform in Vermont: A Conversation with Jim Douglas." *Health Affairs* 26 (6): w697–w702.

McCall, Nelda, C. William Wrightson, Lynn Paringer, and Gordon Trapnell. 1994. "Managed Medicaid Cost Savings: The Arizona Experience." *Health Affairs* 13 (2): 234–45.

McDonough, John E. 2004. "The Road to Universal Health Coverage in Massachusetts: A Story in Three Parts." *New England Journal of Public Policy* 20 (1): 57–63.

McDonough, John E., Christie L. Hager, and Brian Rosman. 1997. "Health Care Reform Stages a Comeback in Massachusetts." *New England Journal of Medicine* 336 (2): 148–52.

McDonough, John E., Brian Rosman, Fawn Phelps, and Melissa Shannon. 2006. "The Third Wave of Massachusetts Health Care Access Reform." *Health Affairs* 25 (6): w420–w431.

McGuire, Therese J., and David F. Merriman. 2006. "State Spending on Social Assistance Programs over the Business Cycle." In *Working and Poor: How Economic and Policy Changes are Affecting-Low Wage Workers,* edited by Rebecca M. Blank, Sheldon H. Danziger, and Robert F. Schoeni. New York: Russell Sage Foundation.

McLure, Charles E. 1967. "The Interstate Exporting of State and Local Taxes: Estimates for 1962." *National Tax Journal* 20:49–77.

Merriman, David F. 2006. "A Theoretical Analysis of Medicaid Supplantation." *Public Finance Review* 34 (1): 33–59.

Mettler, Suzanne. 2005. *Soldiers to Citizens: The G.I. Bill and the Making of the Greatest Generation.* New York: Oxford University Press.

Meyer, Bruce D., and Laura R. Wherry. 2012. "Saving Teens: Using a Policy Discontinuity to Estimate the Effects of Medicaid Eligibility." NBER working paper no. 18309.

Miller, Edward A. 2008. "Federal Administrative and Judicial Oversight of Medicaid: Policy Legacies and Tandem Institutions under the Boren Amendment." *Publius: The Journal of Federalism* 38 (2): 315–42.

Miller, Edward A., and Jane Banaszak-Holl. 2005. "Cognitive and Normative Determinants of State Policymaking Behavior: Lessons from the Sociological Institutionalism." *Publius: The Journal of Federalism* 35 (2): 191–216.

Mintrom, Michael. 1997. "Policy Entrepreneurs and the Diffusion of Innovation." *American Journal of Political Science* 41 (3): 738–70.

Mintrom, Michael, and Sandra Vergari. 1998. "Policy Networks and Innovation Diffusion: The Case of State Education Reforms." *Journal of Politics* 59 (1): 126–48.

Mirvis, David M., Cyril F. Chang, Christopher J. Hall, Gregory T. Zaar, and William B. Applegate. 1995. "TennCare—Health System Reform for Tennessee." *Journal of the American Medical Association* 274 (15): 1235–41.

Moene, Karl, and Michael Wallerstein. 2001. "Inequality, Social Insurance, and Redistribution." *American Political Science Review* 95 (4): 859–74.

Moon, Marilyn. 1990. "The Rise and Fall of the Medicare Catastrophic Coverage Act." *National Tax Journal* 43 (3): 371–81.

Moore, Judith D., and David G. Smith. 2005. "Legislating Medicaid: Considering Medicaid and Its Origins." *Health Care Financing Review* 27 (2): 45–52.

Myers, Robert J. 1970. *Medicare.* Homewood, IL: Richard D. Irwin.

Nathan, Richard P. 2005. "Federalism and Health Policy." *Health Affairs* 24 (6): 1458–66.

Nathan, Richard P., Fred C. Doolittle, and Associates. 1983. *The Consequences of Cuts.* Princeton: Princeton University Press.

Nathan, Richard P., Fred C. Doolittle, and Associates. 1987. *Reagan and the States.* Princeton: Princeton University Press.

North, Douglass C. 1990. *Institutions, Institutional Change and Economic Performance.* New York: Cambridge University Press.

O'Toole, Laurence J. 2007. *American Intergovernmental Relations: Foundations, Perspectives, and Issues.* 4th ed. Washington, DC: CQ Press.

Oates, Wallace E. 1972. *Fiscal Federalism.* New York: Harcourt Brace Jovanovich.

Oates, Wallace E. 1982. "The New Federalism: An Economist's View." *Cato Journal* 2 (2): 473–88.

Oates, Wallace E. 2005. "Toward a Second Generation Theory of Fiscal Federalism." *International Tax and Public Finance* 12 (4): 349–73.

Oberg, Charles N., and Cynthia L. Polich. 1988. "Medicaid: Entering the Third Decade." *Health Affairs* 7 (4): 83–96.

Oberlander, Jonathan. 2003. *The Political Life of Medicare.* Chicago: University of Chicago Press.

Oberlander, Jonathan. 2007. "Health Reform Interrupted: The Unraveling of the Oregon Health Plan." *Health Affairs* 26 (1): w96–w105.

Oberlander, Jonathan. 2008. "The Politics of Paying for Health Reform: Zombies, Payroll Taxes, and the Holy Grail." *Health Affairs* 27 (6): w544–w555.

Oberlander, Jonathan, Theodore Marmor, and Lawrence Jacobs. 2001. "Rationing Medical Care: Rhetoric and Reality in the Oregon Health Plan." *Canadian Medical Association Journal* 164 (11): 1583–87.

Ogbonna, Chinyere. 2007. *Tenncare and Disproportionate Share Hospitals.* Lanham, MD: University Press of America.

Olson, Laura Katz. 2010. *The Politics of Medicaid.* New York: Columbia University Press.

Page, Scott E. 2006. "Path Dependence." *Quarterly Journal of Political Science* 1:87–115.

Palfrey, Judith S. 2006. *Child Health in America: Making a Difference through Advocacy.* Baltimore: Johns Hopkins University Press.

Palley, Marian L. 1997. "Intergovernmentalization of Health Care Reform: The Limits of the Devolution Revolution." *Journal of Politics* 59 (3): 657–79.

Patashnik, Eric M., and Julian E. Zelizer. 2001. "Paying for Medicare: Benefits,

Budgets, and Wilbur Mills's Policy Legacy." *Journal of Health Politics, Policy and Law* 26 (1): 7–36.

Patashnik, Erik M., and Julian E. Zelizer. 2010. "When Policy Does Not Remake Politics: The Limits of Policy Feedback." Unpublished manuscript.

Pelrine, Alicia. 1992. "The Art of the Deal: Health Policy Making on the Fly." *Journal of American Health Policy* 2 (3): 23–28.

Perkins, Ellen J. 1956. "State and Local Financing of Public Assistance, 1935–55." *Social Security Bulletin* 19 (7): 3–13.

Persico, Joseph E. 1982. *The Imperial Rockefeller.* New York: Pocket Books.

Peterson, Paul. 1995. *The Price of Federalism.* Washington, DC: Brookings Institution Press.

Pierson, Paul. 1993. "When Effect Becomes Cause: Policy Feedback and Political Change." *World Politics* 45 (4): 595–628.

Pierson, Paul. 2000. "Increasing Returns, Path Dependence, and the Study of Politics." *American Political Science Review* 94 (2): 251–67.

Pierson, Paul. 2000. "Not Just What, but When: Timing and Sequence in Political Processes." *Studies in American Political Development* 14 (1): 72–92.

Pierson, Paul. 2004. *Politics in Time: History, Institutions, and Social Analysis.* Princeton: Princeton University Press.

Posner, Paul L. 1998. *Politics of Unfunded Mandates: Whither Federalism?* Washington, DC: Georgetown University Press.

Quadagno, Jill. 2005. *One Nation, Uninsured: Why the U.S. Has No National Health Insurance.* New York: Oxford University Press.

Reagan, Ronald. 1990. *An American Life.* New York: Simon & Schuster.

Rivlin, Alice. 1992. *Reviving the American Dream: The Economy, the States and the Federal Government.* Washington, DC: Brookings Institution Press.

Rockefeller, Nelson. Public Papers of the Governor. State of New York.

Romney, Mitt. 2010. *No Apology: The Case for American Greatness.* New York: St. Martin's Press.

Rosenbaum, Sara. 1993. "Medicaid Expansions and Access to Health Care." In *Medicaid Financing Crisis: Balancing Responsibilities, Priorities, and Dollars,* edited by Diane Rowland, Judith Feder, and Alina Salganicoff, 45–82. Washington, DC: American Association for the Advancement of Science Press.

Rosenbaum, Sara. 2009. "Medicaid and National Health Care Reform." *New England Journal of Medicine* 361 (21): 2009–12.

Rosenbaum, Sara, Anne Markus, and Colleen A. Sonosky. 2004. "Public Health Insurance Design for Children: The Evolution from Medicaid to SCHIP." *Journal of Health & Biomedical Law* 1 (1): 1–47.

Rosenbaum, Sara, and Colleen A. Sonosky. 2001. "Medicaid Reforms and SCHIP: Health Care Coverage and the Changing Policy Environment." In *Who Speaks for America's Children? The Role of Child Advocates in Public Policy,* edited by Carol J. De Vita and Rachel Mosher-Williams. Washington, DC: Urban Institute.

Rosenthal, Donald B., and James M. Hoefler. 1989. "Competing Approaches to the Study of American Federalism and Intergovernmental Relations." *Publius: The Journal of Federalism* 19 (1): 1–23.

Rowland, Diane, Barbara Lyons, and Jennifer Edwards. 1988. "Medicaid: Health Care for the Poor in the Reagan Era." *Annual Review of Public Health* 9:427–50.

Sabato, Larry. 1983. *Goodbye to Goodtime Charlie: The American Governorship Transformed*. 2nd ed. Washington, DC: CQ Press.

Sardell, Alice, and Kay Johnson. 1998. "The Politics of EPSDT Policy in the 1990s: Policy Entrepreneurs, Political Streams, and Children's Health Benefits." *Milbank Quarterly* 76 (2): 175–205.

Satterthwaite, Shad B. 2002. "Innovation and Diffusion of Managed Care in Medicaid Programs." *State & Local Government Review* 34 (2): 116–26.

Savage, Robert L. 1985. "When a Policy's Time has Come: Cases of Rapid Policy Diffusion, 1983–1984." *Publius: The Journal of Federalism* 15 (3): 111–25.

Schattschneider, E. E. 1935. *Politics, Pressures, and the Tariff*. New York: Prentice-Hall.

Schneider, Saundra K. 1997. "Medicaid Section 1115 Waivers: Shifting Health Care Reform to the States." *Publius: The Journal of Federalism* 27 (2): 89–109.

Schottland, Charles I. 1956. "Social Security Amendments of 1956: A Summary and Legislative History." *Social Security Bulletin* 19 (9): 3–15.

Shapiro, Robert Y., and John T. Young. 1989. "Public Opinion and the Welfare State: The United States in Comparative Perspective." *Political Science Quarterly* 104 (1): 59–89.

Skocpol, Theda. 1992. *Protecting Soldiers and Mothers: The Political Origins of Social Policy in the United States*. Cambridge, MA: Harvard University Press.

Skocpol, Theda. 1997. *Boomerang: Health Care Reform and the Turn against Government*. New York: W. W. Norton.

Sloan, Frank A. 1984. "State Discretion in Federal Categorical Assistance Programs: The Case of Medicaid." *Public Finance Review* 12 (3): 321–46.

Smith, David G. 2002. *Entitlement Politics: Medicare and Medicaid 1995–2001*. New Brunswick, NJ: Transaction Publishers.

Smith, David G. 2011. *The Children's Health Insurance Program: Past and Future*. New Brunswick, NJ: Transaction Publishers.

Smith, David G., and Judith D. Moore. 2008. *Medicaid Politics and Policy: 1965–2007*. New Brunswick, NJ: Transaction Publishers.

Sommers, Benjamin D., Katherine Baicker, and Arnold M. Epstein. 2012. "Mortality and Access to Care among Adults after State Medicaid Expansions." *New England Journal of Medicine* special article, July 25.

Soss, Joe, and Sanford F. Schram. 2007. "A Public Transformed? Welfare Reform as Policy Feedback." *American Political Science Review* 101 (1): 111–27.

Sparer, Michael S. 1996. *Medicaid and the Limits of State Health Reform*. Philadelphia: Temple University Press.

Sparer, Michael S. 2009. "Medicaid and the U.S. Path to National Health Insurance." *New England Journal of Medicine* 360 (4): 323–25.

Sparer, Michael S., George France, and Chelsea Clinton. 2011. "Inching toward

Incrementalism: Federalism, Devolution, and Health Policy in the United States and the United Kingdom." *Journal of Health Politics, Policy and Law* 36 (1): 33–57.

Starr, Paul. 1982. *The Social Transformation of American Medicine.* New York: Basic Books.

Steinmo, Sven, and Jon Watts. 1995. "It's the Institutions, Stupid! Why Comprehensive National Health Insurance Always Fails in America." *Journal of Health Politics, Policy and Law* 20 (2): 329–72.

Stephens, G. Ross, and Nelson Wikstrom. 2007. *American Intergovernmental Relations: A Fragmented Federal Polity.* Oxford: Oxford University Press.

Stevens, Robert, and Rosemary Stevens. 2003. *Welfare Medicine in America: A Case Study of Medicaid.* New Brunswick, NJ: Transaction Publishers.

Stimson, James A. 1999. *Public Opinion in America: Moods, Cycles, and Swings.* 2nd ed. Boulder, CO: Westview Press.

Stockman, David. 1986. *The Triumph of Politics: Why the Reagan Revolution Failed.* New York: HarperCollins.

Stostky, Janet. 1991. "State Fiscal Responses to Federal Government Grants." *Growth and Change* 22 (3): 17–31.

Swank, Duane. 2002. *Global Capital, Political Institutions, and Policy Change in Developed Welfare States.* Cambridge: Cambridge University Press.

Tanenbaum, Sandra. 1995. "Medicaid Eligibility Policy in the 1980s: Medical Utilitarianism and the 'Deserving' Poor." *Journal of Health Politics, Policy and Law* 20 (4): 933–54.

Teaford, Jon C. 2002. *The Rise of the States: Evolution of American State Government.* Baltimore: Johns Hopkins University Press.

Thompson, Frank J. 2011. "The Medicaid Platform: Can the Termites Be Kept at Bay?" *Journal of Health Politics, Policy and Law* 36 (3): 549–54.

Thompson, Frank J. 2012. *Medicaid Politics: Federalism, Policy Durability, and Health Reform.* Washington, DC: Georgetown University Press.

Thompson, Frank J., and Courtney Burke. 2007. "Executive Federalism and Medicaid Demonstration Waivers: Implications for Policy and Democratic Process." *Journal of Health Politics, Policy and Law* 32 (6): 971–1004.

Thompson, Frank J., and John DiIulio. 1998. *Medicaid and Devolution: A View from the States.* Washington, DC: Brookings Institution Press.

Thompson, Frank J., and James W. Fossett. 2008. "Federalism." In *Health Politics and Policy,* edited by James A. Morone, Theodor J. Litman, and Leonard S. Robins. New York: Delmar.

Thorpe, Kenneth E. 2007. "Vermont's Catamount Health: A Roadmap for Health Care Reform?" *Health Affairs* 26 (6): w703–w705.

Tsebelis, George. 1995. "Decision Making in Political Systems: Veto Players in Presidentialism, Parliamentarism, Multicameralism and Multipartyism." *British Journal of Political Science* 25 (3): 289–325.

Vladeck, Bruce C. 1979. "The Design of Failure: Health Policy and the Structure of Federalism," *Journal of Health Politics, Policy and Law* 4 (3): 522–35.

Vladeck, Bruce C. 1995. "Medicaid 1115 Demonstrations: Progress through Partnership." *Health Affairs* 14 (1): 217–20.

Vladeck, Bruce C. 2003. "Where The Action Really Is: Medicaid and the Disabled." *Health Affairs* 22 (1): 90–100.

Walker, Jack L. 1969. "The Diffusion of Innovations among the American States." *American Political Science Review* 63 (3): 880–99.

Walker, David B. 1991. "American Federalism from Johnson to Bush." *Publius: The Journal of Federalism* 21 (1): 105–19.

Waxman, Henry. 1989. "Kids and Medicaid: Progress but Continuing Problems." *American Journal of Public Health* 79 (9): 1217–18.

Weaver, R. Kent. 1986. "The Politics of Blame Avoidance." *Journal of Public Policy* (6) 4: 371–98.

Weaver, R. Kent. 1996. "Deficits and Devolution in the 104th Congress." *Publius: The Journal of Federalism* 26 (3): 45–85.

Weil, Alan R. 2003. "There's Something about Medicaid." *Health Affairs* 22 (1): 13–30.

Weil, Alan R., and Louis F. Rossiter. 2007. "The Role of Medicaid." In *Restoring Fiscal Sanity 2007: The Health Spending Challenge,* edited by Alice M. Rivlin and Joseph R. Antos. Washington, DC: Brookings Institution Press.

Weingast, Barry R., Kenneth A. Shepsle, and Christopher Johnsen. 1981. "The Political Economy of Benefits and Costs: A Neoclassical Approach to Distributive Politics." *Journal of Political Economy* 89 (4): 642–64.

Weir, Margaret. 1992. *Politics and Jobs: The Boundaries of Employment Policy in the United States.* Princeton, NJ: Princeton University Press.

Weissert, Carol. 1992. "Medicaid in the 1990s: Trends, Innovations and the Future of the 'PAC-Man' of State Budgets." *Publius: The Journal of Federalism* 22 (3): 93–109.

Wilentz, Sean. 2008. *The Age of Reagan.* New York: HarperCollins.

Williams, Lucy. 1994. "The Abuse of Section 1115 Waivers: Welfare Reform in Search of a Standard." *Yale Law & Policy Review* 12 (1): 8–37.

Williamson, Richard S. 1983. "The 1982 New Federalism Negotiations." *Publius: The Journal of Federalism* 13 (2): 11–32.

Wilson, James Q. 1973. *Political Organizations.* Princeton: Princeton University Press.

Wright, Deil S. 1978. *Understanding Intergovernmental Relations: Public Policy and Participants' Perspectives in Local, State, and National Governments.* North Scituate, MA: Duxbury Press.

Zelizer, Julian. 1998. *Taxing America: Wilbur D. Mills, Congress, and the State, 1945–1975.* Cambridge: Cambridge University Press.

Zuckerman, Stephen, Genevieve M. Kenney, Lisa Dubay, Jennifer Haley, and John Holahan. 2001. "Shifting Health Insurance Coverage 1997–1999." *Health Issues* 20 (1): 169–77.

Index

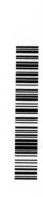